Mary Breckinridge

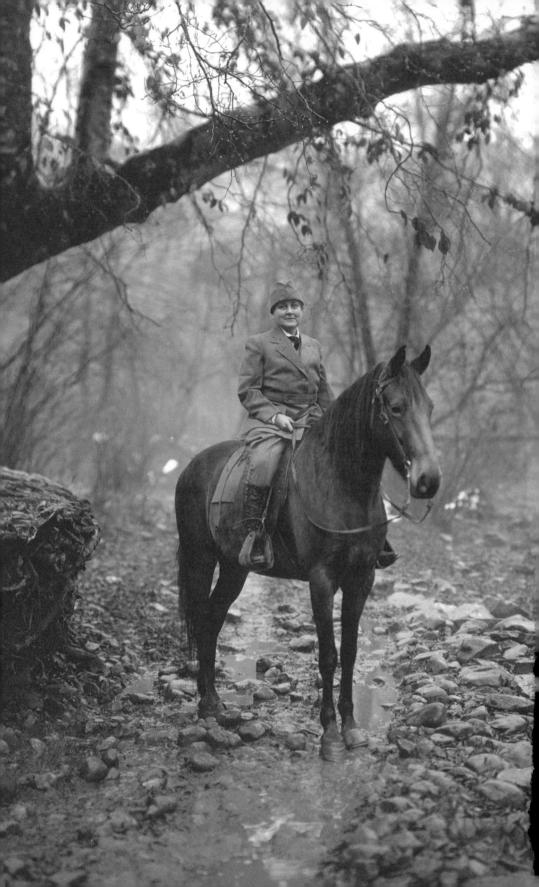

MELANIE BEALS GOAN

Mary Breckinridge

The Frontier Nursing Service & Rural Health in Appalachia

The University of
North Carolina Press
CHAPEL HILL

*Publication of this book was supported in part by a
generous gift from Anne W. and William W. McLendon.*

Designed by Heidi Perov
Set in Ehrhardt and Bureau Grotesque
by Keystone Typesetting, Inc.

The paper in this book meets the guidelines for permanence and
durability of the Committee on Production Guidelines for Book
Longevity of the Council on Library Resources.

Part of this book has been reprinted in revised form from "Establishing
Their Place in the Dynasty: Sophonisba and Mary Breckinridge's Paths
to Public Service," *Register of the Kentucky Historical Society* 101
(Winter–Spring 2003): 45–73.

Library of Congress Cataloging-in-Publication Data
Goan, Melanie Beals, 1972–
   Mary Breckinridge : the Frontier Nursing Service and rural health in
Appalachia / Melanie Beals Goan.
      p. ; cm.
   Includes bibliographical references and index.
ISBN 978-0-8078-3211-0 (cloth: alk. paper)
1. Breckinridge, Mary, 1881–1965. 2. Nurses—Appalachian Region—
Biography—History. I. Title.
   DNLM: 1. Breckinridge, Mary, 1881–1965. 2. Nurses—Appalachian
Region—Biography. 3. History, 20th Century—Appalachian Region.
4. Nursing Services—History—Appalachian Region. 5. Rural Health
Services—History—Appalachian Region. WZ 100 B829g 2008]
RT37.B72G63 2008
610.73092—dc22 2007049300
[B]

12 11 10 09 08   5 4 3 2 1

For my children
Addison, Eli, & Grayson

Contents

A section of photographs appears after page 115.

Acknowledgments

At each step in the process of preparing this manuscript, my skills as a historian have been sharpened and my list of debts has grown. As an undergraduate student at Slippery Rock University, I benefited from the guidance of John Craig and John Nichols. They first convinced me that I could become a professional historian and sent me on my way with the preparation I needed to succeed. Kathi Kern and Patricia Cooper, my dissertation directors, picked up from there, welcoming me as a very green graduate student at the University of Kentucky. They watched as I became acquainted with Mary Breckinridge, and they, along with Ron Eller, Francie Chassen-Lopez, and Ellen Rosenman, the other members of my dissertation committee, encouraged me to move beyond a simple view of Breckinridge and to see her as a complex individual. Fellow graduate students offered helpful criticism and became good friends. Debbie Blackwell, Ed Blum, Carolyn Dupont, Chad Gregory, Caroline Light, Jeff Matthews, Kristen Streater, and Kat Williams all read drafts of this work. My good friend Dana White read a late draft of the manuscript and offered excellent suggestions on how to sharpen the prose. Sian Hunter and the rest of the editorial staff at the University of North Carolina Press have shown great patience throughout the process, and the press's two anonymous readers offered criticisms that substantially improved this book. Ellen Goldlust-Gingrich painstakingly copyedited the manuscript, significantly cleaning it up and catching a number of errors. In spite of these extra sets of eyes, I still remain responsible for any mistakes.

I am grateful for the assistance provided by the late Katherine Breckinridge Prewitt. By sharing stories and memories, she offered a unique personal glimpse of her Aunt Mary. Kate opened her home to me and graciously allowed me to sift through letters, photos, and family memorabilia. She and John Marshall Prewitt have served as careful stewards of the historical records entrusted to them and have assisted a number of historians in their quest to examine the past. Susan Schaefer shared her research on Eureka Springs, Arkansas, with me and very generously dug up information about Breckinridge's second husband and the couple's time there. Dr. Anne Wasson, former medical director of the FNS, also shared useful documents.

A visit to the Frontier Nursing Service in Hyden, Kentucky, provided needed context and allowed me to understand better the culture of Breckinridge's organization and the geography of the area she served. I benefited greatly from being able to stay in Breckinridge's home (in her room, no less), and I thank Jeremy Bush, Barb Gibson, Marylin Hoskins, and other members of the FNS staff for their hospitality. The food at Wendover is delicious!

The vast, impeccably organized and cataloged archival collection housed at the University of Kentucky Special Collections made this book possible. Bill Marshall, the manuscripts curator, has followed this project from its initial stages to its completion and in the process has become a good friend. He and his colleagues, notably Kate Black, Lisa Carter, Gordon Hogg, Claire McCann, Frank Stanger, and Jeff Suchanek, have pulled hundreds of boxes and provided invaluable assistance. Photographic archivist Jason Flahardy tracked down images from an impressive, in-process collection.

The University of Kentucky Department of History and the University of Kentucky Women's Studies Program provided me with research grants. A research assistantship I held through the UK College of Nursing provided additional financial support, and Carolyn Williams, former dean of the college, served as a useful resource. The UK history department has enabled me to teach part time while my children are young, and I am grateful not only for the steady adjunct work but also for the encouragement my colleagues there have offered.

Having three children during the years that I was writing this book has both enriched my perspective and considerably slowed my progress. Giving birth—once under the care of a physician, once with the support of a midwife, and once (unintentionally) with no trained care present—has given me a new appreciation for the care Breckinridge's nurses provided their patients. I could have never finished this book without the help of a number of individuals who have assisted with child care. My in-laws especially have gone above and beyond, adjusting their schedules to allow me concentrated blocks of time during which to work. I also thank the staff at St. John's Lutheran Preschool, Ashlie Beals, Kim Chaffer, Blythe Duckworth, Millye McAtee, and Carla Tabeling. I know Addison, Eli, and Grayson are in great hands with them.

My parents, Dave and Kay Beals, always made education a priority in our home. Neither attended college, yet they assumed that their daughters would earn degrees and financially enabled us to do so. Though they questioned the practicality of pursuing a Ph.D. in history, they have fully supported my decision and have exhibited unwavering albeit unspoken faith in my abilities. My sisters, Ashlie Beals and Courtney Ansell, have followed me through this long process. Finally, my deepest appreciation is reserved for my husband, Brad Goan. He is the model of a supportive spouse. Trained as a historian himself, he understands the research process, and his intelligent questions and keen insight are woven into the fabric of this book. Even as I write these acknowledgments, he is picking up toys and tending to the kids while asking, "What can I do to help?" This book would not have been possible without him.

Introduction

In her were combined the tender healing arts of a
dedicated nurse, the hard-headed acumen of a prac-
tical business man, and the rich charm of a wise
and cultured personality. —ALLAN M. TROUT,
"Nurse and Angel of Frontier Dies," 1965

She was one of the most remarkable women I've
ever known. She had the mind of a man and heart
of a mother. —MARGARET GAGE, interview, 1978

She would undoubtedly have been a four-star
general—a bishop—a prince of finance—had she
been a man. —KATHARINE ELLIOTT WILKIE AND
ELIZABETH R. MOSELEY, *Frontier Nurse,* 1969

Words of praise commemorating Mary Breckinridge's forty years of service to eastern Kentucky and her noble, untiring efforts on behalf of rural women and children appeared in newspapers across the country following her death on May 16, 1965. Many of the tributes highlighted the paradoxical way that the Frontier Nursing Service's fallen leader had possessed the best qualities of both genders. As a trustee of the organization explained, she had the heart of a woman, "with tireless tenderness and concern for anyone in pain or need." Yet she also demonstrated the "swift, logical clarity and scope of a man's mind."[1] Others noted the irony that Breckinridge, a member of one of the nation's most accomplished families, should outshine her male relatives. The *Hazard Herald* declared, "While the deeds of her famous ancestors live on in musty history books, her deeds live on in whole generations of living people."[2]

In the eighty-four years that had passed since Mary Breckinridge's birth in 1881, options for women had expanded considerably. But for her and for other members of her generation, society's expectations were clear: women were made to be wives and mothers. Breckinridge internalized this cultural message and believed firmly that females possessed a natural capacity to nurture and thus belonged in the home. Still, she constantly battled her craving for adventure and her desire to distinguish herself in public affairs, like so many of her male relatives. Eager to "have it all" but raised in a period when doing so was not possible, Breckinridge sought creative ways to fulfill both her private and her public aspirations. She found her outlet when she created the Frontier Nursing Service (FNS) in 1925, and as the tributes written after her death reveal, she performed a careful and very successful balancing act throughout her life.[3]

MARY BRECKINRIDGE needed four decades and endured more than her share of tragedy to find her calling. When looking back on her childhood, she had few positive memories, dwelling instead on her loneliness as a constantly uprooted politician's daughter, on the poor quality of her education when compared to that offered her brothers, and on her failure to really fit in. For Mary, like so many young women of her generation, the years following graduation from high school left her struggling to combine her longing for adventure with her desire to become a wife and mother. Finally concluding that it would be impossible to have both a family and a career, she committed herself to marriage, but every time it seemed she chose a path, she hit a roadblock that required her to regroup. After the death of her first husband, she trained as a nurse. She then put aside her career plans to remarry, and two children followed. Their unexpected deaths and the resulting dissolution of her second marriage again left her unsure of where her future would lead. Following stints as a touring speaker with the U.S. Children's Bureau and as a relief worker in France after World War I, she founded the FNS.

Breckinridge devoted the remaining years of her life to running this public health organization. Through the FNS, she proved that nurse-midwives could provide practical and cost-effective trained medical care in rural areas where physicians were often unavailable. She began work in Leslie County, Kentucky, one of the nation's poorest, most remote regions, establishing a network of nursing clinics, a central hospital, and eventually a school to train midwives. By the 1930s, her mission expanded beyond simply providing health care to addressing the region's economic needs. At the time of Breckinridge's death, the FNS had delivered more than 14,500 babies with only 11 maternal deaths. In all, FNS nurses had treated nearly 58,000 patients.[4]

IN THE public imagination, Breckinridge and the nurses who came to work with her in eastern Kentucky became "angels on horseback," bravely attacking death and disease on the "battlefield" of motherhood.[5] Breckinridge commanded a large national following. Audiences thrilled to hear tales of FNS nurses risking life and limb to ensure the safe delivery of mountain babies. A charismatic figure, she won supporters' devotion not with her physical appearance—except for her piercing blue eyes, her looks were rather nondescript—but with her magnetic personality. Acquaintances described her as charming and witty, possessing the spellbinding public speaking ability for which her male ancestors had been famous. Those who heard her speak rarely forgot her or her mission. The *Louisville Courier-Journal* noted, "She touched consciences and loosened purse strings wherever she went."[6]

As the FNS's reputation spread, Breckinridge found herself showered with honors. During the 1930s and 1940s, the University of Louisville, the University of Rochester, Berea College, and the University of Kentucky granted her honorary doctoral degrees. The Kentucky Press Association named her Kentuckian of the Year in 1952, the first woman recipient of a prestigious award that had previously gone to the likes of Vice President Alben Barkley, Senator John Sherman Cooper, and University of Kentucky football coach Paul "Bear" Bryant.[7] The FNS director's accomplishments were broadcast coast to coast two years later when Bob Hope named her Woman of the Week on his radio show.[8]

Breckinridge received many accolades during her lifetime, but today her work is largely forgotten outside of the small area of eastern Kentucky still served by her organization. In the past half century, Breckinridge's heroic cause has disappeared from American memory. This oversight may have resulted from the rise of Medicare and Medicaid, whose introduction in the 1960s undermined the need for the service and certainly changed the way it did business. The death of Breckinridge, an energetic, compelling spokesperson, may bear some of the blame for the organization's loss of public recognition. More likely, Americans forgot about the FNS simply because times changed. Health care is now big business, Appalachia is no longer isolated from the rest of the nation, and the factors that inspired Breckinridge to create the FNS and drove her donors to support it so generously have largely disappeared. Breckinridge anticipated these changes and fought them in her later years, but in spite of her efforts to secure her legacy, her service has faded into obscurity.

Breckinridge would be disappointed that historians have not paid more attention to her and her organization. This work represents the first full-length treatment of the FNS, though several authors have published articles that provide quick overviews of its work.[9] Breckinridge and the FNS play a key role in Laura Ettinger's *Nurse-Midwifery: The Birth of a New American Profession* (2006). This study, however, like several dissertations written about the service, investigates its work from a very specific angle—in this case, Breckinridge's role in introducing nurse-midwifery to the United States. Arlene W. Keeling includes a chapter on the FNS in *Nursing and the Privilege of Prescription, 1893–2000* (2007). Breckinridge also finds a place in the spotlight in Sandra Barney's *Authorized to Heal: Gender, Class, and the Transformation of Medicine in Appalachia, 1880–1930* (2000), but here again, Breckinridge's work factors in as only part of the larger stories about nurses' role in dispensing medicine and the medical establishment's quest for hegemony in the mountains.

The majority of studies written about the FNS share a significant weakness—they tend to rely heavily on its founder's autobiography, *Wide Neighborhoods: A Story of the Frontier Nursing Service* (1952), taking it as a straightforward historical account instead of as the carefully constructed and highly edited memoir that it represents. When writing *Wide Neighborhoods*, Breckinridge was constantly aware of her audience and naturally strove to present her work in the best light possible. She sifted through memories, some of events more than fifty years in the past, and filtered them in an attempt to provide a cohesive story. *Wide Neighborhoods* remains a key source on Breckinridge's life, and I too use it, but I am careful to critique it, viewing it as a tool to uncover the public persona Breckinridge sought to create.

Because Breckinridge saw her work as historically important, she preserved a wealth of archival material, and the Frontier Nursing Service Collection, housed in Special Collections at the M. I. King Library at the University of Kentucky in Lexington, is massive.[10] But like her autobiography, she carefully selected the material she wanted to save and omitted documents that contradicted the image she wished to present. Despite her very public role, Breckinridge was an intensely private person. As she was writing *Wide Neighborhoods*, she asked friends to return letters she had written, warning that she intended to reference them and then destroy the correspondence when she finished writing. She also destroyed her journals, believing that her book would serve as the definitive source for information about her life.[11] I have attempted to look beyond the FNS Collection to capture a fuller portrait of Breckinridge's work, relying when possible on alternate archival sources, newspapers, and oral history interviews.[12]

IN SEEKING to understand Breckinridge and her organization, I have turned to the growing body of secondary literature produced by women's historians, Appalachian scholars, and medical historians. In many ways, Breckinridge's story stands apart from those of the female reformers who have attracted scholarly attention. She married when many chose to remain single, and she chose to work in a remote rural spot instead of in a northern city. Breckinridge was clearly influenced by the Progressive Era's sense of optimism that an individual could change his or her world and that society was moving steadily toward an improved state. Like the many women before her who committed themselves to ending child labor, outlawing lynching, promoting temperance, or demanding suffrage, Breckinridge focused on an issue that she believed had the power to transform lives, and she made it her sole purpose.[13]

As a maternalist—one who justified women's political participation by emphasizing their unique, innate qualities as caregivers and who celebrated the "socially vital" work women performed—Breckinridge preferred to operate within rather than to challenge the prevailing gender system that designated the home as women's sphere. Maternalists' influence is undeniable. Their lobbying efforts led to the creation of federal bureaus to advance women's and children's interests, resulted in the creation of first mother's pensions and later a welfare system based on gender distinctions, and led to labor restrictions that centered on the special needs of female workers. Historians have documented the important role that maternalists played in the creation of the welfare state and the key ways that they shaped early-twentieth-century public policy. While all of these scholars see maternalism as simultaneously "liberatory and limiting," they vary in which assessment they choose to emphasize.[14] Some scholars underscore maternalists' positive impact, arguing that women helped to soften industrialization's harsher edges.[15] Others dwell on maternalists' class and race prejudices and criticize them for building a welfare state that marginalizes and stigmatizes poor (often black) women, for promoting unrealistic middle-class standards of parenting, and for offering moral critiques of those mothers who failed to live up to maternalist standards.[16]

Both Breckinridge's work with the FNS and her earlier reform efforts were clearly rooted in maternalist ideology. Placing her within the context of this historical literature sheds light on her motivations and ultimately helps to explain the limitations she faced. By claiming that she was just a mother serving other mothers and their children, she protected herself from charges that she was stepping beyond her proper sphere. She shielded herself from scrutiny by creating a woman's organization—that is, a group staffed by women and working primarily on behalf of women. She took advantage of the exalted status assigned to mothers, relying heavily on maternalist rhetoric in her fund-raising materials. By painting Appalachian women as providing a valuable and often dangerous service to the nation, Breckinridge built considerable support for her organization.

Her insistence that women deserved medical care because as mothers they made a unique contribution to the nation equal to that made by soldiers set limits on how far her organization could go in revolutionizing health care, however. Like labor advocates who called for using women and children as an "entering wedge" to gain better working conditions for all workers, Breckinridge began her quest to make health care accessible and affordable for all Americans by focusing narrowly on society's most innocent and helpless members.[17] She could have argued that her patients deserved health care simply because they were human; instead, she attempted to explain why they were "worthy." While this strategy certainly brought success and necessary financial support, it undermined her more ambitious goals.

BRECKINRIDGE IS perhaps best understood within the context of other female Appalachian reformers, the "fotched-on" women who attempted to uplift the mountains in the early twentieth century by creating schools, organizing folk craft programs, collecting ballads, and providing health care.[18] Women such as Katherine Pettit, May Stone, Olive Dame Campbell, and Alice Lloyd came to the area looking for an outlet for their talents and driven by a missionary zeal to introduce the benefits of progress while protecting the region's celebrated traditional values. Breckinridge did not arrive until several decades after these pioneering figures, but she shared many of her predecessors' goals and assumptions.

Debate has raged over the motivations that inspired Appalachian reformers and the impact of their efforts. For nearly twenty-five years, David Whisnant's seminal *All That Is Native and Fine: The Politics of Change in an American Region* (1983) has framed the discussion. Whisnant issues a scathing critique of fotched-on women, who failed to attack industrial exploitation and the underlying factors to blame for Appalachian poverty and instead engaged in "cultural politics." Projects such as Hindman Settlement School, he asserts, "were based upon a flawed reading of local culture, as well as upon a naïve analysis of the relationship between culture, political and economic power, and social change."[19] "Do-gooders" brought a selective, romanticized understanding of folk culture, and armed with this image, they focused on remaking the region into what mainstream America deemed "native and fine." Whisnant acknowledges that "cultural interveners may be on the whole decent, well-meaning, and even altruistic people," but this "does not (indeed must not) excuse them from historical judgment."[20] In the end, he concludes, they did more harm than good.

Whisnant's harsh criticism has elicited a flurry of responses, and many scholars since have attempted to refute his "mean-spirited" portrait of these women.[21] The most recent, best articulated responses to Whisnant criticize him for placing Appalachian residents in the role of victim. In her history of Hindman Settlement School, Jess Stoddart rejects Whisnant's suggestion that the institution was founded on one-sided, top-down relationships. Rather, she emphasizes the "exciting and satisfying cultural exchange" that took place, allowing organizers and students alike to learn from each other. Stoddart directly addresses Whisnant's accusation that reformers encouraged women to adapt their folk crafts to make them more marketable to a northern audience, stressing that local women chose chemical over natural dyes for convenience. She infers that unlike Whisnant, who holds a romantic, unchanging impression of mountain culture, Hindman residents "did not view their designs or techniques as static or sacred."[22] P. David Searles's 1995 study of Alice Lloyd likewise takes Whisnant to task for failing to assign mountain residents agency. According to Searles, Whisnant characterized the efforts of Appalachian reformers as "conspiratorial" and their mountain neighbors as "unsuspecting and defenseless." In response, Searles seeks to tell a story in which the actors are "real flesh and blood, not . . . straw men constructed to further a particular world view."[23]

Whisnant's critics also note that he fails to acknowledge fully the positive changes Appalachian reformers brought to their communities. Stoddart rejects Whisnant's assertion that Pettit and Stone had a narrow view of culture "that focused only on manners and dress, diet, and home decoration."[24] She instead emphasizes the real improvements that resulted from Hindman's educational and community development efforts and the enthusiastic response they received. Searles stresses that conditions were bad in Knott County when Lloyd arrived—residents coped with poor schools, rudimentary health care, poverty, and malnutrition. All the while, community and political structures proved incapable of dealing with the problems. He likewise notes that local residents had the choice of accepting or rejecting Lloyd's ideas, but the community on the whole recognized and appreciated her contributions.[25]

Karen Tice offers the most balanced and articulate response to Whisnant in "School-Work and Mother-Work: The Interplay of Maternalism and Cultural Politics in the Educational Narratives of Kentucky Settlement Workers, 1910–1930" (1998). Like his other detractors, she criticizes him for oversimplifying and pigeonholing female reformers and for denying the agency of the mountain people. She notes that his assumption that Appalachian residents did not share the values middle-class reformers brought to their work is unfair and largely incorrect. In some cases, mountain clients embraced the ideas promoted by reformers, seeking class status or scientific knowledge, but many did so simply because they trusted that new ideas had the power to improve their lives and agreed that "some things needed changing."[26] She rejects social control theorists' tendency "to cast the poor and marginalized as merely placid —putty in the hands of reformers rather than active agents."[27]

Tice emphasizes that we need to get beyond oversimplified assessments that regard reformers as either "relentless villains" or "benevolent" and "heroic" rescuers, and her study begins this process.[28] While she identifies many flaws in Whisnant's work, she does not dismiss it out of hand. She acknowledges that publicity materials prepared by mountain settlement workers often reinforced stereotypical images of their clients, particularly through a tendency to "oscillate . . . between sympathetic images of the mothers as tired drones and harsher images of them as rigid opponents of progress."[29] Even though the women she studied tended to communicate a sympathetic and in many ways realistic picture of life in the mountains, they "contributed to reductive readings of the region and its people by furthering a sense of difference and deviancy" by drawing attention to its problems.[30]

This study of Mary Breckinridge and her organization provides another attempt to complicate Whisnant's oversimplified portrait of Appalachian reform. Breckinridge's story offers an important reminder that the female reformers who came to Appalachia, while often initially naive, developed an increasingly sophisticated understanding of the region's problems as time went on. When she arrived in 1925, Breckinridge assumed that her patients would embrace her and her nurses and willingly adopt their ideas. She quickly discovered that local residents were not as eager to accept modern medicine as she had anticipated. Likewise, Breckinridge at first failed to recognize the challenges that the area's rugged environment and lagging economy posed for its residents and instead focused on the romantic images emphasized by the national media. By the 1930s, however, as her familiarity with Leslie County and its residents grew, she moved beyond her stereotypical assumptions and became an advocate for economic development.

Taking a presentist view, Whisnant asks Appalachian female reformers to step beyond their place and time to expose structural inequality and essentially to declare war on capitalism. One wonders how realistic this expectation is considering the era in which these women worked and the restrictions they faced as females in a male-dominated society. Whisnant fails to consider the achievements of female reformers within the full context of their limitations, and he thus too quickly dismisses figures such as Mary Breckinridge.

THE FNS provides a useful case study through which to view Americans' perceptions of Appalachia in the twentieth century and to understand better the class dynamics and power relationships that historically have driven social reform. Likewise, situating Breckinridge's organization within the larger story of the history of American medicine allows one to view the ways in which scientific medicine established its supremacy over folk healing and to witness the struggles that developed as competing groups of medical practitioners sought legitimacy and fought to gain patients' trust.

Appalachia provides a useful backdrop against which to study the professionalization of medicine. The timing of doctors' quest to elevate and define the boundaries of their profession corresponded to the industrial transformation and the consequent social upheaval taking place in the mountains at the turn of the twentieth century.[31] Barney's *Authorized to Heal* traces how physicians in Appalachia began to view mountain residents as potential patients—or, more specifically, potential customers—in the wake of the coal boom. Barney argues that female grassroots activists and reform-minded women (she specifically points to Breckinridge) assisted doctors in their effort to establish the hegemony of scientific medicine. Although Barney notes that clubwomen and reformers were motivated by self-interest, this point gets lost in her larger narrative, which emphasizes physicians' dominance and ultimate victory.[32]

Breckinridge's story complicates our understanding of the changes taking place in health care in the early twentieth century.[33] The transition from folk to scientific medicine was more than simply a case of greedy, powerful physicians wrangling control from lay and sectarian caregivers and poor, marginalized clients. As her story reveals, the struggle for professional legitimacy depended in large part on patients' recognition that seeking trained medical assistance not only benefited their health but also advanced their class aspirations. The battle for control of health care in Leslie County was more than just a male-versus-female fight; rather, it pitted nurse-midwives against lay midwives and raised the ire of female doctors who saw nurse-midwives as illegitimately claiming professional status.

The story of the FNS gets to the heart of what it means to be a professional. Sociologists identify very specifically the criteria that distinguish professionals from other workers. To be considered a professional, members of a given field must control the production and dissemination of knowledge. Professionals are careful gatekeepers, regulating who can and cannot join their ranks through examinations and licensure. Finally, autonomy and an expressed commitment to ethics are essential markers of a professional.[34] When Breckinridge established her organization, she attempted to carve out space for a new type of professional. Childbirth became increasingly medicalized as first male general practitioners and later obstetric specialists replaced lay midwives.[35] Challenging this emerging model, which dismissed midwives as ignorant, dirty, and backward, Breckinridge argued for the existence of a place for caregivers who, while not as highly trained as doctors, demonstrated their own brand of expertise and offered a needed skill by handling normal deliveries. Rural areas across America lacked access to primary care providers, and nurse-midwives—carefully distinguished from lay midwives by their training and their respect for science—could fill this gap.

Working in a rural setting both opened doors for this new type of practitioner and ultimately restricted the field's development. Situating her efforts in Appalachia enabled Breckinridge and her nurses to claim the mantle of professionalism. Largely out of the sight of doctors who challenged any threats to their authority and empowered by the practical considerations of their remote location to do work that under normal circumstances fell squarely into the realm of a physician, the FNS's nurse-midwives claimed a degree of autonomy and professional respect. But as Ettinger so rightly argues, Breckinridge's decision to establish her "demonstration" in a rural area and her insistence that she was serving only women who would otherwise exist outside of the reach of trained medical care laid the groundwork for nurse-midwifery to become a marginalized field serving only marginalized women. In 2003, nurse-midwives attended only 7.6 percent of U.S. births, even though statistics show that such births are at least as safe as those attended by obstetricians, even among high-risk populations.[36]

WHEN SHE established the FNS, Breckinridge had grand aspirations of improving conditions for women and children around the world. She never created the satellite organizations that she intended, and nurse-midwifery never achieved the legitimacy she hoped, but the creation of the Frontier Graduate School of Midwifery in 1939 ensured that many of her ideas would be carried to the far corners of the globe. One of her coworkers argued that Breckinridge was fifty years ahead of her time when she established the FNS, and in many ways, this assessment is correct.[37] In a period when few recognized the value of such an investment, Breckinridge proved the efficacy of disease prevention. Today, of course, not only is maintenance care widely recognized as a key aspect of better treatment, but the medical industry also has come to see it as an important cost-cutting mechanism.

The thorough preventive services the FNS offered were possible only through the use of auxiliary personnel—first nurse-midwives and later nurse-practitioners. Breckinridge challenged physicians' attempts to monopolize health care. While she firmly believed in scientific medicine and had a deep

respect for professional credentials, she argued that not every situation necessitated a doctor's attention. Lesser-trained practitioners could handle many
normal health issues as long as a physician was available to manage abnormal
situations. This arrangement, she contended, was not only more cost-effective
but better for patients because it allowed for more personalized individual care.

MARY BRECKINRIDGE came to eastern Kentucky in 1925 with a simple goal.
She wanted to make the world safer for other women's babies now that she
could no longer care for her own. She dedicated the remaining years of her life
to addressing not only health care issues but also the economic and social ills
that plagued Appalachia. If the picture of the director and her organization
that emerges in the following pages seems complicated and at times inconsis-
tent, this is intentional. Estelle Freedman argues that "historians too rarely
acknowledge either the complications or contradictory and competing identities in their subjects."[38] Not all of Breckinridge's ideas initially make sense to a
modern audience. She was eager for supporters to admire and fund her work;
therefore, she constantly tried to represent her nurses, her patients, and herself
in the best light possible. This incessant concern for her public image led her
to contradict herself frequently in service publications and especially in *Wide
Neighborhoods*.

Modern observers tend to place reform-minded individuals such as Breckinridge on pedestals, but doing so downplays the challenges they faced and
instead depicts them as predestined for success. Breckinridge fought throughout her life to overcome guilt, lapses of faith, and grief. Her struggles deserve
just as much recognition as her many successes. She was the first to admit that
she was not a saint—she smoked too much and was prone to cursing, qualities
unbecoming of the lady she strove to be. Contemporary critics may justifiably
condemn her for being an elitist and a racist who sought power and in the
process impeded change as she grew older. When criticizing her decisions, I
have attempted to take into account the limitations she faced, always considering her actions within the context of the era in which she lived. I hope a
balanced, complicated picture of a dynamic and enigmatic woman emerges.

part one **Choosing a Path**

one Origins and Obligations

In the late nineteenth century, most Americans and certainly all southerners were familiar with the name Breckinridge. To be born a Breckinridge in the late nineteenth century brought with it a "birthright of advantages," but it also carried a pressing sense of duty.[1] Since arriving on the shores of the New World 150 years earlier, the family's patriarchs had forged one of the nation's most powerful political dynasties.[2] Their dedicated, visionary contributions to the process of state building in Kentucky and to the development of the United States ensured the wide recognition of the Breckinridge surname. Male family members gained notoriety through politics as well as through their work as religious leaders, soldiers, educators, and newspaper editors. As an admiring supporter wrote in 1884, "The name of *Breckinridge* seems to fill the minds of the people."[3] Several years later, another ally remarked that the Breckinridge family represented an "aristocracy of courage and character, the only aristocracy possible in our country."[4]

Possessing the Breckinridge name certainly opened doors, but this advantage came at a cost, placing tremendous pressure on young family members to perpetuate the tradition of service. Starting in infancy, Breckinridge children were "fed a steady diet" of their heritage to the extent that one claimed it "made life almost a burden."[5] Solemn portraits of renowned ancestors peered down on descendants as they scampered through the hallways of their homes. Letters and papers carefully preserved and shared provided instructions from beyond the grave as to how family members should behave.[6] The idea was clear: a Breckinridge strove not simply to succeed but to excel.[7]

For female family members, to whom society offered limited options, the message that Breckinridges must prove themselves as outstanding members of society could be contradictory and frustrating. Born on February 17, 1881, Mary Carson Breckinridge was named for a long line of strong but submissive women.[8] She grew up imbued with the message that Breckinridge males led while the women of the family, in their capacities as wives, sisters, and mothers, played nurturing and supportive roles behind the scenes. But at the turn of the twentieth century, when Mary came of age, options for women were beginning to expand. As a gifted, highly motivated member of the famous Breckinridge family who happened to be female, Mary felt driven to use her talents in a meaningful way and to capitalize on the opportunities being offered to the "New Woman." The message that women belonged in the home, however, continued to weigh heavily on her. She would spend much of her life searching for creative ways to fulfill her obligation to advance the family name and to satisfy her driving ambition while still upholding her duty to remain within women's appropriate sphere.

THE MIGRATION that brought the first Breckinridges to Kentucky started nearly two centuries before Mary's birth. Seeking religious freedom, the family moved from England to the Scottish highlands in the late nineteenth century and relocated soon thereafter to Ireland. Their displacement continued when the first Breckinridges sailed for the American colonies in 1728. They followed the path many Scots-Irish immigrants took, settling first in eastern Pennsylvania before moving down Virginia's Shenandoah Valley. The first generations of American-born Breckinridges distinguished themselves as part of the frontier elite and quickly made their mark in local affairs. They accumulated great tracts of land in Augusta County, Virginia, and purchased slaves to work this land. Throughout the eighteenth century, Breckinridge males advanced through the ranks of the colonial gentry, holding influential positions such as sheriff and justice of the peace. An auspicious marriage to a member of the powerful Preston family further increased the value of the family's stock. Although their future in Virginia appeared bright, some members of the family remained restless and began to look farther west.

The availability of cheap, high-quality land and the opportunities for political leadership within an infant state attracted John Breckinridge to Kentucky.

Having sent his slaves ahead to clear land and build a comfortable home, he packed up his family and set out for the frontier in 1792.[9] Kentucky in the late eighteenth century was an inviting though notoriously dangerous place. The Native Americans who used this region as a hunting spot and a travel corridor referred to it as a "dark and bloody ground." Unfortunately for many settlers who tried to make it their home, this description proved accurate. Between 1783 and 1790 alone, an estimated fifteen hundred white individuals lost their lives in the Indian Wars. The hostile landscape and roaming white outlaws made the chance of death even greater. Still, many ambitious and optimistic individuals, lured by promises such as that made by one excited clergyman that heaven was "a mere Kentucky of a place," were willing to overlook the risks. The region's abundant resources proved too great a temptation to ignore.[10]

More fortunate than many, John Breckinridge's gamble paid off. He and his family survived the dangers of the frontier, and his political connections and legal knowledge allowed him to establish himself quickly. Having served in the Virginia House of Delegates, Breckinridge became an active player in the developing Kentucky government. He helped revise the state constitution in 1799 and introduced the Kentucky Resolutions, which articulated an early version of the states' rights philosophy. A loyal Jeffersonian Republican, he served as speaker of the Kentucky House of Representatives, as U.S. senator, and as U.S. attorney general before his death from tuberculosis cut short a promising career in 1806.[11]

John's son, Joseph Cabell Breckinridge, appeared poised to spread the family's political influence even farther, but he too died suddenly. Instead, his only son, John C. Breckinridge, was left to carry on the legacy. Family members trained the future statesman from infancy with this goal in mind. His grandmother, Polly, better known within the family as Grandma Black Cap, introduced young John C. to his grandfather's ideals and philosophies. Thus, as he grew into adulthood, he displayed a clear sense of direction rare for a man his age. When combined with striking good looks and a gift for public speaking matched by few, this political grounding allowed him quickly to scale the ladder of local and state politics.[12]

Elected vice president of the United States on the Democratic ticket in 1856 at just thirty-six years of age, John C. Breckinridge took the national stage at a critical moment when the country struggled to solve the slavery crisis. He became the champion of states' rights and the protection of slavery in 1860 when he ran unsuccessfully for president as the Southern Democratic candidate. Abraham Lincoln's election triggered the secession of southern states. Though Breckinridge hailed from Kentucky, a state that at first declared neutrality and later chose to remain loyal to the Union, he pledged his support to the cause of Dixie. In the fall of 1861, the former vice president accepted a commission in the Confederate army as brigadier general. In so doing, he became the highest-ranking U.S. official to lead troops for the southern states, and he ultimately became Jefferson Davis's secretary of war. The defeat of the Confederacy led to his exile, first to Cuba and subsequently to Europe and then Canada. Although he eventually returned to Kentucky, his political career had come to an end.[13]

THE CIVIL War irrevocably influenced the lives of the family's future generations. More than any other factor, the legacy of the Civil War would shape Mary Breckinridge's upbringing. Both of her parents, Clifton Rodes Breckinridge and Katherine Breckinridge Carson, came of age during the war, and they found themselves forever changed by their experience during these watershed years. Throughout his life, Clifton sought the success his father and great-grandfather had achieved, but he never attained the status expected of a man of his lineage.

When war broke out in 1861, Clifton Breckinridge, like many young men of his generation, welcomed the excitement and glory he expected the conflict would bring. Clifton was the second of six children born to John C. Breckinridge and Mary Cyrene Burch Breckinridge. Clifton was born in Lexington, Kentucky, in 1846 but spent much of his childhood at Cabell's Dale, the family's purebred horse farm located seven miles outside the city. Just fifteen when his father rode off to join the Confederate army, Clifton soon followed, enlisting as a private in a cavalry unit. He was eager to win glory on the battlefield but instead spent much of the war performing mundane tasks and running errands for his father.[14]

At the end of the war, nineteen-year-old Clifton stood on the brink of manhood, but he lacked a clear sense of direction. Now in exile, his father could not directly advise him, so family friends provided guidance and financial support. Following the Confederate surrender, Clifton worked for a time in a Cincinnati dry goods store before enrolling at Washington College in Lexington, Virginia. He was welcomed to campus in 1868 by hero and family friend Robert E. Lee, who had recently assumed the presidency of the institution, which was later renamed Washington and Lee College. Breckinridge was a diligent though mediocre student. He never earned a degree, but his time at "one of the most virulent rebel institutions in the land" further reinforced his identity as a southerner. Throughout his life, he took very seriously Lee's advice to "stay with the South."[15]

When he left school, Clifton was eager to establish himself, but the disfranchisement of former Confederates combined with the family's reduced financial situation to leave him with limited options. In 1870, he moved to New Orleans and set himself up as a cotton merchant. He struggled for a time, serving as a middleman between planters and textile producers, before moving to Pine Bluff, Arkansas, to join his older brother as a cotton planter. This venture also proved unprofitable. He found the years 1870 to 1883 marked by economic uncertainty.

Despite his financial difficulties, Clifton won the hand of distant cousin, Katherine Breckinridge Carson. The couple married on November 21, 1876, in Memphis in what one historian has described as "an Old South wedding in a New South city."[16] The impressive heritage of both the bride and groom certainly was not lost on those in attendance. The son of former Confederate president Jefferson Davis served as best man, reminding guests that this ceremony was significant not only because it joined the lives of two individuals but also because it linked two prominent southern families. Guests undoubtedly found the occasion an opportunity to reminisce about the Confederacy's past glories.[17]

Katherine Carson Breckinridge, like her husband, boasted an impressive pedigree. Born in 1853, she was the daughter of a wealthy Mississippi Delta cotton planter. Her father, James Green Carson, was the only son of an only son and consequently inherited a sizable estate comprising several thousand acres of prime land near Natchez, Mississippi, and nearly six hundred slaves to work it. Though the family later claimed that Carson morally opposed slavery and sought medical training to provide an alternative income that would allow him to free his chattel, evidence suggests that he manumitted only one bondsman during his life. Instead, Carson expanded his holdings in humans and land by purchasing Airlie Plantation on the Louisiana side of the Mississippi River in 1846.[18]

Katherine Carson grew up in the luxury so often romantically ascribed to the Old South. Visitors to her family's estate traveled down a long tree-lined avenue, finally coming upon a mansion overlooking acres of well-manicured gardens.[19] Reflecting their status within the community, Dr. Carson and his wife, Catherine Waller Carson, entertained "often and charmingly," as one neighbor later recalled.[20] Their close proximity to Natchez, a "bustling river town" with a "reputation for high living and notorious characters," provided them ready access to the luxuries and conveniences of the day.[21] On the eve of the Civil War, Natchez and its aristocratic nabobs boasted a higher concentration of wealth than any other town in the South.[22]

The war, however, took its toll. The Carson family's fortune, like that of many white southerners, evaporated during the course of the conflict. Between 1860 and 1865, southern wealth declined by 43 percent, even excluding the value of slave property. During that period, cotton production fell to only one-tenth of its 1860 level. Fewer than 25 percent of antebellum planter families in the Natchez District retained title to their estates by 1870.[23] Life would never be the same for the Carsons following the war. When federal troops launched their siege of Vicksburg in 1863, Dr. Carson fled with his family to Texas, bringing little besides the slaves, who would soon be emancipated. During the relocation, Dr. Carson fell ill with diphtheria and died suddenly, leaving his wife and several young children to start over alone.[24] A chronic invalid, Catherine Carson could not face returning home without her husband. Instead of rebuilding her life in the Delta, the widow settled in Memphis. To provide a better environment for her only daughter, Catherine Carson sent the girl to live with Susanna Preston Lees, a wealthy New York aunt.

Only twelve in 1865, Katherine took from the wartime experience a fierce loyalty to the Confederacy, which Aunt Lees encouraged. Young Katherine named her pony Rebel and her cat R. E. Lee and vowed always to remain "unreconstructed." In a further display of her southern pride, Katherine expressed hope that she would one day marry a "soldier who had lost a leg or been shot through the lungs."[25] Clifton Breckinridge never got close enough to battle to face danger, but his young bride apparently found his Rebel experiences sufficiently glorious to overlook his poverty and commit her life to his. Katherine gave birth to the couple's first child, James Carson, less than a year after their 1876 wedding; Mary arrived four years later. Two more children eventually followed—Susanna Preston Lees in 1883 and Clifton Rodes Jr. in 1895.[26]

BY THE time Mary was born, Clifton had been trying to earn a living as a cotton planter for more than a decade. Instead of rebuilding the family fortune, he found himself struggling daily to survive, able to afford only a small, rented house "in an unfashionable quarter" of Pine Bluff.[27] Now with a wife and two small children to support, he looked for another vocation. Like so many of his male relatives, Clifton found himself drawn to politics. After Confederate soldiers regained their full political rights, he ran for a seat in the U.S. House of Representatives.[28] His victory ensured that the Breckinridge political dynasty would survive the catastrophic war years.

From 1882 to 1894, Clifton Breckinridge represented Arkansas's Second District in Congress. The stocky, bespectacled politician with the drooping mustache flourished in his new role, gaining the respect of voters and his fellow representatives alike. Referring to his political success and in jest to his short stature (he was only five feet, five inches tall), his colleagues affectionately nicknamed him the Little Arkansas Giant. His popularity in Congress gained him an appointment on the prestigious and powerful Ways and Means Committee.[29] Political life was good to Clifton Breckinridge, but his family suffered the strain of his busy schedule and frequent travel. Mary later recalled that she spent much of her early life on trains, resulting in an "unsettled" existence. Because the family moved several times each year between Washington, D.C., and Arkansas, the Breckinridge children found it difficult to establish ties within the community. Her parents did not own a home and moved often, adding to her feeling of instability.[30]

Without a family home of her own, Mary's best childhood memories came from time spent in the homes of her extended family. She enjoyed visits each summer to Hazelwood, her great-aunt Lees's estate in High Bridge, New York, where cow pastures, wide lawns, and wonderful climbing trees brought hours of pleasure. Mary also fondly remembered yearly trips to her uncle Joseph Carson's Mississippi Delta plantation, Oasis. There, she and her cousins spent their days fishing and hunting deer, learning to ride horses, and exploring old Indian mounds.[31] Mary loved the outdoor life and recalled with pride that her talents as a hunter won her several prized "trophies."[32] Each evening, the members of the younger generation gathered to hear the older folks tell stories. Mary recalled learning about the hard times that followed the Civil War and hearing frightful tales of "strange negroes, inflamed with carpetbag teachings," who descended on the cities during Reconstruction.[33] More often, older relatives nostalgically let their minds slip back to the happier time before the war. Growing up among the ruins of the Confederacy, the Breckinridge children came to see the antebellum period as a golden age. The poverty, corruption, and racial unrest that plagued the New South appeared in sharp contrast to the idyllic accounts of life in the Old South.[34]

DURING THE long, hot summer days spent in Mississippi, the Breckinridge children gained a sense of their place in the social hierarchy. With traditional power structures seemingly under attack from all angles, white southerners harkened back to the prewar days when every individual—male or female, black or white—had a clearly defined role. Clifton and Katherine Breckinridge, like so many of their peers, enthusiastically embraced the myth of the Lost Cause and reared their children to view the past within this framework. Offering both a justification for secession and a condemnation of Reconstruction, the Lost

Cause provided southerners a means through which "to fashion new selves and a new society from the materials of the old."[35] According to historian Charles Reagan Wilson, adherents of this "civil religion" celebrated a "good society" that was "paternalistic, moralistic, well-ordered and hierarchical."[36]

Proponents of the Lost Cause argued that rather than an evil, barbaric system, slavery had actually been a positive, civilizing force that worked to the benefit of masters and slaves alike. Clifton Breckinridge described the antebellum master-slave relationship as the high point of race relations. During the prewar years, the two races had lived together peacefully with "the aggravated crimes of later days . . . absolutely unknown." Before emancipation, black and white children grew up side by side, cared for each other in later life, and submitted to the "refined and elevated rule" of the period. Reconstruction, by contrast, brought "social and civic disorder." Bitterness and racial strife reigned as the "Negro was taught to hate the Southern white man [and] to reject his influence."[37] Now that the protective bonds of slavery that had always kept blacks in check had been broken, Clifton and Katherine Breckinridge embraced segregation as the best option to prevent racial disorder and taught their children to do so as well.[38]

Southern elites not only lamented the breakdown of racial boundaries that followed the war but also resented the blurring of traditional class structures. Disdainful of the "new money" that emerged as a result of industrialization, southern families who had lost their fortunes during the Civil War took comfort in knowing that their genteel heritage continued to set them apart from the nouveau riche.[39] To prove their superior status, many turned to genealogy. As eminent historian C. Vann Woodward has explained, through genealogy, the "fabled Southern aristocracy, long on its last legs, was refurbished, its fancied virtues and vices, airs and attitudes exhumed and admired."[40] Money would always be a little tight for the members of Clifton's family, but their bloodlines and good breeding entitled them to membership in this "fabled Southern aristocracy." The Breckinridge children were taught to believe that personal qualities such as honesty, integrity, and service to others rather than a large financial fortune determined their worth. "Genteel poverty," in their minds, became a badge of honor, while extreme wealth elicited suspicion and disdain.[41]

Southern whites struggled to regain the upper hand in race relations and to reinforce their class status in the wake of Reconstruction, yet they found that they could hold onto one dimension of their past lives by maintaining traditional gender roles. Southern men and women alike in the postwar years fondly recalled the days when chivalry was in full bloom. They eagerly read the novels of Sir Walter Scott and worked to protect the patriarchal society this romantic literature extolled. Southern men might no longer claim the ultimate respect of their former slaves, but they could still expect women to defer to their authority. In this one area, life could remain unchanged.[42]

Nineteenth-century women of all social classes and to some extent all races felt the pressure to uphold the "cult of true womanhood" by exhibiting the cardinal virtues of piety, purity, submissiveness, and domesticity.[43] However, historians agree that white southern women remained wedded to the system of separate spheres longer and more enthusiastically than their counterparts in other areas of the country.[44] In the bleak days of Reconstruction, southern women exaggerated their submissive status as a way to reassure Confederate veterans that their military defeat had not left them emasculated. By emphasizing their sustained dedication to true womanhood, southern ladies provided a sense of continuity in a society turned upside down by political and social turmoil.[45] In return for deferring to the men in their lives, southern women received financial support and protection and preserved their spot on the pedestal described by Anne Firor Scott in her classic study, *The Southern Lady: From Pedestal to Politics, 1830–1930* (1970).

Adolescent girls in the South at the turn of the century received clear lessons on how to behave, and Mary Breckinridge was no exception. Parents and family members instructed young women to be demure and self-sacrificing, focused always on the needs of others. Advice manuals, ministers, and mass circulation magazines further reinforced this message, providing constant, clear lessons on the qualities young women needed to cultivate as future wives. Although women's actual behavior often diverged from the ideal proclaimed by such sources, the archetypal southern woman looked down from her pedestal over the society into which Mary Breckinridge and her young contemporaries were born, casting a shadow they could not ignore.[46]

Clifton and Katherine Breckinridge taught their children that God had created men and women to hold opposite but complementary roles in society. Men's reasoning abilities and aggressiveness, members of the Breckinridges' class assumed, naturally equipped them to hold leadership positions in government and business, while women were ideally suited to care for the home and children since they were inherently more nurturing, intuitive, and moral. The Breckinridges did not simply pay lip service to these gender norms: their daily behavior provided a model of how men and women should behave. Clifton held a public position of power, while Katherine served as a dedicated helpmate, working behind the scenes to make his goals into realities. As intended, Mary learned to see this public-private division of labor as customary and comfortable. By watching her parents as well as her extended family, Mary came to regard white supremacy and male authority as normal, providing a much-needed sense of order in a society shaken to its core.

CLIFTON BRECKINRIDGE continued to serve in the House of Representatives until 1894, when he lost the primary to his Populist opponent. He did not have long, however, to contemplate his next career move. Almost immediately after the election, President Grover Cleveland appointed Breckinridge minister to Russia, in recognition of his devotion to the Democratic Party. Excited about his new position, the family members prepared to move to the Russian capital in the fall of 1894.[47]

Their excitement, however, quickly dissipated. Their three years in St. Petersburg proved a stressful and dreary period for all the Breckinridges. They found themselves surrounded by unfamiliar people, strange customs, and a much harsher climate. Accustomed to the mild weather of the U.S. South, they were not prepared for the raw, cold days that seemed to follow one after another without relief. Writing to Susanna Lees, Katherine complained that "no one who has not experienced it can realize what it means to be without a ray of real sunshine for weeks—especially to a Southern woman."[48]

Financial difficulties compounded the family's unhappiness. The U.S. government at this time provided only the sparsest of resources for its foreign delegations. From his own small salary, the minister was expected to rent a building to serve as the embassy and to entertain guests in a fashion that would reflect favorably on his government. Tradition dictated that ambassadors dip into their personal savings to cover costs when necessary.[49] Katherine did all she could to streamline their budget. The Breckinridges even moved the embassy from its traditional location to a less convenient spot to economize. Still, they continually ran short of funds. Throughout their marriage, Clifton and his bride had lived comfortably but never ostentatiously. They had little savings and therefore found it difficult to make up for the shortfall they faced. Katherine often had to turn to her wealthy Aunt Lees for money during this period. To add to their worries, their economizing did not go without notice. Critics scoffed at Breckinridge, claiming that he lacked the sophistication and the personal wealth to serve as minister.[50]

Preoccupied with their own worries, Clifton and Katherine failed to see how unhappy their older daughter had grown. Only thirteen years old when the family arrived in the Russian capital, Mary spent the next few years feeling more alone than ever before. She missed her many American cousins. In her new home, she found very few girls her age. Her sister, Lees, was only two years younger, but she provided little companionship. A tremendous gulf seemed to separate the young woman from the small girl who remained caught up in childish pursuits. Mary looked to her mother for attention, but Katherine was busy carrying out her official duties and caring for her youngest son, born after the family's arrival in Russia.[51] For Mary, Clifton Jr.'s birth was the only bright spot in these long, lonely years. While in Russia, Mary suffered physically and emotionally and demonstrated perhaps the first signs of a lifelong battle with depression. The family's physician recognized that she was unwell and thus limited her food intake, believing that fasting could improve nearly any condition. Not surprisingly, Mary found that over the course of the two years she spent under this doctor's care, she grew increasingly weak. Feeling that she had no one with whom to share her worries and frustrations, Mary sat up at night covering the pages of her journal with tales of the "dullness, loneliness, and . . . wickedness" of her life.[52]

Mary turned to books, especially poetry and literature, as an outlet. She memorized volumes of verse, including Sallie A. Brock's *The Southern Amaranth* (1869), a favorite, which was dedicated "to the memory of the Confederate dead."[53] Mary understood that she had a talent for intellectual pursuits, and she resented her parents for failing to take her education seriously. Her older brother, Carson, attended the finest schools in Washington, D.C., before transferring to a European boarding school. Meanwhile, a succession of governesses who spoke poor English taught Mary and Lees at home. Katherine Breckinridge had been educated in this manner, and it was "the kind [of training] she wanted for her little girls."[54] The idea that their daughters might have to support themselves financially never crossed the minds of women of Katherine's generation and upbringing. Mary and her sister, it was assumed, would marry respectable gentlemen who would fully provide for them.

Mary craved formal training in serious subjects such as math, Latin, and philosophy. She longed to attend school, not only for the mental challenge it would bring but also because doing so would allow her to socialize with other girls her age.[55] She was overjoyed when her parents announced that she would enroll at a Swiss boarding school in the fall of 1896.[56] The experience turned out to be everything she had hoped for and more. During the year and a half she spent in Lausanne, she experienced a profound social and intellectual awakening. Being away from home for the first time initially left her feeling disoriented, but she soon made friends and adapted well to her new, cosmopolitan environment. She developed close bonds with her classmates, who encouraged her to set aside her naturally serious nature and dance, play games, and "cut up out of sight of the teachers watchful eyes."[57] Faculty planned frequent day trips that allowed students to take in cultural events held in nearby towns, and the school often sponsored excursions to the surrounding countryside, where the girls were allowed to pair up and search out "caves with hidden streams and waterfalls" and "shy little lakes tucked into faraway places."[58] During these years at Rosemont, Mary later claimed, she developed her strong affinity for mountains and their inhabitants.[59]

These years away from home allowed her to "pluck [her] first edelweiss"; more important, however, the experience exposed her to serious, challenging academics.[60] At first glance, Mary and her classmates appear to have received the type of frivolous education so in vogue for upper-class young women in the nineteenth century. She described Rosemont as a "first-class school of the old-fashioned kind."[61] Administrators designed the curriculum around subjects that would prepare students to serve as charming and informed wives to politicians and businessmen. Rosemont emphasized writing, literature, and languages while paying much less attention to mathematics and science. Students were encouraged to read on their own, but their library was restricted to works appropriate "pour les jeunes filles" (for young ladies). Studying was limited to one hour each evening.[62] Despite the intentions of parents and school officials, however, students found their time at Rosemont to be intellectually stimulating and in some cases an invitation to explore further. Even within the tightly regulated curriculum, individual faculty members incited passion for their subjects. In the upper school, professors from the University of Lausanne provided instruction.[63] In awe of these "masters in their fields," Mary threw herself into her studies, eager to earn their praise.[64]

Mary excelled academically at Rosemont, but in Victorian fashion, her parents expressed continual concern that she was exerting herself too much. Her experience, she reported, had "opened up whole areas of [her] mind" and left her thirsting for more opportunities to learn and study. At the start of her second year away, Mary assured her mother, "I do not find the classes too difficult for me, and *so* interesting. I have been growing fonder of my studies every day since I came to Rosemont but I never loved them like I do now."[65] Though her mother celebrated upon hearing that her daughter had been promoted to the first class, Katherine urged Mary not to push herself too hard and always to consider her health first. "You have plenty of time to cultivate your mind, but if your body is weak you cannot accomplish anything."[66]

Mary remained in Switzerland through the fall of 1897, when her father's assignment as ambassador ended and her family returned to the States. With two years of high school remaining, she transferred to Miss Low's finishing school in Stamford, Connecticut. She found the transition difficult. The girls at Rosemont had come from countries around the world—only two were Americans—while most of Miss Low's students hailed from the local area. These Yankees seemed to Mary "like a new race of people." To combat her discomfort, she immersed herself in her studies, taking particular joy in learning Latin.[67] With time, as she became involved in more activities, she adjusted to her new surroundings. She joined the Literary Committee and served as editor of the yearbook. In February 1899, she assured her mother that she was "never sad now."[68] Although she actively participated in school clubs, classmates still described her as a distant and somewhat intimidating figure. The school yearbook reported that with her in-depth knowledge of philosophy, Breckinridge "completely silenced" her peers.[69]

FOR MARY, the decade following her graduation from Miss Low's left her struggling to reconcile "the life [she] longed to live" with the "life allowed [her]."[70] In 1899, she stood at a crossroads. She could choose a life of independence and adventure, or she could take the more predictable route that society advocated and embrace women's traditional domestic role. She found herself torn. She had great dreams of continuing her education and of "wander[ing] through the most difficult and inaccessible parts of the world." However, another side of her longed to marry, to establish a comfortable, stable home and raise eight children.[71]

As a young girl, she imagined ways she could have both domestic bliss and the adventure that she craved. She envisioned herself crossing glaciers and taming jungles, carrying her children with her when they were small. She knew of course that there would come a day "when their little legs could not keep up with so active a mother. Then a good grandmother could take over."[72] But with graduation came a sense of reality and profound recognition of the limitations society placed on young women. She wanted to have it all in an era when combining motherhood with a career was not an option.

In the late nineteenth century, as Mary and her parents planned her future, options for women were increasing as the True Woman began to slip into the shadow of the New Woman. At the turn of the century, "the middle-class Victorian cultural image of the 'angel in the house' remained the ideal, but as historians have shown, the distance between that image and the reality of women's lives was growing rapidly."[73] The years 1870 to 1920 marked an important period of transition for white privileged females, bringing expanded education and career opportunities as well as new possibilities for voluntary public service. The Industrial Revolution helped to make possible these changes. As mechanization eased the burden of household chores and transformed the home from a productive to a consumptive unit, middle-class daughters now found themselves free to pursue interests outside the home and did so in growing numbers.[74]

During these years, the nation's college campuses offered clear proof that woman's role was changing. In the half century following the Civil War, the number of females pursuing higher education increased nearly 400 percent. By World War I, women made up almost half of the postsecondary student body. But women's pursuit of higher education did not come without resistance. Critics, the most outspoken of whom was Dr. Edward Clarke, warned that higher education would physically and emotionally damage delicate females, causing "neuralgia, uterine disease, hysteria, and other derangements of the nervous system." As late as 1904, psychologist G. Stanley Hall predicted that educated women would "become functionally castrated [and] unwilling to accept the limitations of married life." Undeterred by these dire admonitions, young women found college a rewarding and uplifting experience. Not only did colleges offer academic challenges, but single-sex institutions in particular created tight-knit female communities that encouraged social and civic growth.[75]

Female college graduates left campus inspired to improve their world, but they often encountered a gulf between the training they received and the options they found available. They had learned new skills but soon discovered that these skills could not be utilized while continuing to conform to "expected patterns of behavior."[76] The separate spheres mentality that suggested that men and women were naturally equipped for different purposes continued to hold sway even as the shift from True Woman to New Woman was occurring. Some Americans were beginning to support women's decisions to use their special female qualities through either voluntary or professional service, but not even the most progressive questioned the assumption that career and family were mutually exclusive lifestyles. College graduates found themselves forced to make a choice—would they marry, or would they pursue professions?[77]

Mary, like so many of her peers, experienced a crisis as she struggled to plan her future.[78] She found her decisions further complicated by her family heritage. Growing up surrounded by so many famous public servants, she could not help but conclude that an individual of her station had a responsibility to lead. This expectation helped fuel her deep-seated desire "to do something useful."[79] Yet the family's endorsement of traditional gender roles encouraged Mary's conservative tendencies, which suggested that happiness could come only from being a wife and mother.

To reconcile these two competing messages, Mary understandably looked to the examples set by female family members. The experiences of the two most significant women in her life—her mother, Katherine Carson Breckinridge, and her great-aunt, Susanna Preston Lees—clearly illustrated that women's proper place was in the home. Both women were active in charity work, but they chose to volunteer their time only to causes that concerned mothers and children. Katherine did help to establish the Daughters of the American Revolution and served for a time as state regent of the Arkansas chapter, but she always made it clear that her husband and children were her top priority and that their needs came first.[80] In the eulogies that followed her death in 1921, admirers frequently noted her self-sacrificing nature. As one relative recalled, "She uniformly set her preference aside and chose what seemed best for [her family], finding her happiness in doing so."[81]

Susanna Lees's life choices further drove home this message to her young impressionable great-niece. Lees, whom Mary called Grandmother, impressed on the girl that family should be a woman's primary focus. Even though Lees could not bear children, she found other ways to serve as a mother by taking in orphaned southern children following the Civil War. She also acted as a surrogate mother to mountain schoolchildren by corresponding with them and paying their tuition. Lees's example taught Mary that motherhood was not a choice but an imperative that all women must embrace.[82]

Conversely, Mary's cousin, Sophonisba Breckinridge, provided a very different example of what a woman could choose to be and do during this period. Among the first wave of American women to enroll in college, Nisba earned a degree from Wellesley College in 1888. Following graduation, she studied law with her father and became the first woman to pass the bar exam in Kentucky. The young attorney, however, struggled to establish a successful practice due to her gender. Seeking a more fruitful outlet for her talents, she enrolled at the University of Chicago, where she earned a doctorate in political science and a law degree. After completing her studies, she accepted a position on the university's faculty. Sophonisba's greatest achievement was in professionalizing the infant field of social work. She played a key role in carving out a spot for the fledgling specialty within the academy and helped shape the nation's developing welfare state. Sophonisba never married. Instead, until her death in 1948, she worked tirelessly and very publicly on behalf of African Americans, women, immigrants, and the poor.[83]

Although it was unusual to hold such progressive views in Kentucky in the nineteenth century, Sophonisba's parents, Issa and W. C. P. Breckinridge, a member of the U.S. Congress, were enthusiastic advocates of women's education, and they fully supported their daughter's intellectual pursuits. In one of the many affectionate, encouraging letters Sophonisba received from her father while attending Wellesley, he recommended that she study chemistry, electricity, and botany rather than literature and needlepoint, arguing that the sciences could provide "a great field of profitable and honorable work for women."[84] Issa and W. C. P. offered similar encouragement when another daughter, Curry, decided to train as a nurse.[85] The congressman believed that women should involve themselves with "honest toil" rather than live the typical "aimless life" so many young girls pursued.[86]

Clifton and Katherine Breckinridge did not share their relatives' progressive stance on women's education and pointed to Sophonisba specifically to discourage Mary from continuing her education. Katherine accused her kinswoman of forsaking her duty to home and family. The lure of learning had enticed her away from her ultimate womanly calling. Katherine Breckinridge felt that the only acceptable place for a woman was in the home—either that of her father or that of her husband. Although middle-class women were attending college in larger numbers by 1900, Mary's parents did not want their daughter to take such a bold step into the public arena. Mary later claimed that a lack of funds prevented her from pursuing additional schooling, but the fear that it would lead her, like her cousin, to choose a career over marriage surely figured more heavily in the decision.[87] Through the generations, the Breckinridge family had heartily endorsed higher education, at times sacrificing heavily to cover the cost of tuition. This attitude that education was not a luxury but a necessity extended only to males, however, and Mary's parents remained convinced that higher education would lead their daughter down the wrong path.[88]

Unwilling directly to challenge her parents and society, Mary shied away from the choices that her bold cousin had made and assumed the role of the dutiful daughter. In her correspondence with her parents, she frequently noted her desire to please them, "not so much in lessons even, as in life."[89] Unlike Issa, who encouraged Sophonisba to make choices different from the ones her mother had made, Katherine emphasized Mary's obligation to uphold her parents' and society's expectations. Katherine reminded her young daughter that happiness gained from doing her "duty" would "far outweigh" any "pleasures" she had to forgo. She reinforced the message, adding, "You have always been conscientious and I always feel sure you will do your duty."[90]

AFTER GRADUATING from Miss Low's in June 1899, Mary rejoined her family in Arkansas, not knowing what her future would hold. His appointment as ambassador over, Clifton carefully considered his options. He could return to cotton planting, write a biography of his famous father, or assume the presidencies several small southern colleges were offering, but none of these choices appealed to him.[91] Instead, he accepted a federal appointment on the Dawes Commission for Indian Affairs in June 1901. In this role, he would work with the Cherokee to compile a list of legitimate citizens to aid in the division of tribal land that would soon take place as the Oklahoma area prepared for statehood.[92] Katherine frequently accompanied her husband in his travels through the Indian Territory, but the couple deemed such trips unsuitable for their young, unmarried daughter; much to Mary's dismay, they rarely allowed her to accompany them.

Aside from infrequent sojourns to Oklahoma, Mary Breckinridge spent the first five years after her high school graduation living the life of a sheltered southern debutante, moving often among the homes of relatives in Memphis, New York, Mississippi, and Canada. She craved adventure and longed for the opportunity to explore new areas. Instead, social calls filled her days, while parties and dances occupied her evenings.[93] She recalled that she "chafed at the complete lack of purpose in the things [she] was allowed to do," but when she petitioned her parents to continue her education, she met with resistance. After much pleading, her parents permitted her to take summer classes at the University of Tennessee, where her brother was enrolled. They preferred, however, that she devote her energy to more ladylike pursuits such as courting beaux. Although she was frequently outside her parents' careful watch, concerned relatives accepted the role of chaperone in their place. As was typical for the time, these surrogate guardians closely monitored their charge's actions to protect against the slightest suggestion of impropriety.[94]

During this time, Mary remained uncertain that she could devote herself fully to a husband, as marriage required. She felt called to continue her education and to pursue a career, though doing so would clearly violate her parents' wishes.[95] She understood that her parents and society expected her to marry a "gentleman" from a "good family" and to have several children. Throughout her young adulthood, she constantly felt pulled by these two incompatible options. Would she follow the path of the New Woman, or would she take the more predictable route and embrace women's traditional domestic role?

Mary vividly portrayed the dilemma she and many of her contemporaries faced in *Organdie and Mull* (1948), an autobiographical short story. She provided two possible endings to this story, allowing readers to determine the future of the main character. They had to decide whether Cynthia, whose mother had recently died, would obey tradition and wear a white mull dress to a party, or whether she should go with her impulse and break her period of mourning by wearing a colorful, green organdie dress. Cynthia recognized that her decision would make more than just a fashion statement; her future hinged on the chosen garment. She knew that each of the two competitors for her hand would admire a different dress. Thus, her choice of attire would signify her preference for a husband and a lifestyle. In the first possible ending, Cynthia selects the organdie garment and agrees to marry Ronald, the adventurous world traveler who approves of expanded roles for women. In the second ending, Cynthia chooses the mull dress and decides to marry Leigh, the safe, devoted friend of the family who has protected her throughout her adolescence.[96]

Mary intentionally never disclosed which ending she preferred. When responding to an admirer of the story, she observed that Cynthia faced a difficult choice: "Whichever one she married, there would always be a longing ache in her heart for the other one." According to the author, "therein [lay] the tragedy in the lives of so many young girls of Cynthia's vintage." Cynthia and women like her—including, by extension, Mary—were forced "to take on all of a man's life and give up all of their own."[97] As a young girl trying to plan her future course, Mary, like Cynthia, felt "torn this way and that."[98] She resented the restrictions placed on women and dreamed of ways to break free from traditional expectations, but she also desired to marry and have children, not only to please her parents and society but also to fulfill her own needs.

For five years following her high school graduation, Mary sought a way to reconcile her conflicting goals, but in the end, she recognized that she could not have both a family and a career. Having met a man who offered her all she wanted in "married friendship," she chose the domestic path and accepted his proposal. Mary writes little about her first marriage in her autobiography; she does not even reveal her husband's name. She does, however, convey the care with which she made the life-changing decision to wed. In a scenario heavily imbued with symbolism, embellished consciously or unconsciously, Mary relates the events leading to her marriage. She met her future husband in 1904 at Oasis, the Mississippi plantation owned by her uncle, Joseph Carson. Carson, whom she describes as her "beau ideal," had recently died, and she was making her final visit to the haven that in her memory most closely represented the carefree days of childhood. Rather than being a completely sorrowful occasion, the trip was marked with the joy of "love-making" and the thrill of a difficult decision. Still struggling to overcome her "longing for exploration" and a career of her own, Breckinridge sought comfort and reassurance at her uncle's graveside. According to her account, this experience marked a turning point in her life, reconciling her to the fate that lay ahead. It was as if she had buried a piece of herself in that small family plot. She "rose comforted," confident that she could put aside her dreams once and for all and embrace those of her husband.[99]

Breckinridge explained that having made this difficult decision, "the seasons of [her] aimless girlhood" came to an end in 1904 when she married. Her husband was Henry Ruffner Morrison, a twenty-nine-year-old lawyer from Hot Springs, Arkansas. To honor Mary's parents, they chose to exchange vows on November 21, Clifton and Katherine's twenty-eighth wedding anniversary.[100] The twenty-three-year-old bride looked forward to a long and happy marriage blessed with many children, but the couple had trouble conceiving. Seeking expert medical care, Mary traveled to New York in 1905, remaining there for four months. Morrison met her to escort her back to Hot Springs, but on the way, he developed appendicitis. Doctors operated when he arrived home, but treatment came too late, and he died shortly after their first anniversary, leaving Mary feeling guilty and heartbroken.[101]

A WIDOW at twenty-four, Breckinridge wondered "what to do with the years of life that lay before" her. Having had a taste of independence, she decided that returning to her parents' home would be "impossible."[102] She dabbled in poetry and wrote an article, "The Women of Thackeray," published in the *Westminster Review* in 1907.[103] She longed, however, to do something more meaningful. At her family's urging, she spent the summer of 1907 at the Elisabeth McRae Institute, a settlement school for girls in the mountains of North Carolina. Grandmother Lees had donated a large sum of money to the school, and Mary had grown up hearing about the children her aunt helped to educate.[104]

When accounting for the reasons that led her to create the Frontier Nursing Service, Mary recalled that her experience that summer played a key role in her eventual plans. Watching a child die of typhoid fever at the institute led Breckinridge to conclude that improved health care was one of the nation's greatest needs. She was dismayed to find that despite her desire to help alleviate the victim's suffering, her lack of education made her "not fitted to be of service to anyone."[105] Following her stay in North Carolina, Mary decided that caring for the sick could provide the outlet she sought following the tragic end of her marriage. Soon thereafter, she announced her plan to attend nursing school.

Mary chose to study nursing because she, along with many Americans at the time, saw it as one of the few careers appropriate for a woman. Nursing, she recognized, allowed women to demonstrate their nurturing, self-sacrificing temperaments.[106] Nursing traditionally had been viewed as an acceptable job for women even when their employment outside the home had generally been frowned upon. Nursing provided women a safe, respectable avenue to the excitement, autonomy, and independence a profession could offer while permitting them to preserve their softer, feminine side.[107] Of all the careers Mary could have pursued, nursing seemed the most appropriate because it fit well with her view of acceptable roles for women.

With the help of a family friend, Dr. William Polk, who attested to her moral and physical fitness, Mary applied to the St. Luke Hospital School of Nursing in New York City.[108] One of the first schools to offer nursing training, St. Luke's program was among the nation's finest, turning away hundreds of applicants each year who could not meet its stiff criteria.[109] Superintendents carefully reviewed applications, selecting only the most "sober, honest, truthful, trustworthy, punctual, quiet, orderly, clean, neat, patient, kind, cheerful, and obedient" candidates. Mary's family heritage and social connections helped to set her apart from other applicants. Confident of her integrity and virtue, administrators admitted her along with twenty-nine other "respectable" women.[110] Eager to make a fresh start, Mary moved to New York and began classes in the spring of 1907.

As long as illness has existed, women have served as nurses. In 1907, however, professional nurse training was a relatively new concept. Before the Civil War, few Americans sought treatment in hospitals. The sick remained in their homes, cared for by family members, neighbors, or servants. Most Americans considered hospitals suitable only for the poor and insane.[111] But during the Industrial Revolution, as Americans began to migrate to cities and nuclear family living arrangements became standard, the need for care options outside the home arose. New medical knowledge in the late nineteenth century made hospitals a more attractive and certainly safer option. Institutions that critics had previously condemned as "sinks of human life" became an integral part of city landscapes.[112] In 1873, fewer than two hundred hospitals existed in the United States. By 1910, more than four thousand were in operation.[113]

The growing number of hospitals required a new source of labor, a need filled by the opening of nurse training schools. By 1910, one out of every four hospitals in the nation operated a training program.[114] As Susan Reverby notes, "Nursing education was called training; in reality it was work."[115] Students worked twelve-hour shifts, six days a week. Long hours on the wards required students to develop both physical and emotional stamina. Over the course of a shift, nurses found themselves walking miles through hospital corridors and continually pushing, pulling, and lifting patients and equipment.[116]

Student nurses provided the bulk of nursing care at St. Luke's Hospital, where Breckinridge enrolled, but like their colleagues throughout the country, they received no wages. However, their tuition, blue-and-white-checked gingham uniforms, textbooks, and room and board were provided free of charge. Graduate nurses, superintendents, and physicians closely observed students' actions and could dismiss them at any time for misconduct or inefficiency. Student nurses were required regularly to attend religious services and could leave the hospital only for short periods during daylight hours unless they had special permission.[117] In her mid-twenties, Mary was older than most of her fellow students, and she was the only one who previously had been married. As a widow used to making her own decisions, the degree of oversight to which she found herself subject surely required her to swallow her pride on many occasions.

Students who chose nursing because it would allow them to demonstrate their womanly gifts often found themselves taken aback by how physically and intellectually demanding their training proved. Mary and her classmates routinely found themselves pushed beyond their comfort zones and forced to expand their views of acceptable work for women. Any romantic notions that women had upon arriving quickly evaporated. Instead of holding hands and wiping brows, probationers found themselves emptying bedpans and changing dressings. Highly regimented nursing schools empowered women to become more confident and to reject the idea that women were naturally weaker than men. Hospital training served as a "powerful rite of passage," causing nursing students "to see delicacy and refinement as mere squeamishness, and to view emotional expressiveness as suspect."[118] This experience further convinced Mary that women could and should use their special qualities to make meaningful contributions outside the home.

Despite the strict rules of the training program and the physically demanding work, Breckinridge enjoyed her time in New York. She particularly liked working with infants at the city's Lying-In Hospital. While she found the loss of her husband painful, the realization that she might never have children struck her even harder. Unsure of whether she would ever marry again, she rather impulsively adopted an abandoned baby suffering from spina bifida. She believed that hospital supervisors had approved the adoption, but when she took home the infant, whom she named Margaret, administrators temporarily suspended her, thinking that she had stolen the baby. Arriving for her shift the next morning, "the biggest cyclone that ever swept over [her] head" greeted her. She was reinstated within a few hours, but the disciplinary board denied her petition to keep the baby. When Margaret died several days later, Mary paid the burial costs, recognizing that the only thing she could do now for her "little friend" was to save her from a pauper's grave.[119]

MARY GRADUATED from nursing school and passed her state boards with honors in 1910, but she decided to forgo any immediate career plans.[120] "Yielding to the pull of family," she joined her parents in Fort Smith, Arkansas, at their request. The summer passed quickly as she nursed her mother through a brief illness, oversaw household affairs, and entertained frequent guests.[121] She also found time to write another article for the *Westminster Review*, examining "The Poetry of the Southern United States."[122] As a trained nurse, she now had a skill she could share with others and an opportunity to pursue the life of adventure she had always longed to lead, but when it came down to it, obligation to family won out and the daughter who promised always "to do her duty" returned home.[123]

two Motherhood—A Career

M ary Breckinridge seemed to epitomize the New Woman with her advanced training in nursing and the independence that widowhood offered, but she remained convinced that motherhood was woman's highest calling, and she did not wait long before embracing domesticity once again. She met her second husband in 1911 while staying with her parents in Fort Smith, Arkansas. Her dream of having a house full of children, which she had abandoned after her first husband's death, rekindled the following October when she married educator and businessman Richard Ryan Thompson.

The couple celebrated their union in a small, private ceremony held at the Brackens, the Breckinridge family's Canadian summer home. Following the festivities, the newlyweds settled in Eureka Springs, a bustling resort town located in northwestern Arkansas in the Ozark Mountains. This area had become a popular vacation spot for health seekers beginning in 1879, when local residents discovered that its waters had healing powers. By 1881, the town featured fifty-seven boardinghouses and hotels to serve visitors. Home to an estimated five thousand permanent residents, it soon became the sixth-largest city in the state. The area's growth would eventually slow, but in 1912, when Mary moved there to join her husband, it remained a popular tourist draw, combining the charms of a rural setting with the conveniences of urban living.[1]

Dick Thompson had moved to Eureka Springs in 1908 to teach languages at Crescent College and Conservatory, an exclusive two-year women's college that served between eighty and one hundred well-to-do students. Born in 1878, he hailed from Mayfield, Kentucky. Before moving to Arkansas, he had earned a bachelor's degree from Union University in Jackson, Tennessee, and a master's degree from the University of Michigan. In 1910, Crescent College named him vice president, and in 1914, he assumed the presidency, a position he would hold until 1923.[2]

When the new Mrs. Thompson had married for the first time, she claimed that she had completely discarded her own ambitions in favor of her husband's career and interests. This time, however, she was considerably more mature and less willing to shrink into the shadows. She envisioned herself a full partner in her husband's work at Crescent College and in his larger efforts to improve Eureka Springs. The Progressive Era reached its apex in the years preceding World War I, and the Thompsons reflected the energy and opti-mism of the movement, establishing themselves as prominent reform-minded members of the community. Besides joining the college's faculty as a French instructor, Mary used her position as the wife of a college president to promote issues such as literacy, child welfare, and suffrage. Her name appeared fre-quently on the editorial pages of local newspapers as she publicized her causes and weighed in on controversial political topics.[3]

Nursing—always in a voluntary capacity—absorbed most of her time imme-diately following her marriage. Rather than seeking a paid nursing position, she worked behind the scenes to advance the young profession's status.[4] In the early twentieth century, nurses across the nation were fighting to institute licensure laws designed to elevate the status of their field. Nurses hoped to pass laws similar to those that had successfully standardized the medical profession by distinguishing "regular" physicians from "quacks." Beginning in 1903, nurses lobbied for practice acts on a state-by-state basis. These laws, designed to separate the trained from the untrained, varied in their scope but as a rule required any individual who claimed the title of registered nurse to hold a diploma from an accredited school and to pass a state-sponsored examination.[5]

Breckinridge played a key role in pushing for a nurse practice act for Arkan-sas. Her diploma from a well-respected program, combined with the weight her family's name carried, made her a perfect spokesperson to lead the cam-paign to professionalize nursing. In 1914, as a member of the state board of nursing, Mary headed a study of nurse training schools. She was happy to report that Arkansas's sixteen existing programs provided sufficient opportunity for aspiring nurses to earn the proper credentials. Reassured that a registration act would not interfere with the profession's growth, the state board endorsed a licensure law, which the Arkansas legislature easily passed.[6]

In addition to her attempts to professionalize nursing, Breckinridge held leadership roles in the public health movement, work that would foreshadow her later involvement with the Frontier Nursing Service. She joined several key health committees, including the newly founded National Organization for Public Health Nursing, serving as Arkansas's professional nurse representative. In this role, she corresponded with federated women's clubs in the state to publicize the goals of the public health movement and to persuade club members to volunteer to help with the organization's projects. She also worked closely with the National Organization for Public Health Nursing's Standing Committee on Tuberculosis and held several leadership roles in the Arkansas Public Health Association.[7]

By adopting such a visible role during this period, Mary joined a new generation of women who were invoking the traditional linkages among femininity, self-sacrifice, and moral superiority to justify taking on new responsibilities outside the home. Labeled "municipal feminists" or maternalists by historians, these women did not seek to escape the confines of separate spheres but instead used their special responsibility to nurture others as a springboard to new forms of professional and voluntary service. Female reformers such as journalist Rheta Childe Dorr, for example, argued that "home" was anywhere women and children were. Writing in 1910, Dorr eloquently illustrated the need for women to adopt a more public role. "Woman's place is Home," she explained, "But Home is not contained within the four walls of an individual house. . . . The city full of people is the Family . . . and badly do the Home and Family need their mother."[8] Similarly, Mary Breckinridge viewed her activities outside the home as an extension of her natural domestic role. Invoking her position as a woman and as a potential mother to legitimize her public activities allowed her to use her talents in a meaningful way and to serve as she was taught a Breckinridge should do while protecting her from the scrutiny society often leveled against women who stepped beyond their proper sphere.

EVEN AFTER she learned that she was pregnant with her first child, Mary Breckinridge did not retire from the spotlight. Instead, she defended her volunteerism, arguing that although it required her to leave the confines of the home, her efforts would ultimately benefit her children by improving the world they would one day inherit.[9] Her first child, Clifton Breckinridge "Breckie" Thompson, was born on January 12, 1914. A sturdy baby with deep-set violet eyes, fair skin, and curly blonde hair, Breckie became the center of his parents' world.[10]

Mary maintained her interest in nursing issues and local reform after Breckie's birth, but she increasingly turned her attention to maternal and child welfare issues that corresponded more closely to her new role as a mother. In seeking to improve the health of mothers and babies, Mary Breckinridge joined a powerful national movement led by public health reformers, social welfare advocates, and concerned women who argued that the nation's future rested on its mothers' ability to raise healthy and productive citizens. Baby saving became one of the most popular crusades of the early twentieth century. As historian Robert Wiebe asserts, "If humanitarian progressivism had a central theme, it was the child."[11] The activities of child welfare advocates included organizing pure milk stations, endorsing mothers' pensions, condemning child labor, establishing kindergartens and playgrounds, and working to reduce infant and maternal death rates.

Around 1900, experts began to apply scientific theories to child care, ushering in the birth of the child-study movement and the rise of "educated motherhood."[12] This national obsession with children reflected a significant shift away from earlier attitudes toward parenting. Americans traditionally had failed to see childhood as a distinct life stage. Instead of treating children like fragile creatures in need of special care and guidance, parents during the colonial period saw children largely as a supplemental labor source. This is not to say that parents did not feel real affection for their offspring; they grieved intensely over their children's too-frequent deaths. Most, however, viewed the high infant mortality rate as God's will and therefore as beyond their control.

During the nineteenth century, the belief that children's deaths resulted from divine providence gave way to a growing recognition that mothers played a key role in ensuring their offspring's health and welfare. The mother-child bond, however, remained predominantly a private relationship throughout this period. Women learned how to mother by watching female neighbors and relatives. Those who sought reassurance that they were fulfilling their role could consult advice manuals written by clergy or could join mothers' clubs, but most continued to believe that mothering skills were innately bestowed rather than learned.[13]

By the turn of the twentieth century, Americans' ideas concerning child rearing and children's place in society had changed considerably. Society no longer viewed parenting haphazardly but rather saw it as a skill that mothers must study and perfect. Mothers increasingly shared responsibility for their children with public health officials, physicians, and the state. Experts—most of them male—became the arbiters of what constituted "normal" and "abnormal" child development and encouraged women to "raise baby by the book."[14] Mothers no longer left the well-being of their children to chance but instead facilitated the rise of a "maternal commonwealth" by demanding that the government work as their ally to ensure that all young Americans grew up to be happy, industrious adults.[15]

Several factors account for why child welfare issues came to dominate the national agenda when they did. The Industrial Revolution, which helped to transform childhood into a distinct phase of life, was one important factor. As production moved out of the home, children became a drain on rather than a supplement to the family income. Consequently, birthrates declined significantly over the course of the nineteenth century. The nation's fertility rate dropped steadily, falling from an average of 7.04 children per white woman in 1800 to just 3.56 children one hundred years later.[16] This reduction in family size led parents to pay more attention to the welfare of each individual child. In the colonial period, as Laurel Thatcher Ulrich explains, "mothering meant generalized responsibility for an assembly of youngsters rather than concentrated devotion to a few." As time went on and as family sizes decreased, a shift from "extensive" to "intensive" mothering occurred.[17]

As Americans embraced the machine age, they began to place more faith in humans' ability to control their own destiny. Many parents were no longer willing to chalk up children's deaths to God's will and instead sought ways to protect their sons' and daughters' health. Parents turned to the developing medical profession to provide healing when illness struck but preferred to try to ward off disease by applying scientific theories to child care. Just as household engineers recommended that women conduct time and motion studies to determine better ways to perform repetitive tasks such as dishwashing, proponents of scientific motherhood urged caregivers to scrutinize their day-to-day activities.[18] As historian Sara Evans explains, "No longer could a 'good mother' simply feed and clothe her little ones and send them off to school on time. Now she weighed her babies and visited doctors on a regular schedule, oversaw children's clubs and music lessons, studied nutrition, and participated in the PTA."[19] Experts urged women to learn as much as they could about the "wonderful little mechanisms" in their care. The belief that individuals' careful efforts could keep children safe and healthy helped draw followers to the child welfare movement.[20]

Turn-of-the-century attitudes concerning race and the fear of national deterioration further fueled Americans' interest in children's health and well-being. Influenced by Darwinian evolutionary theory, many people expressed fear that the nation was becoming "soft." Leaders, most notably Theodore Roosevelt, warned that inferior races would soon surpass white Anglo-Saxons in the quest to be most fit. This fear became particularly acute during World War I as news reached the public that draft boards had rejected many army recruits as a consequence of poor health. In this climate, children became the nation's most precious resource, and child saving became a patriotic mission.[21]

Interest in protecting America's youth reached a peak in 1912 with the creation of a federally funded children's bureau. Florence Kelly and Lillian Wald had first proposed a national agency dedicated to women and children's health in 1903. They developed this idea one day at breakfast after running across a story detailing the federal government's attempts to combat the South's boll weevil infestation. Outraged that Washington leaders undertook such a vigorous campaign to protect farmers' profits while doing nothing to prevent the deaths of three hundred thousand babies each year, Kelly and Wald sketched out a plan for the new government department. After lobbying for almost nine years, they finally convinced President William Howard Taft to sign a measure creating the Children's Bureau.[22]

The agency's funding never matched the enthusiasm it generated, however. Constrained by a tight budget, the bureau's chief, Julia Lathrop, enlisted grassroots support to accomplish its ambitious goals of banning child labor and of lowering maternal and infant death rates. Members of the General Federation of Women's Clubs worked with the bureau to form a network of state and local child welfare committees. Female volunteers were central to the bureau's efforts to collect vital statistics by expanding the nation's Birth Registration Area and to teach women mothering skills through the distribution of pamphlets and the organization of annual Baby Week celebrations.[23]

Mary Breckinridge was one of thousands of women who enlisted in the Children's Bureau's campaign to protect mothers and babies. This movement attracted her and women like her for several reasons. First, child rearing remained a precarious enterprise in the early twentieth century, and the child welfare movement promised to reduce the risks. Between 1915 and 1919, seven out of one thousand pregnancies ended in the death of the mother, and ninety-five out of one thousand babies born did not live to see their first birthdays.[24] Although an individual's economic class could provide a slight degree of protection from these dangers, all women faced a significant threat. Second, by treating motherhood as a vocation mothers must practice and master rather than as an innate skill, the child welfare movement validated the work women performed in the home. Women were drawn to a cause that showcased their contributions to society.

HAVING SPENT so many years searching for an outlet for her talents and a way "to do something useful" without undermining her femininity, Mary Breckinridge enthusiastically embraced both the public and private dimensions of her new role as a mother.[25] She took every step possible to prepare for the "profession of motherhood."[26] She believed her training as a nurse provided her an important foundation from which to execute her duties. Still, she voraciously read the most up-to-date literature from child experts and carefully followed their recommendations.

Psychologist G. Stanley Hall's ideas particularly intrigued Breckinridge. His "recapitulation theory" posited that to grow into well-adjusted adults, children had to relive each stage of their ancestors' evolutionary development. Parents, he warned, should not interfere with children's natural tendencies. He encouraged mothers of young boys to allow their sons to express their primitive, animal urges through play.[27] To understand and minister to their children's needs, mothers had to be familiar with the stages of human development and had to keep track of where their children were in this process. To this end, Hall recommended that women turn their homes into "laboratories for child study" and that they create "life books" in which they could meticulously enter their children's weight and height and the details of their social development.[28]

Mary followed Hall's advice, scrupulously tracking Breckie's growth. She admitted that "the lives of few young children have been recorded in such detail as was his."[29] She weighed her son every week during the first year of his life, every month the second year, and every three months thereafter. She first weighed his clothing then weighed him, "deducting always the weight of his clothes before charting the pounds and ounces on his record."[30] She kept close tabs on his mental development as well by periodically administering the Binet-Simon intelligence test.[31] She viewed the data she collected not only as a measure of Breckie's physical development and mental maturation but also as proof of her success as a mother.

Breckinridge did not subscribe to Hall's argument that parents should submit completely to their children's will. Instead, she balanced his advice with that of behaviorists such as L. Emmett Holt, who argued that mothers needed to restrain children's natural urges through habit training. In his popular advice manual, *The Care and Feeding of Infants*, which went through seventy-five editions, Holt urged readers to regulate the young children's meals, rest, and playtime. Only then could they could grow up to be disciplined, successful adults.[32] Breckinridge heeded Holt's advice, paying close attention to Breckie's daily routine. For example, she served his food, which came mainly from their own small garden, on a regular schedule, in his own chair in the "food laboratory" she set up in the family's suite of rooms at Crescent College.[33]

Breckinridge felt confident that raising her son in rural Arkansas, in the middle of the Ozark Mountains, would enhance his development. Like Hall, she believed that cities disrupted natural impulses and stunted babies' growth. Living in a rural area, however, was not enough. She took Hall's theory even further, making sure that Breckie was outdoors as much as possible. He was "never far from natural things even in sleep," she recalled. Except for the coldest winter nights, Breckie slept on the balcony so the winds could sweep "over his little crib." Breckinridge credited his time outdoors for "making his body sturdy and his nature sweet."[34]

In the spring of 1916, when Breckie was two years old, Mary learned that she was expecting her second child. She recognized that her daily activities would have a direct impact on the health of her unborn baby and thus took precautions to ensure a good outcome. She cut back on her volunteer work and sought the best medical care possible. Nevertheless, Mary, now thirty-five years old, had a difficult pregnancy, feeling "discouraged and ill" much of the time.[35] In early July, Mary fell sick and retired to bed for the next five days. In spite of careful attention to her health, a daughter—"an exquisite baby with a well-shaped head"—arrived prematurely and lived only six hours.[36] Breckinridge poignantly recorded her grief in her journal: "For nearly seven months I had carried her and now my body felt so still since she had left it and my very breasts were to throb for the lips which could never suckle them."[37] Breckinridge silently mourned the death of the child she called Polly for years to come.

PERHAPS AS a way of coping with the acute grief she felt after her miscarriage, Mary renewed her efforts to promote child welfare with even greater vigor. As her son sat in her lap, playing with her typewriter and adding his notes to her letters and reports, she attempted to teach other women to be "proper" mothers.[38] Drawing on her experience and on her training as a nurse and relying on child care provided by Breckie's mammy, she enthusiastically spread the gospel of scientific motherhood.[39]

From November 1916 to June 1917, Breckinridge published a series of seven articles in *Southern Woman's Magazine* under the title "Motherhood—A Career."[40] In these monthly articles, she provided specific suggestions regarding how to properly feed, bathe, and discipline children; more important, however, she outlined her theory of motherhood, which she described as a "business" for which women needed to carefully train. She encouraged young ladies to prepare early by questioning and studying before they became pregnant. She urged those who knew they would one day bear children to take care of their bodies during adolescence and to carefully select their mates. She recommended that girls judge suitors by their potential to be good fathers. Genetics, she explained, was one of the most significant factors in the creation of healthy, intelligent children.[41] In keeping with the eugenic arguments popular at the time, Breckinridge contended that only women of good blood who married men of good blood should reproduce.[42]

A course in child welfare that she offered at Crescent College provided Breckinridge another outlet through which to spread her ideas on motherhood. Disturbed that women spent hours studying mathematics and Latin while they "knew next to nothing about themselves and absolutely nothing of the babies that most of them would one day bring into the world," she developed a curriculum that would combine "the most useful aspects of nursing and kindergarten training." Course work consisted of reading current literature on child psychology as well as hands-on instruction using her "own little son."[43] Before introducing her course in the fall of 1917, she sought input from several nationally renowned experts. She received responses "heartily endorsing" her plan.[44] For example, Lathrop praised Breckinridge's efforts, expressing a wish "that such work could be put into every school for young women in this country." Students too responded favorably to the new course, with twenty-six enrolling during the first year.[45]

While sharing theories on scientific motherhood consumed much of her time, Breckinridge was careful not to allow this work to interfere with her domestic responsibilities. She stressed that her family was and would always be her top priority. She dutifully turned down assignments that would require her absence from home. When asked to join the Arkansas Public Health Association's board of directors, she accepted but stipulated that she would leave her family only "for matters of special importance."[46] For Breckinridge as for so many women of her generation, motherhood would provide a fitting route to power and influence, but the nature of their calling would always require a careful balancing act.

IN LITERATURE describing the goals of her child welfare course, Breckinridge explained that she hoped to "give [students] an intelligent grasp of the general conditions affecting all children." Students could thus "contribute to the public life of the State . . . the same devoted and wise maternity we expect of them in their homes."[47] This statement illustrates how far her view of women's appropriate sphere had stretched by the 1910s. The line separating the public and private domains had blurred in her mind, drawing her into politics to an extent that she would have formerly judged indecent and unacceptable.

By 1917, largely as a consequence of the influence of her cousin, Sophonisba Breckinridge, Mary reversed her position on women's suffrage.[48] While at one time she opposed extending the franchise to women, arguing that political participation would distract them from their primary responsibilities, she now argued that it was imperative that the nation's mothers cast their votes. Like many female Progressive reformers, she came to believe that only through politics could she accomplish her goals for change. Women initially found ways to influence government without directly participating in the corrupt rough-and-tumble male arena. For example, in 1906, women secured passage of pure food and drug legislation by bombarding Congress with telegrams and letters. However, indirect methods such as petitioning allowed them to push only so far regarding the issues they deemed important. The ballot was essential to protect the future health and welfare of their families.[49]

Breckinridge supported the suffrage movement because she believed that the franchise would empower mothers to improve children's lives. As corresponding secretary for the Eureka Springs Equal Suffrage Committee, she wrote to the local *Daily Times-Echo*, announcing that she supported women's right to vote because she was "first and foremost and above all for babies." She urged other concerned mothers to join the fight. The benefits, she noted, would be great. The expansion of the electorate, according to Breckinridge, would ultimately lead to lower infant mortality rates and would result in the production of more intelligent children.[50]

Although she endorsed women's suffrage, Breckinridge would have by no means considered herself a feminist. Historian Nancy Cott defines feminists as individuals who supported the abolition of gender hierarchies and who presupposed that women's inferior condition was socially constructed rather than ordained by God.[51] On one hand, Breckinridge, like feminists, critiqued society's tendency to accord more respect to men's contributions than to those of women. She believed that both sexes had unique but essential roles to play in society. She compared mothers' service to that of soldiers fighting to defend their country. As she saw it, both men and women performed courageous, essential work.[52] On the other hand, unlike feminists, Breckinridge believed that the division between men and women's spheres was natural and ideal. All women, she claimed, were innately suited to have children. She believed this gift, which "springs up anew in every girl baby," to be both universal and timeless.[53] Women should not feel restricted by the obligations of motherhood, she insisted, but instead should consider them a privilege.[54] Like other maternalists, Breckinridge believed that female empowerment would come not from abandoning the home but from making society respect women's unique gifts.[55]

AS BRECKINRIDGE and her fellow child welfare advocates were waging war against the dangers threatening America's children, the nation was bracing itself to fight an even greater enemy overseas. Dick and Mary Thompson closely followed news of the conflict in Europe. The "overtones of war" dominated conversation in their home, especially after the United States announced in the spring of 1917 that it had joined the fight to make the world safe for democracy. With two brothers in the armed services and a sister working with the YMCA in France, Mary anxiously prayed that the war would end quickly.[56]

Unable to contribute directly to the war effort by serving as a nurse, Breckinridge actively recruited other trained women to volunteer overseas and taught local women to prepare surgical supplies according to the American Red Cross's specifications.[57] In keeping with her belief that mothers had a responsibility to protect not only their own children but those of women everywhere, she raised money for the Belgian Children's Relief Fund.[58]

While he could not understand fully why the world was at war, Breckie too tried to do his part. His parents encouraged him to buy Liberty Bonds with the change from his piggy bank, and he helped tend the family's victory garden. As he played, he would often pretend that his teddy bear ended the war by killing the kaiser. He idolized his uncles, Clifton and Carson, who were members of the U.S. Army, and Mary encouraged his fascination with the military.[59] Seeking to live vicariously through her son, she dreamed that Breckie would one day get to experience the "adventure" of war. Her brother, Carson, however, sternly cautioned against such a hope, noting that "adventure" was "only interesting for others to read about" and that he had "already had enough 'adventure' to last [the] family a generation."[60]

Breckie turned four on January 12, 1918, and his parents celebrated with a cake made from war flour and covered with powdered sugar icing. "With hands trembling," Breckie lit his own candles and cut the cake himself, his mother proudly recalled. The joy of this milestone, however, would be short-lived.[61]

MARY BRECKINRIDGE had more advantages than most early-twentieth-century mothers. She was financially secure, she lived in a home outfitted with modern conveniences, and she was a trained medical professional. Still, in the end, she was unable to protect her son. Five days after his fourth birthday, Breckie grew ill. He had awakened "in his accustomed splendid health," so Mary was only mildly concerned when he refused dinner, although she admitted she was "perplexed as to what could have upset his perfect digestion." The illness that "seemed so light" turned out to be quite serious. The doctor could not make a clear diagnosis when he visited the next morning, but he nevertheless booked an operating room. Surgery revealed an obstruction in Breckie's large intestine. Aware that Breckinridge was a nurse, the doctor summoned her to the operating table to see "where the trouble lay." She was devastated to find that infection had begun to set in.[62]

In the days before antibiotics, Breckie's caregivers could do little but wait. Several days of alternating hope and "sinking" fear followed. Finally, on January 23, 1918, Breckie's weakened heart gave way. The Eureka Springs newspaper announced his death, reporting sadly that although "every care and scientific method were used in making Breckinridge a sturdy, strong man . . . it was not to be." The Fort Smith paper suggested that "had he lived, with the intellectual gifts inherited from both his parents and grandparents, he would have had a brilliant career." Clutching his teddy bear, Breckie was buried the following day. The Thompsons chose not to hold a memorial service because, as his mother explained, "God didn't need to be told about Breckie."[63]

INSTEAD OF forcing Mary to reevaluate the scientific methods she so enthusiastically advocated, Breckie's death inspired her to commit herself more fully to promoting child welfare. Fearing that her son's death might plant seeds of doubt in the "minds of the uninformed," Breckinridge enlisted a sympathetic doctor to write an editorial in the local newspaper. In this piece, he provided a detailed explanation of the factors that had led to Breckie's death and reiterated the value of scientific child care methods. In this way, she sought to insure that the movement she helped to inaugurate in Eureka Springs would not perish along with her son.[64]

Breckie's death required Mary to make a "complete readjustment" as she watched her vision for her future crumble.[65] She viewed herself first and foremost as a mother and only secondarily as an activist. She wanted to improve conditions for women and children but saw herself playing an indirect role. Her ultimate contribution to the child welfare movement would come, she had reasoned, not through her own efforts but through the work her son would one day do. She had humbly insisted that she could only help "a little here and there," while Breckie, "in his manhood a leader of men, would strike at the roots of poverty, ignorance, and vice and rescue childhood."[66] She had felt certain that she was raising "a man child who would emerge some day to lead the crisis of his age."[67]

Now he was gone, leaving her to carry on alone. In the days following Breckie's death, she reconciled herself to the fact that she would have to find a new way to "rescue childhood." Thirty-seven years old, Mary again had to decide how to spend the remaining years of her life. When she had first contemplated her future at eighteen, she had abided by her parents' and society's expectations and chose marriage and family over adventure and a career. Much had changed in the intervening years. New options were open to women. In 1917, a contributor to *Good Housekeeping* reported that "in the lifetime of girls even twenty years old, the tradition of what girls should be and do in the world has changed as much as heretofore in a century."[68]

Despite the new options open to females, Breckinridge remained wedded to the assumption that God made women to be mothers. Particularly now that her children were gone, she identified herself with her maternal destiny. Following Breckie's death, she immediately began to search for a new way to use her mothering skills. Although there was "no longer any need for [her] in [her] nursery," she did not feel that her duties as a mother had ended. A proponent of "spiritual motherhood," she argued that women had an obligation to use their nurturing skills to benefit others after their own children died or left home.[69] Writing soon after her son's death, she observed that children's lives "from pole to pole of this planet" could be improved "if every one who had ever loved a child would but do his part."[70] Now that she was no longer able to care for her own babies, she committed herself full time to improving the health of disadvantaged children and to educating their mothers. The thought of helping other women's babies even if she could not save her own would help her to cope with her grief and ultimately would give her life new purpose.

By turning her private sorrow into public action, Breckinridge followed the lead of other child welfare reformers in the United States whose losses similarly inspired their work.[71] For example, Dorothy Reed Mendenhall, a physician who lost two children under the age of four, explained that her work with the Children's Bureau "came out of agony and grief" and stressed that "a mother never forgets."[72] Likewise, Breckinridge's sorrow and her desire never to forget would compel her to devote the remaining years of her life to advocating the special interests of women and children.

AS LONG as she remained in Eureka Springs, Mary was surrounded "every hour by the reminders of . . . motherhood." She needed to leave—soon.[73] In 1918, Europe seemed a logical place to escape. Trained nurses were in short supply, and Breckinridge's country needed her. Fluent in French and German, she was the perfect candidate to serve overseas. She immediately submitted notice to the American Red Cross that she was available for service. On February 4, 1918, only twelve days after her son's death, Breckinridge received a telegram from Jane A. Delano, the director of the Red Cross's Department of Nursing, offering her a position with the organization's overseas bureau. Breckinridge immediately accepted, committing herself for as long as the Red Cross needed her.[74] Dick Thompson, recently named state highway commissioner for Arkansas, supported her decision, hoping that by seeking to relieve "some part of the world's overwhelming grief," his wife could begin to "forget her little handful of grief." Her parents, whose consent she still felt the need to secure, likewise approved.[75] When describing her new assignment to her cousin Sophonisba, she expressed relief that she had skills that she could use on behalf of others. "What an unspeakable blessing it is to be equipped with a profession of real use to which to turn at a time like this," she confided.[76]

Breckinridge intended to begin work with the Red Cross in May 1918, after the courses she was teaching at Crescent College finished, but government regulations interfered with her plan. She was disappointed to learn that a State Department ruling prevented women with brothers in the army from serving in war theaters. Since Carson Breckinridge was fighting overseas, she had to wait until the government rescinded the "brother/sister rule" (also known as the "sister exclusion").[77]

While wrapping up loose ends in Arkansas, Breckinridge began writing a book to memorialize her son's short life. She dedicated this book to all who had "relinquished a loved child." When she finished, she had *Breckie: His First Four Years* privately published. By writing this tribute, which she distributed to family and friends, she attempted to come to terms with her grief. She reassured herself and her readers that Breckie was doing well "on the other side." She had gained this knowledge by communicating with friends who had already "crossed." The proud mother announced that Breckie was "with his sister and impressing all who meet him over there."[78]

Breckinridge found comfort in Spiritualism following her son's death, and she was not unusual in doing so. Americans first became interested in Spiritualism in the 1850s when two sisters from Rochester, New York, claimed that they heard rapping noises coming from the walls and furniture of their home. The movement spread "like a prairie fire" throughout the nation, winning endorsement from well known-figures such as William Lloyd Garrison, Horace Greeley, and Mary Todd Lincoln. It is impossible to estimate the number of Americans who participated in the movement at its height since its adherents rejected formal organization. One way to measure Spiritualism's popularity is to consider the number of publications directed at its followers: more than one hundred Spiritualist newspapers and magazines appeared between 1850 and 1900.[79] Grief-stricken individuals, particularly mothers, were drawn to Spiritualism's promise of life after death and were soothed by the thought that although their physical bonds with loved ones had been broken, their spiritual bonds persisted.[80]

Perhaps trying to convince herself that she was capable of moving forward, Breckinridge claimed that she had "accepted Breckie's death from the first" and that she was "not tortured about him at all." In reality, however, she spent the next ten years trying to overcome her devastating pain, seeking solace through psychiatry and conventional religion as well as Spiritualism. When she finished writing her account of Breckie's life, Mary burned her journals from those years. Refusing to dwell in the past, she threw herself into her work.[81] She reminded herself that she must be brave, as "her little soldier" had been when he faced death, and put her grief behind her. But by burying her sorrow, she subjected herself to future periodic emotional breakdowns. Memories of her son haunted her for the rest of her life.

WHILE WAITING for clearance to begin work overseas in the summer of 1918, Breckinridge accepted a position as a traveling lecturer with the U.S. Children's Bureau.[82] During the war, the Children's Bureau spearheaded a campaign to educate mothers across the country. As head of the bureau, Lathrop "milk[ed] the war for all it was worth," constantly reminding the nation that saving babies was "a vital part of fighting the war."[83] With the end of the war now in sight, the Children's Bureau hoped to maintain the excitement it had generated during the conflict by sending representatives who would promote its agenda into communities throughout the nation.

During her intensive three-month sweep of the country, Breckinridge visited at least ten states, traveling as far west as Montana, Wyoming, and New Mexico. She made several speeches each day in a variety of venues, including churches, county fairgrounds, town halls, and even her car when necessary. Fliers beckoned "patriotic intelligent citizen[s] . . . interested in future welfare of the community and nation" to attend the free community events.[84]

Blessed with her family's renowned gift for public speaking, Breckinridge enthralled audiences with her impassioned message. She encouraged spectators to take motherhood more seriously. She emphasized that at least when children were thrown into the Nile in Egypt, their deaths were quick and easy, unlike modern children, who faced "drawn-out torture" at the hands of well-intentioned but untrained mothers.[85] She criticized a system that took so lightly the fate of the nation's most precious resource. "We would not allow women to experiment on a typewriter without a knowledge of its use, nor would we allow a woman to run a tractor without knowing something about its mechanism," she pointed out. "Yet we will allow American women to kill their babies every year without asking why."[86] She stressed that child welfare work should not be solely the duty of mothers but that every citizen should make it a priority. According to Breckinridge, "One need not even be fond of children" to participate.[87]

Breckinridge's travels allowed her to witness firsthand the plight of rural mothers. The lack of adequate medical care outside of cities particularly appalled her. While speaking in South Dakota, she traveled through areas that had only one doctor to answer calls as far as seventy-five miles away. She was incensed that the state government was doing nothing to improve rural mothers' predicament. "South Dakota is much more interested in its livestock and crops than its babies," she reported to Lathrop in disgust.[88]

As September neared and her term with the bureau approached its conclusion, Breckinridge had to decide whether to extend her speaking tour or to begin her assignment with the Red Cross as scheduled. She had found her experience with the Children's Bureau rewarding because it allowed her to reach a broader audience than ever before with her message that women needed to be trained to be effective mothers. The positive responses to her speeches contributed to her indecision. One listener from the Minnesota Council of National Defense encouraged her to continue her work as a speaker. "There are others who can nurse," she noted, "there are others who can speak French, but there is no other who can bring the Child Welfare appeal to the people of our United States as you can." Another spectator, moved by Breckinridge's presentation, reported that "she created a real furore in regard to Child Welfare." She rejoiced that after hearing Breckinridge speak, "all the slackers who had been beseeched to have children weighed and measured and treated the matter indif[f]erently are now clamoring for meetings."[89]

Breckinridge was unsure where she would go next, but she was certain that she would not return to Eureka Springs. Although records on the subject are scarce, her letters to her mother during this period reveal that at some point, she and Richard Thompson became estranged. He asked to meet her in September 1918, but she refused. To ensure that she would not have to see him, she advised her mother not to share her travel plans with Dick.[90]

DESPITE THE urging of women who had been touched by her presentations, Breckinridge ultimately decided to honor her original plan to join the war effort. She traveled east in the fall of 1918 to secure her passport and loyalty papers. Arriving in Washington, D.C., at the height of a devastating influenza epidemic, however, she again found herself detained. Learning of the desperate shortage of nurses, she made her services available to the U.S. Public Health Service. Over the next several months, she cared for some of the city's one hundred thousand flu-stricken residents.[91] During that time, world leaders signed the armistice that ended World War I, and the Red Cross soon stopped deploying nurses overseas.

The war's end brought much to do in the way of reconstruction. Breckinridge applied to work with the Comité Américain pour les Régions Dévastées de la France (CARD, the American Committee for Devastated France). A privately funded relief organization established by Anne Morgan, the daughter of American financier J. P. Morgan, CARD sought to heal the "shattered human souls" of French peasant families who had endured years of German occupation.[92] CARD's female volunteers transported and delivered supplies, replanted fields, and even hosted Christmas parties. Because they lived on site, committee workers shared the poor living conditions their clients faced, including harsh weather, scarce food, and rudimentary lodging.[93]

When she finally arrived in France in February 1919, Mary began work in Vic-sur-Aisne, serving as director of child hygiene and district nursing. Before the war, this area, located in the northern section of the country, had more than six hundred residents, but by the time she arrived, only twenty-three suffering people remained. In keeping with her training, Breckinridge immediately assessed her clients' needs. She witnessed children who were two to four years behind in their growth as a result of prolonged starvation, mothers left weakened from forced labor, and men recovering emotionally and physically from war wounds.[94]

Still grieving the deaths of her own children, the condition of the French youth struck Breckinridge hardest. In the days following the war, malnourishment was the most pressing problem. She lamented that she lacked the supplies necessary to alleviate their suffering. Writing to her mother, she casually remarked that she could significantly improve the health of the children if only she had a goat for every family. Seeing the opportunity to aid her daughter's work, Katherine Breckinridge enlisted the help of friends and relatives. Within a short time, twenty-nine goats arrived in France for distribution. Each time her "circle of goat givers" expanded, Mary sent a note to the donors, describing the difference their gift, named for them, had made.[95]

Breckinridge thrilled at the fast pace of her days in France and the new experiences and challenges the work entailed. She found the adventure she had long been seeking as she sped across the countryside, overseeing her terri-tory.[96] Breckinridge's experience in France allowed her to develop the admin-istrative skills that would later make the Frontier Nursing Service so success-ful. During her two and a half years with CARD, Breckinridge built a well-oiled visiting nursing service that provided both general and maternity care to the men, women, and children who resided in scattered villages. She excelled as an administrator. In only one year, she expanded her staff from one to eleven nurses and enlarged the region they served from one village to seventy-two.[97] Recognizing that France needed trained nurses to continue her work after CARD withdrew, she conducted a study of the Paris hospital system and devel-oped a plan to establish a nurse training school in the nation's capital.[98]

Despite the victories she was experiencing in France, personal difficulties back in the United States left Mary emotionally exhausted. Witnessing con-stant suffering wore on her, but the breakup of her marriage proved an even greater source of anxiety. Dick had been a devoted and "tenderly kind father" to Breckie, but he had not shown an equal level of faithfulness to his wife.[99] With their beloved son gone, Mary could no longer bear the "indignities" committed by Thompson.[100] After seeking the advice of her parents as well as of several trusted aunts and uncles, she initiated divorce proceedings against Richard Thompson in the spring of 1920.[101] Divorce, although increasingly common in the early twentieth century, carried a strong stigma, particularly for a woman of her class, and she did not pursue such a course lightly.[102] In the suit, Breckinridge alleged that Thompson's infidelity had begun within a few months of their marriage and continued throughout.[103]

Breckinridge took a brief leave of absence from her work in France in April 1920 to travel to Fort Smith, Arkansas, to secure a "quick" divorce. Distrustful of Thompson, Mary instructed her mother to inventory Mary's belongings to ensure that he returned everything.[104] Perhaps the most telling description of her second marriage is the listing of her ex-husband in a family genealogy she compiled in 1948. She hesitated to even mention him as part of her past but concluded, "I suppose I have to include my second marriage because of the children."[105]

To signify her separation from Thompson, Breckinridge took back her maiden name "like a pair of comfortable old shoes" immediately following her divorce.[106] Her compatriots in CARD were surprised when she announced that they should now address her as Mrs. Breckinridge. Her decision to be known as Mrs. rather than Miss Breckinridge was a calculated move. She recognized that her child welfare efforts would have more credibility if she retained the married title. She also understood that the name "Breckinridge" was widely recognized and would thus provide her instant respect and authority.[107]

Breckinridge returned to France after resolving her "difficulties in Arkansas," but she remained emotionally and physically drained. Writing home in the spring of 1921, she remarked, "I . . . am so tired, not in my body, but in my head, which doesn't seem to be my head but somebody else's which I am carrying around on a platter like the daughter of Herodias."[108] A vacation in Cannes in March did little to restore her energy. She continued to lack her usual "zest and enthusiasm."[109] Concerned about her daughter, Mary's mother suggested that she retain her position with CARD but visit home more often. Recognizing the impracticality of her mother's advice, Breckinridge tersely replied, "The Director of a department of Child Hygiene in a great international committee can't jump in and out of Europe like a tennis ball."[110]

Mary grew increasingly homesick throughout the spring. In April 1921, after a great deal of contemplation and prayer, she concluded that she was "not the person for this larger work in France."[111] She loved the French people and desired to serve children throughout the world, but she felt that her real duty was to those living in her native land, where Breckie and Polly were born and buried. "I can forward things better with my own people," she explained to her mother. "I know and love my own people best."[112] Confident that "some very special thing [was] waiting for [her] on the other side of the ocean," she sailed for home in September 1921.[113]

Breckinridge did not have a plan fully formulated when she decided to return to the States, but she knew that she was destined to serve American children in some capacity. Writing to her mother, she explained, "I dream dreams and see visions and tens of thousands of children, mostly very little ones, are dancing always across the visions and the dreams."[114] Breckinridge had learned a great deal during her time in France. Administering a vast network of clinics allowed her to meet important health officials both in the United States and in Europe, and through her goat project, she learned important fund-raising strategies. She planned to continue serving as secretary to CARD's subcommittee on nursing while she worked out the details of her plan, but she eagerly looked forward to the day when she would use her skills to address the suffering of American mothers and babies.

MARY RETURNED from France physically exhausted but relieved to have a new sense of direction. She retired to the Brackens to catch her breath before resuming work. The sudden death of Katherine Carson Breckinridge one month later, however, sent her reeling. With its lush evergreens, lapping waves, and big stone fireplaces, the Brackens had traditionally provided an escape from the pressures of the outside world, but with her mother, its manager, gone, being there served to intensify Mary's sorrow.[115] Her divorce and now her mother's death were too much for her to handle in her exhausted state. After Breckie's death, she had temporarily overcome her grief by throwing herself into reform activities, but this time, she could not face work. Mentally drained, she suffered a debilitating breakdown.[116]

Breckinridge never discussed this breakdown, so one can only speculate on its causes. Perhaps her incapacitating bout of depression stemmed from feelings of guilt that she had not been home to care for her aging mother. Their relationship had never been particularly close, but like other "dutiful daughters" of her era, Mary recognized that she had a primary obligation to her family.[117] Her mother had asked her to spend more time at home, but she had refused her request, intent on completing her work in France. Mary may have felt that her mother's death was a punishment for her disobedience. Her cousin Sophonisba experienced a similar breakdown after her mother died in 1892. Sophonisba was in Europe when she received word of her mother's death, and though her parents had fully supported her decision to leave home, she still felt as though she had forsaken her duty to her family. For Mary, trained as a nurse, the feelings of guilt were surely even more intense.[118]

Katherine Breckinridge's death may also have caused her daughter to question her future plans. Mary had only recently decided that her true calling was to establish a public health organization in the United States, much like the one she had administered in France. Her mother's sudden death, coming just after Mary had finally selected a path that she believed would lead to personal fulfillment, surely caused her to question her intentions. Her father was now alone with no one to care for him. She was the only unmarried daughter. Perhaps God intended for her to return home after all.

Acting on doctors' orders, Mary did not resume work for six months following her mother's death. She wrote to Anne Morgan that she would be taking a leave of absence. Mary explained that she would be prone to "another and more disastrous breakdown" if she resumed work too soon. However, she assured Morgan that if she took time off to recover, she could once again "become as vigorous as anyone."[119]

AS SHE attempted to put her mother's affairs in order and to prepare the family's summer home for sale, she sought the emotional support not of her siblings but of her close friend, Lucille "Pansy" Turner. Mary had met Pansy ten years earlier, shortly after arriving in Eureka Springs. Pansy had been Breckie's godmother, and the two women remained close after his death despite the miles separating them. Pansy joined her friend in Canada during the spring of 1922.[120]

Pansy's emotional support helped Mary cope with her grief and begin to look toward to the future once again. Pansy could relate to her friend's feeling of emptiness and need for direction. Following the death of her husband, Jesse, she had felt a similar lack of purpose. She overcame her depression, she recalled, by trying to make "every hour worthy to be looked upon by God." Pansy advised Mary likewise to turn to God for comfort. She also encouraged Mary to seek comfort through their shared belief in Spiritualism. Pansy confidently claimed that her beloved Jesse watched her from heaven and insisted that they would one day be reunited. Consequently, she devoted herself to "working every minute" so that he would not be ashamed of her when she eventually joined him. Pansy reassured her grieving friend that her loved ones too were watching from heaven and encouraged Mary to find a way to make them proud.[121]

By late 1922, Breckinridge was ready to embark on her plan to serve American mothers and babies. She decided to emphasize rural children since children in the cities had received more attention from Progressive Era reformers. Her experience in Europe and contact with British nurse-midwives led her to believe that a similar system could work in the United States. As she saw it, the period from before birth to age six was the most formative and precarious in a child's life, and she decided to focus on this crucial period. Many questions, however, remained for her to answer: What exactly would the organization she created look like? How would it be funded? And where specifically would it operate? Much work lay ahead, but Mary was ready to begin.

THINKING BACK on this period of her life, Mary insisted that Breckie's death would have "altogether crushed" her had she not had important work to do.[122] From the moment her son died, Breckinridge felt an obligation to work on behalf of other women's babies. Several years passed before she determined how best to utilize her talents, and dealing with her grief remained a continual burden, but her experiences with the Children's Bureau and CARD helped provide her a sense of direction. January 23, 1923, marked the fifth anniversary of Breckie's death. Mary reflected on her loss that day, as she did every day, but she had reason to celebrate. She was preparing for the work that lay ahead by taking classes in public health at Columbia University.[123] Her plans for the future were beginning to come together. She was certain Breckie would be proud.

"Until our maternal and infant death rates are reduced we shame the place we hold in civilized society." In the spring of 1923, with this dramatic call to action, Mary Breckinridge outlined her plan for a rural public health service designed to serve women and children.[1] The U.S. failure to care for its most vulnerable citizens, she concluded, was a "national disgrace" and must be fixed immediately. She deemed it unacceptable that a country that so enthusiastically embraced progress and promised justice for all allowed its "little ones, by the hundreds of thousands, [to] pass from one dark cradle to another with hardly a gap between."[2] Convinced that the nation could and must do something to prevent future needless deaths, Breckinridge committed herself to finding a solution.

Although reformers had been calling attention to the problem for more than two decades, maternal and infant death rates remained disturbingly high in the United States in the early 1920s. U.S. Children's Bureau officials had done much during World War I to address the situation, but statistics continued to paint a grim picture. Instead of decreasing, the maternal death rate actually increased during the first quarter of the twentieth century. Medical advances had led to a decline in deaths from infectious diseases, but childbirth remained extremely risky.[3] American women of childbearing age had a greater chance of dying from childbirth than from any other medical condition except tuberculosis. In 1923, the U.S. maternal mortality rate of 6.7 per 1,000 live births was one of the highest in the Western world.[4] The campaign to prevent infant deaths had shown slightly more success, but thousands of babies still died needlessly every year.[5]

Public health reformers felt certain that they could reduce death rates by establishing prenatal clinics and pure milk stations. To prove their point, they set up a number of these "demonstration" programs in northeastern cities in the first two decades of the twentieth century.[6] After World War I, however, many reformers began to shift their attention to rural women and babies. To a large degree, the Children's Bureau sparked this growing interest in rural women and children's health. In 1921, after lobbying Congress for several years, the bureau celebrated the passage of the Sheppard-Towner Maternity and Infancy Act, a revolutionary bill that specifically targeted rural women. Its main function was to provide matching grants to states that created maternal and child health care programs. The states then used these funds to print and mail educational pamphlets, to sponsor prenatal and child health clinics, to establish midwife training programs, and to send nurses into women's homes to offer expert advice. The act remained in effect for seven years, during which time hundreds of thousands of women in all corners of the United States benefited from its services.[7]

Reformers' concern for rural women and children corresponded to a more general focus on the advantages and disadvantages of rural living. As the nation became thoroughly industrialized, many people began to look back nostalgically on a way of life that was quickly being lost. In contrast to urban areas, where filth, disease, and crime supposedly proliferated, farming communities seemed to offer a haven where traditional values survived. Writers such as dramatist Percy MacKaye celebrated the virtues of country life. According to MacKaye, rural areas provided not only beautiful scenery but also a slower pace of life and a greater degree of autonomy. While city dwellers were trapped in "cages of steel and marble and cement," rural Americans did not "chase the dollar . . . serve machines [or] learn their manners from the movies."[8] Progressive reformers hoped to preserve these positive qualities while bringing to the nation's hinterland the benefits of modern life—roads, education, farming technology, community development, and of course medical care.[9]

Critics viewed the poor health of rural Americans as a threat to the nation's vitality. The residents of these areas reputedly possessed pure bloodlines, in contrast to the cities, which teemed with African Americans and immigrants from southeastern Europe. Many proponents of eugenics looked to the sturdy old stock living on the nation's farms and frontier to lead the United States into the future. Mary Breckinridge herself stressed the rural roots of the nation's corporate leaders, claiming that "fully eighty percent, I am told . . . came from rural regions, mainly in the West and South." As she explained, "Mother Nature has a way of reaching over rich nurseries to her own rough bosom and picking great men from the soil."[10] She believed that future leaders currently being born in lonely, isolated regions would reinvigorate a nation that many claimed was losing its vitality.

Experts agreed that the high disease rates among rural Americans stemmed not from genetics or inherent weakness but from the lack of trained health care providers. As one public health reformer pointed out, in "great areas of sparsely settled plains, prairies, deserts, and mountain country," the nearest doctor could be as far as one hundred miles away.[11] The problem was not that America did not produce enough doctors but that they tended to be concentrated in the cities, with few choosing to practice in remote areas where financial rewards were not as great.[12] Giving birth far removed from a physician's care was particularly dangerous. Most expectant mothers in rural regions found themselves forced to deliver with only the assistance of untrained neighbors or in extreme cases to give birth alone. Child welfare advocates viewed rural America as new, uncharted territory, full of deserving individuals, and as a place where they could reduce mortality rates simply by increasing the availability of professional care.[13] The question was how such changes could be accomplished and who should bear the cost.

MARY BRECKINRIDGE was vitally concerned with these questions. She believed that her son, Breckie, would not have died had she lived in a bigger city with greater access to medical care.[14] She wanted to ensure that every mother and child had the finest medical care available, no matter where they happened to live. Drawing on her nursing training, her work with the Children's Bureau, and her time in Europe, Breckinridge developed a plan to bring high-quality, low-cost care to rural mothers and babies. She submitted this proposal to the American Child Health Association in February 1923.[15] While the name she initially selected for her project, the Children's Public Health Service, was not particularly flashy, other aspects of her plan were quite innovative.

Long before "universal health care" became a political hot button and a commonly heard phrase, Breckinridge envisioned such a program. The medical service she outlined would make health care not only "practical and cheap" but most importantly accessible. Each child living within her organization's territory would receive free health care, beginning in the womb and continuing until he or she graduated high school. Mothers similarly would receive the best medical care available, with professionals overseeing their pregnancies every step of the way. She hoped that a network of organizations patterned after her pilot program would eventually exist to serve every American mother and child.[16]

Central to her plan to make health care affordable and accessible was a new brand of practitioner with whom few Americans were familiar—the professional nurse-midwife. Breckinridge had first witnessed nurse-midwives in action while serving overseas with the Comité Américain pour les Régions Dévastées de la France. She was impressed with the practicality of the British health care system, which employed caregivers trained in both general nursing practice and specialized obstetric care. Nurse-midwives could handle normal deliveries and knew when to call physicians for difficult births. Such an arrangement made childbirth safer yet kept costs low. Breckinridge left Europe convinced that her native country could solve its rural health care dilemma by adopting a similar system.[17]

In calling for the introduction of this new type of caregiver, Breckinridge entered a heated debate that had engaged the American medical community for more than a decade.[18] Beginning in 1908, discussion of the nation's "midwife problem" filled prestigious medical journals. As medical professionals debated the present and future status of the midwife, the general public also began to view the untrained "granny" midwife as a threat to the safety of the women and children she served. The granny midwife, who not coincidently was often of African or eastern European descent, became a symbol of backward, superstitious, dangerous care. Reformers singled her out for causing the nation's high infant and maternal mortality rates and called for her eradication as a step toward progress.[19]

American women traditionally had controlled every aspect of childbirth. When it came time to deliver, prospective mothers sought the assistance of midwives while female friends and relatives gathered around to offer encouragement and support. Custom dictated that men remain outside home birthing rooms. When "man midwives" began to advertise their services in the mid–eighteenth century, opponents protested their presence in the lying-in chamber as immoral. However, in seeking to reduce the risks of childbirth, women gradually invited male practitioners, later called obstetricians, to attend deliveries and welcomed the new procedures and technology. Historian Judith Walzer Leavitt documents the "medicalization of childbirth," showing how labor went from being a female social ritual to a potentially pathological condition requiring the careful oversight of a male physician and increasingly the amenities of the modern hospital.[20]

This transition occurred naturally for the most part, as women themselves demanded the most advanced methods of care. Still, physicians intent on shoring up their professional status took active steps to convince the American public that their techniques were superior to those of lay midwives. Obstetricians in particular sought to discredit midwives as a way of earning respect for their young field. Specialists argued that their profession would never get the credit or the remuneration it deserved as long as midwives continued to practice.[21] They attacked midwives' lack of formal training as well as their noninterventionist approach to childbirth. Unlike midwives, obstetricians stressed that they were prepared to "do something" when labor slowed or crises occurred.[22] Physicians' warnings that midwives were old-fashioned and unscientific inspired a significant reduction in the number of women seeking the care of lay women. From 1900 to 1930, the number of American women whose babies were delivered by midwives dropped precipitously from 50 to 15 percent.[23]

The midwife debate concerned not whether lay midwives should be eliminated but how and when it should happen. Many physicians argued that doctors must immediately replace midwives. Such advocates claimed that more than enough physicians existed to care for every American mother. Banning midwives would allow the increasing supply of doctors to find sufficient cases to support their practices. Other critics logically pointed out that it would be impossible immediately to bar midwives from practicing. To do so would leave thousands of rural and poor women without any means of care.[24] Instead, they described lay midwives as a "necessary evil" and called for new means of training and regulating these women until they could be phased out.[25]

While Mary Breckinridge agreed with others in the medical community that lay midwives posed a threat to American mothers and babies, she offered an alternative solution. Like her fellow public health workers, Breckinridge insisted that it was "useless to condemn the ignorant midwife when there is no one to take her place." However, she believed that training and licensing lay midwives, as some observers encouraged, would not solve the problem in the long run. To do so would be a "heartbreakingly long task with the outcome only a makeshift."[26] Ideally, a qualified physician would attend every delivery, but this goal remained impossible in too many of the nation's rural areas. Instead, Breckinridge recommended that public health nurses who were willing to settle permanently in rural communities receive three months of intensive training in labor and delivery. These professionally trained women, she argued, would fill the gap in rural health care.[27]

The centrality of nurse-midwives to Breckinridge's proposed project was not the only way the Children's Public Health Service resembled the British health care system. Breckinridge planned to assign her nurses to specific districts, in much the same way the services she had witnessed in London were organized. The district health movement had originated in Liverpool, England, in 1859. Reformers divided the city into eighteen districts and assigned each a nurse who would live in the center of her territory and provide routine health care to her patients. Other English cities soon copied this successful arrangement. The potential of this system so impressed Queen Victoria that she donated funds to create a nursing school and to place district nurses throughout the United Kingdom; district nurses thus also became known as the queen's nurses.[28]

The district nursing concept was not new to the United States in the 1920s, when Breckinridge considered its possibilities. In the late nineteenth century, wealthy women in several northern cities, including Boston and Philadelphia, had established what became known as visiting nurses' associations. Lillian Wald's Henry Street Settlement, established in 1896 to serve poor New York City residents, provides one of the best examples of the application of the British district nursing concept to an American community.[29]

Breckinridge believed that the thorough type of care offered by the visiting nurses' associations had great potential not just for the urban poor, who up to that point had been its primary recipients, but also for anyone, anywhere in the nation who lacked access to health care. The service she proposed, like its British and American predecessors, would rely on a team of nurses scattered throughout its territory to provide patients with in-home care. Breckinridge suggested that each nurse assigned to a rural district could cover an area between six and seven square miles. Ideally, each would be responsible for no more than sixteen hundred patients.[30]

A small nurse-to-patient ratio was necessary if the Children's Public Health Service was to accomplish its goal of offering comprehensive care to every woman and child in its territory. The organization's nurses of course would treat acute illness, but more important, they would strive to prevent illness by frequently examining and educating healthy patients.[31] Although the public health movement stressed the need for preventative care, most medical practitioners were just beginning to recognize its importance in the 1920s. Insurance companies and industry had pioneered preventative health care as a cost-cutting measure, but doctors were slower to abandon their illness-centered approach.[32] The American Association for the Prevention of Infant Mortality passed a resolution in 1911 encouraging infant welfare workers to make prenatal instruction and examination a priority; still, as historian Richard Meckel explains, such care remained "the stepchild of the infant welfare movement."[33] Even in the most progressive, affluent communities, fewer than 25 percent of parturient mothers received prenatal care in the early 1920s.[34] Breckinridge's organization would serve its patients not simply by making medical care available but also by providing a level of cutting-edge, thorough care available to few Americans at the time.

The most innovative aspect of Breckinridge's plan was her proposed method of funding. She solicited the American Child Health Association for interim financial support, but she ultimately expected the federal government to assume the cost.[35] She viewed health care not as a privilege but as a basic human right. Mothers, by bearing and rearing children, performed a national service equal to that of soldiers, she argued, and society should reward mothers' contributions. By leaving rural women and infants to "drag out a mutilated existence unrelieved," the United States imperiled its collective welfare. She argued that good health was just as essential to the nation's future as universal public education. The whole nation would benefit as the health of its citizenry improved, and thus, she insisted, taxpayers should foot the bill.[36]

Few of the ideas undergirding Breckinridge's proposal were new. British and American health care models that had already proved successful on a limited basis heavily influenced her plan. What was innovative was the way she combined these ideas to attack the poor distribution of health care and the nation's persistently high maternal and infant mortality rates. She was confident that the program she proposed would offer a cost-effective, practical solution to the dilemma so many Americans acknowledged but did not know how to solve. As she mailed her proposal to the American Child Health Association in the spring of 1923, she felt optimistic that its representatives would recognize her plan's potential.

WHILE BRECKINRIDGE waited for the American Child Health Association's seal of approval, she looked for the perfect place to locate her demonstration. Though she had lofty ambitions for transforming health care across the nation, she recognized that she first needed to start work in a small area and prove her plan's effectiveness on a limited scale. Perhaps more than any other factor, the decision about where to begin would determine her organization's success. She considered locating her project in rural Arkansas, where she had lived for nearly ten years and had been active in community affairs. The Ozarks, however, carried bad memories of her troubled marriage and the deaths of her children. Instead, she began to investigate the possibilities the

Appalachian Mountains could offer as a home for her service. She was perhaps drawn to this area by the recent publication of John C. Campbell's landmark study, *The Southern Highlander and His Homeland* (1921). In his comprehensive survey of Appalachia, Campbell declared lack of health care "the most pressing of the mountain questions" and called for the creation of "a pioneer nursing corps"—a public health service, "national in scope, working so far as possible in cooperation with local and state agencies." The organization Breckinridge eventually created fulfilled Campbell's recommendation.[37]

When one thought of a poor region, cut off from the advantages offered by urban living, Appalachia then as now naturally came to mind. By the 1920s, local color writers, northern missionaries, textile mill owners, and settlement workers had successfully situated Appalachia within the American imagination as a troubling anomaly. While the rest of the nation embraced progress, the mountains, according to observers, offered a "present day picture of pioneer times."[38] Journalists reinforced Appalachian Otherness, describing it as "another world" and as home to a "strange land and peculiar people."[39] Americans celebrated the region's unique folk culture by collecting ballads, coverlets, and dulcimers while simultaneously decrying the area's association with feuds and moonshine. The tourist industry helped to further broadcast stereotypical images of the region as backward, and many economically strapped Appalachian residents played a role in reinforcing the nation's static view in an attempt to profit from the growing fascination.[40] Subsistence farming, high birthrates, outhouses, and horseback travel came to symbolize Appalachia just as these phenomena were dying out in other areas.

Americans found their belief that Appalachia was a land apart reinforced on every front. Stories of moonshine production, strange religious practices, and bloody feuds made good press, with newspapers across the country running stories of quaint mountain customs. The *New York Times* piqued readers' interest with headlines such as "Kentucky Is Still the Land of Murder in Honor's Name" (1895).[41] Following World War I, Sergeant Alvin York, a Tennessee hero, received widespread national attention not only for his military contributions but also because he represented a throwback society that continued to hold dear family values, patriotism, and religious conviction.[42] John Fox Jr.'s numerous and highly popular novels introduced the nation to stock, colorful mountain characters.[43] Between 1904 and 1927, at least 476 films depicted life in Appalachia, helping to solidify its backward image.[44]

Appalachia's emergence as a social construct provided an Other by which Americans could define themselves. At the turn of the century, Appalachia both nostalgically represented something that America had lost and triumphantly symbolized something the nation had overcome. Appalachia reminded Americans of their rural agrarian roots just as the nation grew increasingly urbanized and industrialized.[45] As historian Jane Becker explains, Americans "asked the southern mountaineers simultaneously to embrace the industrial present and future while maintaining, for the benefit of all America, certain desirable customs and values presumably endangered by a standardized, industrial culture."[46] Of course, the portrayal of Appalachia as a backward region further served America at the turn of the century by justifying the economic exploitation that was occurring as industrialists hauled away the area's coal and timber to fuel urban industries.[47]

Many middle-class Americans read accounts of Appalachian Otherness and became inspired to assist the region. Efforts to "uplift" mountain residents began in the 1880s as northern missionary organizations established schools and churches and continued in the early twentieth century as young college-educated women sought outlets for their talents and energies. Mountain reform projects benefited from Americans' growing fascination with the area while helping to reinforce oversimplified images of the region. In seeking support for Berea College, President William Goodell Frost described the region as "a museum of historical survivals—a present day picture of pioneer times."[48] Katherine Pettit and May Stone, the founders of the Hindman Settlement School, helped to introduce Appalachian ballads and folk craft traditions to their supporters. Americans likewise heard about the promise of the mountains from Linda Neville, who sought to eradicate blindness, and Cora Wilson Stewart, who founded the Moonlight School movement to combat illiteracy.[49] Though often in competition with one another for the same funds, these projects and many others like them united in their desire to raise Americans' consciousness of the "mountain problem."

Reformers offered many theories about what needed to be done to assist the people of the region. Some reformers went so far as to argue that the mountains should be cleared and the residents relocated to cities. Most observers took a less drastic view and instead proposed ways to rehabilitate the mountain people and to unlock the area's potential. The trick, they argued, was to find a way to move the area forward without destroying the qualities that made it special.[50] Most champions of the region remained thoroughly committed to maintaining the agrarian lifestyle that characterized the mountains but envisioned a romanticized society in which everyone lived in neat houses with attractive landscaping, traveled on good roads to well-equipped schools, and earned a decent living by doing meaningful work.[51] Reformers carefully constructed an image of the typical mountaineer they were seeking to uplift that emphasized the worth of the mountain people balanced against an account of the area's pressing needs. In reform literature, mountain folk were poor but proud, disadvantaged but eager, left behind but fully redeemable.

Mountain workers paid particular attention to the supposedly pure blood that coursed through the mountaineer's veins, and such claims regarding the area's racial purity proved one of the most compelling fund-raising tactics. For example, Stewart reminded supporters, "these children are . . . not the descendants of the african, the mongolian, or other inferior races, but the sons of the Clays, the Jacksons, the Lees, the Marshalls, and all the nobility of the South."[52] Beginning in the 1890s, Frost entreated Americans to develop the potential of "America's neglected resource."[53] Using population statistics that showed that only 2,000 of 561,881 mountain residents were foreigners and only 13,000 were black, Frost stressed the pure ethnic heritage of his students.[54] He encouraged Americans "who shrink from seeing the Saxon race submerged in the United States" to support Berea's "program of uplift."[55]

Like many Americans living in the early twentieth century, Mary Breckinridge believed that Appalachia was a unique area and particularly worthy of assistance, and she focused on this region when considering locations for her demonstration. She appreciated that the mountains offered a home to "five million native born Americans of homogeneous stock."[56] In spite of its pure blood, however, isolation, poor transportation, and poverty held the area back from fulfilling its potential.[57] Like her contemporaries, Breckinridge idealized and romanticized the mountain people. She praised their honesty, work ethic, independent spirit, and hospitality. She sincerely believed that the native population residing in the mountains possessed above-average natural intelligence, making them "of the greatest possible value to the nation."[58] She explained, "The people there are receptive, responding eagerly to every opportunity from without, and their potentialities are so high that any infant salvaged, any child released, may preserve us a leader among men."[59] The area simply needed access to education and health care services to maximize its potential, and she planned to make the latter possible.

After deciding to begin in Appalachia, Breckinridge still had to pick an exact locale, and she very quickly turned her sights to eastern Kentucky. Although she had never lived in Kentucky, her father was born and raised there, and she found herself drawn to the Bluegrass State. She knew that she could rely on her Kentucky relatives, many of whom were recognized political, educational, and religious leaders, for advice, assistance, and donations.[60] She also felt certain that the Breckinridge name, so well known in the state, would provide instant recognition and acceptance. She had personal connections with many prominent Bluegrass families, related to her and otherwise, and she recognized that she could capitalize on the responsibility they felt to assist their "benighted brethren in the mountains."[61] As she explained, "I would be too doubtful of success to push this project in Vermont or Michigan, but I *know* I can put it across in Kentucky."[62]

Kentucky officials lent their support to Breckinridge's planned project, further convincing her that it was the right place to begin. In the early 1920s, Kentucky's leaders were committed to improving the health of their constituents, particularly that of mothers and babies.[63] Kentucky had joined the federal Birth Registration Area in 1911 and in 1918 had established the country's first full-time county health departments. Despite the state's traditional suspicions regarding federal power, Kentucky leaders enthusiastically endorsed the Sheppard-Towner Act and in 1922 used the matching funds it provided to create the Bureau of Maternal and Child Health. The bureau oversaw the work of four traveling nurses, sponsored clinics to examine preschool children, distributed nutrition information to mothers, and published a weekly column, "Healthy Babies Talks," that appeared statewide in county newspapers. In addition, the bureau attacked the state's "midwife problem" by instituting a program to train and register lay caregivers and to distribute needed supplies such as silver nitrate drops to treat newborns' eyes.[64]

State health officials recognized that Breckinridge's proposed project would nicely augment their attempts to improve the health of mothers and babies and thus offered their cooperation. Dr. Arthur T. McCormack, health commissioner for the commonwealth, promised Breckinridge "carte blanche" to carry out her plan and later issued her a special state license to practice midwifery.[65] Likewise, Dr. Annie S. Veech, head of the state Bureau of Maternal and Child Health, endorsed Breckinridge's plan as an extension of the bureau's work. Veech and Breckinridge shared the goal of educating women to allow them to take better care of themselves and their children, and both women argued that safer parturient and prenatal care must be made available to every expectant mother. "If Kentucky is to hold aloft the high standard of citizenship which we mean that it should," Veech proclaimed, "then we must help our young fathers and mothers to produce physically fit citizens."[66] Her initial endorsement of Breckinridge's proposed Children's Public Health Service praised its potential to lower mortality rates. In the summer of 1923, in a blanket letter mailed to eastern Kentucky physicians and residents, Veech urged cooperation with Breckinridge, describing her as "working in conjunction" with the bureau.[67]

During the summer of 1923, with authorization from the Bureau of Maternal and Child Health, Breckinridge embarked on a comprehensive study of prenatal and midwifery care available to mothers in eastern Kentucky.[68] She zeroed in on Leslie, Owsley, and Knott Counties, intending to pinpoint the area most in need of her service and to obtain a baseline assessment of the problems she would be attempting to fix. With the help of thirteen "pathetic" horses and three mules, she traveled 650 miles over a three-month period. In the course of her travels, she interviewed fifty-three midwives. When she embarked on her study, Breckinridge assumed that she would find a substandard level of care, dangerous practices, and the need for a change, and her report revealed just that. Breckinridge outlined a system in which all women, both those receiving care from lay midwives and the midwives themselves, were victims. Breckinridge's detailed data revealed that the average age of the women providing care was just over sixty years. Most had children themselves —an average of nine each. All had very little if any medical training, and many were illiterate. She emphasized that the vast majority of the midwives did not choose this work; rather, it had been "thrust upon them" as they responded to the needs of their friends and neighbors. Prenatal care, she discovered, was nonexistent, as typically was aftercare. Midwives generally left as soon as mothers were "fixed up" and babies were dressed.[69] From her study, Breckinridge concluded that the care given women and children in this region was "medieval" and that her medical service could significantly lower mortality rates.[70]

While Breckinridge assessed the state of midwifery care in these counties, she hired psychologist Ella Woodyard to administer intelligence tests to the mountain children.[71] Breckinridge had two goals in commissioning this study. First, she wanted to show that the poor health of the area's residents was not a product of inherent weakness but clearly a result of inadequate medical care. Second, she sought reassurance that by locating here, she would be working with some of the nation's finest stock and that her work would have the greatest possible benefit. Woodyard's findings matched what Breckinridge suspected to be true. After testing sixty-six children, "picked up by the roadside quite at random," Woodyard calculated their median IQ to be 99.6.[72] Woodyard concluded that considering the "language barrier," the mountain children were slightly more intelligent than the U.S. population in general.[73]

In deciding where to begin, Breckinridge also sought advice from leaders in the area. She posed three questions: Did residents have access to trained medical care? Would residents show interest in and cooperate with the work? And what rail lines and roads existed? In answer to her solicitation, Berea College president William Hutchins sang the praises of Owsley County, noting that three cooperative physicians worked there. Mechanisms were already in place to make a health service work, and a substation could easily be established at one of the mission schools. Breckinridge could expect a warm welcome and assistance from the hundred-plus Berea graduates living in the county. Owsley, he pointed out, had "unquestionably some of the best blood in Kentucky." In reference to available transportation, Hutchins explained that although the county was off the railroad, a good roads movement was under way, and travel throughout the county could be accomplished with little difficulty. Owsley offered some important modern conveniences yet remained "characteristically mountain."[74]

Breckinridge was clearly looking for a spot off the beaten path. She asked about rail lines and roads not because she hoped to find these conveniences but because she wanted to start in an area that was as remote and difficult to traverse as possible. She was particularly concerned with finding an area where coal was not yet being mined.[75] Breckinridge for a time agreed that Owsley County had great potential, and she tentatively noted it in her plans, but after additional consideration, Breckinridge decided that Leslie County—"a poor little orphan of a county"—would be the best place to initiate her demonstration.[76] She felt sure that if her organization could prosper in this rugged environment, anyone trying to replicate the service's work elsewhere could also succeed.[77] Nowhere, as she explained, were "conditions more remote or more difficult."[78]

Leslie County appeared outside the norm in nearly every way. As the nation became predominately urban, industrial, and affluent, this area remained rural, agricultural, and poor. The 1920 census marked an important turning point for the United States, showing that for the first time more than half of Americans lived in cities. Leslie County, with its population of 271 per square mile, stood out in sharp contrast to metropolitan areas such as Louisville, with its population density of 7,400 residents per square mile.[79] Outside observers saw Leslie County not just as behind the times but as troublingly primitive. A contributor to *Harper's Monthly Magazine*, writing in 1915, claimed that he had "never before seen so dismal and desolate a haunt of human life" as Hyden, Leslie's county seat.[80]

Leslie County lacked the modern conveniences other Americans now took for granted.[81] Even the most contemporary homes in the region lacked indoor plumbing. Model Ts were rolling off Henry Ford's assembly line at a rate of one every ten seconds, but automobiles had yet to make their appearance here. With streambeds serving as roads and horses providing the primary form of transportation, most Leslie County residents rarely traveled far from home. The nearest rail station was located twenty-four miles away, in Hazard, and the state did not complete the first paved road connecting Hazard and Hyden until 1932.[82] The area's geography, combined with the lack of telephones and electricity, resulted in a high degree of physical and cultural isolation.

Unlike neighboring counties, where mining provided a good income if not steady work, coal would not transform Leslie County's economy until the 1940s.[83] In 1920, only thirty-six Leslie County residents worked in manufacturing. Instead, most continued to eke out a modest living through subsistence farming. As inheritance further divided farms and as soil was depleted, it became increasingly difficult for the land to support the population. By 1920, only one-third of Leslie County's farms consisted of more than one hundred acres.[84] Families nevertheless managed to make do, producing most of the goods they consumed at home. Neighbors gathered to make sorghum, kill hogs, pick blackberries, shear sheep, and make soap. Corn, perhaps the most versatile crop mountain families grew, provided a staple food item. Mountain families also distilled corn into whiskey, used it as filler for mattresses, and fed it to livestock. Trapping and hunting provided entertainment as well as needed food and leather. To supplement their income, families cut the area's plentiful walnut and yellow poplar timber and floated it down the river for sale. "Sangin'," or the collection of ginseng, also provided a bit of additional money.[85]

But Leslie County's residents possessed a sense of optimism that the future would bring economic improvement. Area farmers enthusiastically participated in agricultural workshops such as the Farmer's Institute, first held in 1906.[86] Real estate ads ran frequently in the county's newspaper, *Thousandsticks*, offering to buy coal and timberlands, and Leslie County's leaders practically begged developers to invest. In 1908, *Thousandsticks* published an "industrial issue" in which it celebrated individuals who had found success in banking and timber. The paper called for the extension of railroads into the area to allow "public spirited men of the county and capitalists" to "carry out the enormous amount of hardwood timber and the billions of tons of coal." "The mountains of Kentucky have certainly lingered long enough in the somnambulistic stage," the publication declared. It was time "to awaken and set out . . . bait."[87] In their attempt to attract capital investment, Leslie County leaders sought to correct the area's reputation as a violent, lawless place. Editorials frequently challenged stereotypes, reminding readers that in Leslie County, unlike Louisville and other big cities, one did not need to guard his or her life and pocketbook.[88] Despite these efforts at boosterism, however, by 1923, when Breckinridge began investigating conditions in Leslie County, the transformation that leaders had anticipated had not occurred. Cash remained scarce, bartering was common, and the people remained very poor.

Beyond its evident poverty, several factors—most notably, its lack of medical providers—drew Breckinridge to Leslie County. A nurse employed by the state board of health had resided in the county, but she resigned in 1923.[89] While seven physicians had practiced in Leslie County in 1914, no licensed doctors served the area nine years later.[90] Finding trained medical care required residents to travel to Hazard, a trip that could require more than a day in the saddle. Appalachian inhabitants noted that by the time someone reached a doctor, he or she often had either gotten well or died.[91] Physicians from Lexington and Louisville held free clinics from time to time to combat specific ailments such as trachoma, a highly contagious eye disease, but many people in Leslie County could obtain treatment only from untrained practitioners, whom Breckinridge derisively labeled "pseudo-doctors" and whom the medical community dubbed "quacks."[92] Many residents depended on patent medicines such as Dr. Pepper's Mountain Herbs, advertised in *Thousandsticks* as "the Best and Cheapest Medicine on Earth." Dr. Pepper's was available at Ray Brothers Drugstore for just one dollar for one hundred pills, and its makers guaranteed that it would cure rheumatism, constipation, indigestion, dyspepsia, and kidney trouble.[93]

Doctors hesitated to move into Appalachian counties because they recognized that the cash-poor economy would make it difficult to earn a living. Indeed, physicians who attempted to support themselves by practicing in remote areas such as Leslie County faced the challenge of collecting fees from poor clients who were adjusting to the idea that medical care was a commodity that they must purchase. Dr. G. B. Lawrence, one such struggling physician, placed a notice in the Leslie County newspaper in 1906 to explain that contrary to rumors, he was happy to visit patients in either the "country" or the "town," but only if "the money was ready" and he could be confident of payment.[94] Historian Sandra Barney stresses that financial hardship and isolation, not a fatalistic, backward culture, as many have assumed, led mountain residents to continue to rely on treatments that most Americans considered outdated and steeped in superstition. Barney reminds readers that "prayer, folk healing, stoicism, and tenacity were free or could be acquired locally through barter," while "trained doctors seldom lived nearby, and their services were expensive."[95]

The knowledge that Leslie County had no licensed medical doctors convinced Breckinridge of the need for her organization and removed the possibility that members of the medical profession might interfere with her plan. In her proposal to the American Child Health Association, she assured readers that the few physicians practicing in surrounding areas supported her intended venture and that no "friction" would arise.[96] Her fear that doctors might impede her efforts was legitimate. According to Barney, Appalachian residents suddenly gained new appeal as possible clients when coal and timber operations arrived in the early twentieth century. Treating mountain patients, however, could bring financial return only if residents accepted a fee-for-service model of health care. The subsidized treatment that reform organizations provided interfered with doctors' efforts to convince patients that medical care was a commodity that they must purchase. Harriet Butler, the first public health nurse stationed at the Hindman Settlement School, experienced so much interference from local physicians that she wrote to Dr. Joseph Mc-Cormack, the chair of the state board of health, in 1911 to protest and to seek his assistance.[97] However, by choosing a region where the coal boom and consequently doctors had not yet arrived, Breckinridge avoided the opposition that Butler and many of her associates faced.

WITH COMPLETE confidence in the value and potential of her plan, Breckinridge threw every ounce of her being into selling it throughout the state. All the energy she had once devoted to the care of her son was now channeled into her new project. She felt certain that she had the solution to the nation's high maternal and infant mortality rates and that her skills and her connections to influential Americans would lead to a revolution in rural health delivery. Breckinridge sincerely desired to help other women and babies now that her own children had died, but, perhaps unconsciously, she was also looking for an opportunity to gain a platform and a power base for herself. Her need to use the leadership abilities she inherited from her famous family and her desire to further the Breckinridge name led her to seek a position of authority. Having selected a location in which to begin, Breckinridge proceeded with "effervescent enthusiasm" to implement her plan.[98]

Before she could introduce nurse-midwifery to eastern Kentucky, Breckinridge herself first had to become a nurse-midwife. No schools in the United States offered this type of instruction, so she traveled to London in the fall of 1923 to study at the British Hospital for Mothers and Babies. Over the next four months, as she attended lectures and completed shifts on the wards, she was transported back to her days fifteen years earlier as a student nurse. The ringing of a bell to signal that a delivery was about to occur punctuated the daily routine. Breckinridge, like all student nurses, had to oversee twenty normal deliveries before she could take her certification exams.[99]

In her precious time off, Breckinridge continued to work out the final details of her plan so she would be ready to begin when she returned to the States. Her biggest concern remained how to fund her project. Her hopes of gaining the endorsement and financial support of the American Child Health Association faded when she broke ties with the Kentucky Bureau of Maternal and Child Health in the fall of 1923. Her once friendly relationship with the bureau's director grew tense after Breckinridge announced that she planned to publish the results of her midwifery study, against Dr. Veech's advice. While Breckinridge believed that bringing Kentucky's problems to light would lead to solutions, Veech insisted that Kentucky's "distressing midwife problem" did not "concern the great public." In a stern letter forwarded to Breckinridge in London, Veech explained, "Broadcasting such a report as yours is like making public, family skeletons or shouting ones sorrows on the housetops."[100]

Going a step further, Veech criticized Breckinridge for overestimating her ability to improve conditions: "I would very heartily [sic] endorse a program for mountain work, but I do not feel that I can accept the plan as you outline it, because I do not think it practical." Veech viewed Breckinridge as naive and judged her plan as too ambitious to succeed, predicting that "its branches will have to be pruned and well trimmed."[101]

After receiving Veech's letter, Breckinridge quickly penned a polite but terse response. She defended her decision to publish her midwifery study, arguing that it would be of use to those across the nation who were "racking their brains over similar questions." She challenged the accusation that she was exploiting her future clients, reminding Veech that the Breckinridge family had a long-standing tradition of service to the state. Breckinridge tactfully reassured Veech that her intentions were sincere: "Never fear that I shall exploit any section of my country, less the South, least of all Kentucky."[102]

At its heart, the disagreement between Veech and Breckinridge stemmed from issues of power and authority. As head of the Bureau of Maternal and Child Health, Veech had developed a plan to solve Kentucky's "midwife problem" that hinged on training lay midwives from rural counties. In 1924, Veech proudly noted that Kentucky tied for third with North Carolina in a ranking of states having the largest number of registered midwives, and she emphasized that "the midwives attending classes now are eager to learn everything offered to them and gratefully accept all instructions."[103] Unlike the lay midwives, Breckinridge was not willing to defer to Veech's authority. Veech reminded Breckinridge that other organizations had "gladly taken" her suggestions and upheld her "outlined policy for work in the state." They had not "suggest[ed] how we should do things, but knowing our experience here have come asking how they could help to do the things as we thought best."[104] Veech expected Breckinridge to work in an auxiliary fashion, like other women's club members across the state, while Breckinridge saw herself and the nurses that she planned to recruit as primary care providers, blazing a path rather than following one cut by others.[105] Breckinridge was not willing to defer to "experts" and instead saw herself as the true expert since she had studied the problem and had the data to support her position.

Their disagreement also stemmed from the differences in their educational and professional status. Dr. Veech saw midwives as treacherously aspiring to a status legitimately belonging to physicians. Discussing her conflict with Breckinridge with Hutchins, Veech condescendingly declared, "A nurse-midwife is only a midwife." She feared the "tendency among certain groups of nurses towards practicing medicine for which they are in no way prepared without graduating in medicine." She defended her hard-won status, noting, "If high-type young women want to be of real value in isolated areas, why do they not prepare themselves by taking a medical degree?" Veech, a graduate of the Woman's Medical College in Philadelphia, was appalled at a challenge to her expertise from Breckinridge, "only a midwife."[106]

Breckinridge severed all relations with Veech and the Kentucky Bureau of Child and Maternal Health in November 1923. "If you do not want [to support the Children's Public Health Service,] you shall not be importuned again," she promised. Breckinridge also withdrew her request for funding from the Child Health Association.[107] Referring to Veech as "Mr. Ready-to-Halt," Breckinridge rejoiced that she had broken ties with someone who had been "tugging like a ball and chain at my heels from the beginning." She made it clear however, that she was not giving up—she would find alternate funding sources.[108] "It is not usual, I know, for public interests to take the initiative in pushing forward with new ideas. Private initiative nearly always blazes the trail."[109] She confidently predicted, "We will get it financed, somehow, under other auspices—private ones—and though the beginning may be slower it will go more smoothly in the long run."[110] She still hoped that when her project was up and running, the government would provide "recognition and support."[111]

In spite of her funding problems, Breckinridge remained certain of the value of the organization, which she now renamed the Kentucky Committee for Mothers and Babies. Writing to Ella Phillips Crandall, assistant general executive of the American Child Health Association, Breckinridge confidently declared that she had not "the smallest doubt" that her plan would be implemented: "It is unthinkable that it should not be, for the points it emphasizes, which seem radical today, will be the commonplaces of another decade."[112] She did not let Veech's resistance dampen her enthusiasm as she continued to prepare herself for the work that lay ahead. Crandall responded that she had no doubt that Breckinridge, with her "indominitable [*sic*] spirit," would find a way to proceed.[113]

AFTER COMPLETING her course work, taking her final exams, and receiving certification through the British Central Midwives Board, Breckinridge spent the rest of 1924 traveling in the United Kingdom to witness in action medical services similar to the one she proposed. She was especially impressed with the work of the Scottish Highlands and Islands Medical and Nursing Service, run by Sir Leslie MacKenzie. The organization's nurses offered comprehensive care to patients in their homes, traversing their rural districts on bicycle. Breckinridge was impressed with the practicality of MacKenzie's system and eventually copied many of his methods.[114]

The time Breckinridge spent overseas in 1923 and 1924 was important for what she learned about midwifery and running a public health service, but it also allowed her to begin to move beyond the pain and guilt she had continued to carry since her children's deaths and her divorce. During her time in London, she further explored her interest in things of a "psychic nature." She attended lectures sponsored by the English Society for Psychical Research and made new friends through the London Spiritualist Alliance.[115] Spiritualism and messages from Breckie and Polly relayed by mediums brought her a small degree of comfort, but she continued to battle severe depression, struggling "through darkness too thick for a knife to cut."[116]

Maud Cashmore, an instructor at the British Hospital, recognized the pain that threatened to overcome Breckinridge. Seeing her need for peace and deeper answers, Cashmore urged her student to speak with her sister, Adeline, a cloistered nun.[117] Mary at first resisted, finding conventional religion too sterile and its reliance on faith rather than phenomenon too unscientific.[118] She rejected the "rubrics and creeds and holy water and immersions and hair-splitting controversies" that for her represented religion. Churches, she noted, had done little to "still the aching longing of [people's] wayward hearts" and instead had given them stones for bread.[119] By the mid-1920s, as the conflict between fundamentalism and science came to a head in the Scopes trial, many female reformers shunned formal religion, recognizing that its association with benevolence and sentimentality undermined their attempts to earn respect as serious professionals.[120] Breckinridge, like a growing segment of Americans, viewed denominational religion as old-fashioned and resisted the Cashmore sisters' attempts to reunite her with God.

Finally, only weeks before she intended to leave England, Breckinridge agreed to a meeting. Adeline rarely saw visitors, dedicating her days to constant prayer, but made an exception. According to Breckinridge, the sister greeted her with arms outstretched, surrounded by a white light that could be "felt and almost seen."[121] Following their two-hour meeting, Mary claimed she finally found herself free from the pain that had gripped her for seven years.[122] She met Adeline Cashmore in person only four times over the next twenty years, but her influence deeply shaped Mary's personal life as well as her fledgling organization.[123]

In spite of her outward confidence and enthusiasm, Breckinridge was desperate for the reassurance and support that her new spiritual guide provided. Following their initial meeting, Cashmore began writing her new friend as often as twice a week. Her letters at times provided detailed answers to Breckinridge's theological questions but often simply assured her that God found the work she was doing pleasing.[124] Cashmore's promise to pray "every day and many times a day" for Breckinridge's project in the mountains reinforced her resolve.[125] She completely trusted Cashmore and her power to intervene on Breckinridge's behalf. She explained that Cashmore "loved God . . . so utterly that when she lifted causes and people up to Him and held them there, a channel was opened through which God's love could pour unimpeded."[126] Years later, in her autobiography, Breckinridge attributed her success in Kentucky to Adeline Cashmore, claiming that "the story of the Frontier Nursing Service could not be told but for Adeline."[127]

The burden of prayer was not the only weight Cashmore lifted from Breckinridge's shoulders. The sister's counseling helped Breckinridge deal with the sorrows of her past. Cashmore reassured her friend that God "doesn't despise broken and contrite hearts," even when they belonged to divorcées. When Breckinridge told Cashmore that she was thinking of seeing an alienist (a psychiatrist) for counseling because of the guilt that continued to plague her following her divorce, Cashmore advised that doing so would be a mistake. She encouraged Breckinridge to remain faithful to Jesus, "the only Alienist that understands."[128] Seeing the good in every occurrence, Cashmore helped Breckinridge begin to accept Breckie's and Polly's deaths as part of God's larger plan, assuring her grieving friend that she would eventually be reunited with her children. Until then, Cashmore urged, Breckinridge should use her talents to the fullest.[129]

BRECKINRIDGE COMPLETED a postgraduate course in midwifery in London in late 1924 and then welcomed the new year by sailing for the United States. She had spent two years intensively preparing for her new venture. She had thoroughly investigated the problem, pursued additional training, and taken steps to heal her lingering emotional wounds. The time to begin was finally at hand.

part two **The Frontier Nursing Service: The Building Years**

A s she recounted her organization's early history in her 1952 autobiography, Mary Breckinridge questioned whether she would have had the courage to "launch the small movement destined to grow into the Frontier Nursing Service" if she had foreseen all the challenges that lay ahead.[1] When she initiated her project a quarter century earlier, however, Breckinridge had few reservations. She believed completely in the potential of her plan and in the value of the clients she intended to serve. Mothers and children needed her, and she was anxious to heed the call.

After returning from England, Breckinridge spent the spring of 1925 selling her proposal to prominent citizens throughout Kentucky. By May, she proudly announced that she had assembled a committee composed of "men and women of the highest influence and most ability." The individuals she recruited responded to her excitement and expressed their confidence in the project; she was delighted to find that no one she approached turned her down.[2] She enlisted, among others, eight doctors, the presidents of Berea College and the University of Kentucky, a newspaper editor, an officer of the Louisville & Nashville Railroad, several well-respected mountain workers, and a gubernatorial candidate. She looked to this committee to provide wisdom and guidance, but more than anything, she hoped that having the support of so many state leaders would lend respectability to her efforts.[3]

Breckinridge's years of planning finally culminated on May 28, 1925, when her Kentucky Committee for Mothers and Babies met for the first time. Former chief justice of the Kentucky Court of Appeals Edward C. O'Rear called the meeting to order at the New Capitol Hotel in Frankfort.[4] Breckinridge chose to inaugurate her organization in the state capital to demonstrate that her project was broad in scope and to give it legitimacy. Twenty-one men and women, many of them kin to Breckinridge, gathered that day to hear her outline her plan to bring medical care to the women and children of Leslie County.[5] Although she had already worked out the basic details for her organization's functioning, Breckinridge sought the committee's approval on questions of location, staff, publications, and record keeping. As they would in the future, committee members enthusiastically rubber-stamped their leader's suggestions.[6] After electing officers and giving Breckinridge permission to hire two trained nurse-midwives, the committee adjourned.[7]

Breckinridge left Frankfort exhilarated by the level of support and interest she had witnessed. The meeting had come less than a month after the first annual Child Health Day, when stores had set up displays, communities held parades, and movie theaters ran films promoting child welfare.[8] Breckinridge drew on the lingering enthusiasm. Calling the Appalachian people "the seed corn of the world," Judge O'Rear applauded the "sublime audacity" of the project that would bring such important results not only to the individuals served but to the nation as a whole. Mountain reformer Linda Neville told the committee that because she had no children of her own, she had previously failed to recognize the dangers rural mothers faced. Moved by Breckinridge's presentation, however, Neville solemnly pledged that from that point on, "her slogan would be 'save the mothers'" and Breckinridge would have her "whole-hearted assistance."[9]

As Breckinridge took the final steps to implement her plan, one important question remained—how would she turn the interest expressed by several dozen committee members into funding adequate to support what promised to be a very costly endeavor? She did not solicit funds at the group's inaugural meeting but planned instead to underwrite the expenses herself for the first three years out of her inheritance from her mother's estate. She expected that by the time her savings ran out, the value of the project would speak for itself, and money would flow in naturally. She recognized that if her plan was to develop on the scale she hoped, she would need to find a steady funding source, but she was willing to use her money to get the organization off the ground, shrugging it off as "just one of those things" that had to be done.[10]

HAVING SECURED the endorsement of her committee, Breckinridge immediately invited Freda Caffin and Edna Rockstroh to become the organization's first two employees. Native New Yorkers and trained nurses, the women had recently completed their midwifery training in England. Breckinridge enticed them to commit to her venture by emphasizing the innovative nature of the project. To sweeten the deal, she promised each a competitive salary of $150 per month plus living expenses.[11] Rockstroh later admitted that had she known what she was "getting into," she probably would not have taken the position, but at the outset she shared Breckinridge's desire to begin work as soon as possible.[12] The new recruits arrived in Kentucky in late July, eager to open the first nursing center and to begin accepting patients. However, Breckinridge informed them that this task would have to wait.

Instead, she assigned them to help conduct an exhaustive survey of births and deaths in Leslie County. In 1911, Kentucky had initiated a program to collect vital statistics, but Breckinridge doubted the completeness and accuracy of the state's records, especially in mountain areas.[13] Following the recommendation of health commissioner Dr. Arthur T. McCormack, she sought to obtain a valid reading of the existing mortality rate. Looking to the future, she recognized that she could not argue convincingly that her methods worked unless she could present detailed preliminary statistics.[14]

To head up the survey, she hired Bertram Ireland, a Scottish researcher who had done similar work for the Highlands and Islands Medical and Nursing Service. With a staff of four, "Ireland from Scotland," as Breckinridge called her, visited more than sixteen hundred Leslie County families that summer on horseback, canvassing more than 376 square miles in the process. Zilpha Roberts, a Leslie County teacher who donated two months of her time to help Ireland, declared that "the next census should be taken by aeroplane and parachute!" Dismounting from her horse on one occasion, Roberts stepped directly on a snake. Horrified, she jumped back, managing somehow to step on the snake twice more. According to Roberts, she "danced a jubilee on that old snake all the way down the mountain."[15] If such occurrences upset a native of the county, the New York nurses who were new to the region certainly received an abrupt orientation to what was in store.

Ireland and her team of investigators finished their survey in September 1925, leaving, according to Breckinridge, "not one family in Leslie County unvisited." They discovered that there had been 10 percent more births and 17 percent more deaths than had been reported for the fourteen-year period.[16] Armed with this information, Breckinridge became even more certain that her plan had the potential to improve the quality of life for hundreds of women and children.

While Ireland and her team collected data on births and deaths, Breckinridge spent the summer building local support for her project.[17] She traveled through the county, asking those she considered its "leading citizens" to endorse her work. In establishing her local branch, Breckinridge applied the same hierarchical attitude that had led her to recruit the state's best and brightest to serve on her executive committee. She condescendingly believed that wealth, education, and sterling pedigrees determined virtue and that some Leslie County residents were clearly more worthy than their neighbors. The "tone of the community," she argued, was "set by its best men." Therefore, she assumed, she could bring real change to the community only if she enlisted its most prominent residents, who would in turn provide an example for those around them.[18]

After months of recruiting, the Leslie County committee met for the first time in August 1925. Thirty-five of the county's most distinguished men and women attended, including the sheriff, three judges, a banker, a lawyer's wife, a pastor, the school superintendent and his wife, several merchants, and the editor of the county's newspaper, *Thousandsticks*. Members included such individuals as Judge L. D. Lewis, descended from one of the county's "pioneer families," who was educated at Union College and had earned a law degree at the University of Louisville before serving as school superintendent and state representative. His wife, Rebecca, likewise came from a family that valued education, and Breckinridge approvingly described Rebecca Lewis as "a great lady in any place or time."[19] Breckinridge praised the dedication of those who traveled to Hyden for the meeting, dramatically reserving her highest accolade for one of the female members who "rode all day to be present, with her baby over one arm." Unlike urban committee members, who "roll[ed] to . . . meetings in limousines" with "blasé indifference," the members of this committee revealed their deep commitment by traveling long distances on horseback over rough terrain.[20] To maximize the benefits of the attendees' efforts, a good roads meeting followed Breckinridge's event.[21]

Although its members had little input in decision making, the local committee, like its counterpart on the state level, lent respect and legitimacy to Breckinridge's new venture. She believed in the importance of proving to supporters that her organization was working through rather than for the people of Leslie County.[22] In her early proposals for a Children's Public Health Service, Breckinridge recommended that the organization be administered by a local board of "influential citizens who should be led to take all possible initiative themselves." However, Breckinridge's statewide executive board and her local committee ultimately were token gestures, and she expected her advisers on all levels to defer to her ideas.[23]

NOW THAT she had a supportive local committee in place and preliminary data by which to gauge the service's success, Breckinridge and her two nurses were finally ready to begin work. In September, they opened the first clinic at Hyden. Mary's experience in Europe had taught her that a few nurse-mid-wives, dispersed evenly throughout a region, could efficiently care for a large population with minimal physician support.[24] She planned to establish multiple centers, each staffed by two nurse-midwives, positioned around a central hospital.[25] Time and money would be needed to create this decentralized system; in the interim, the three women would work together in Hyden to build a patient base.

A small house rented from the local Presbyterian school functioned temporarily as the first clinic until Wendover, Breckinridge's home and the organization's headquarters, was built. The three women shared the tiny seven-room center with Caffin's mother, Caroline, and Mary's seventy-nine-year-old father, Clifton Rodes Breckinridge. Each resident had clearly defined duties— Caroline Caffin did the cooking and cleaning; Clifton Breckinridge cared for the horses and performed odd jobs around the center; and Mary Breckinridge, Freda Caffin, and Rockstroh focused on nursing. One room, freshly painted and outfitted with linoleum, became the dispensary.[26] Even though the building lacked indoor plumbing and adequate space comfortably to house its residents, Mary described it as "an oasis of modern science" compared to other structures in the area.[27]

In the initial issue of the committee's *Quarterly Bulletin*, Breckinridge painted a glowing picture of her first month of work with her nurses. In all, 233 patients made 561 visits to the center, while the nurses made 46 home visits. Using serum supplied by the state board of health, Caffin and Rockstroh gave 30 adults and 114 children typhoid inoculations. The women also booked twenty midwifery cases and sent four children to doctors in nearby cities for treatment. Breckinridge modestly pointed out that the nurses' patient load appeared even more impressive when one considered that they had not solicited visitors and took only "what fell in their way."[28]

By October, Breckinridge was already making plans to open a second center at nearby Wolf Creek. When local support was not forthcoming, however, she put the plan on hold, arguing that her organization should build clinics only in areas where residents expressed enthusiasm. Asked for input on the matter, the executive committee authorized Breckinridge to "use her own judgment" concerning the Wolf Creek center. The committee members granted her the authority "customarily given to field directors" in all matters concerning the organization. She would continue to solicit advice from her executive committee, but from the start, she had free rein in fiscal as well as day-to-day affairs.[29]

With plans for a center at Wolf Creek indefinitely postponed, Breckinridge focused on construction of the building that would serve as administrative headquarters for the Kentucky Committee. While traveling through the county several years earlier, she had fallen in love with a remote piece of land that overlooked the middle fork of the Kentucky River. From that moment on, she dreamed of constructing a cozy log cabin there. The site, she gleefully reported, was "so picturesque . . . that Little Red Riding Hood and Hop O' My Thumb would find themselves at home if they chanced by."[30] She eventually purchased this parcel of land, and in the summer of 1925, construction began on the two-story lodge that she would name Wendover.[31]

While waiting to move into her envisioned retreat, Breckinridge concentrated on increasing the scope of her organization. She directed the bulk of her efforts in these early years to securing funding for the fledgling service. She spent most of her time outside the mountains, while her growing staff of nurses concentrated on winning the confidence of their patients and on improving the collective health of their adopted community. The builders completed Wendover in the spring of 1926, and from then on, it served as the organization's center of operations. More important, however, it provided a home for the organization's founder, who since her days as an uprooted politician's daughter had been searching for the protection and security of such a place.

BRECKINRIDGE REVELED in the opportunity to retreat from city life and enjoyed the challenge Leslie County's rugged terrain offered, but her fellow workers focused less on the picturesque nature of their remote location and more on the obstacles it imposed. Freda Caffin and Edna Rockstroh and the new employees who joined them quickly discovered that the work for which they had signed on little resembled that for which their training had prepared them. While riding horseback over mountains to come to the aid of helpless patients seemed romantic on first consideration, the reality of this endeavor quickly hit home. Nurses may have expected glamour, but they found themselves confronted by hard work and considerable danger.

Committee nurses maintained rigorous schedules. They spent forty-four hours a week holding clinics and making frequent visits to their expectant maternity cases. Breckinridge established her organization on the idea that nurses would do the majority of frontline care, with doctors providing only backup, emergency assistance. Nurses thus focused on early intervention and hands-on care and closely followed their maternity patients. Nurses saw normal prenatal cases every two weeks until the seventh month and then every week until delivery, checking patients' blood pressure and urine at each visit. This routine work occupied much of the nurses' days, but their time on the clock often extended late into the night when emergencies arose. Any time a maternity case called, be it day or night, a nurse was required to go, and she was expected to stay with the mother no matter how long it took her to deliver. Breckinridge believed that being there for the "long hours of the first stage of labor has a bearing on the outcome," and nurses often spent a day or longer waiting for nature to take its course.[32] After delivery, the nurse continued to provide thorough care, visiting the patient every day for ten days and then at least twice more during the baby's first month of life to ensure that lactation had been successfully established.[33] Because overtime work was so common, Breckinridge allowed nurses six weeks of paid vacation each year.[34]

The extensive paperwork that Breckinridge required her nurses to complete added to their heavy workload. The director reminded her nurses to keep meticulous patient records, which were, after all, the service's "most valuable possessions." Detailed records would not only allow them to recognize "leaks, weak spots, and deficiencies" but also prove to the world that Breckinridge's ideas worked and convince others to adopt her methods. A nurse's legacy lay in the quality of records she kept; incomplete records would stand "against the nurse's name forever," Breckinridge warned. In case of fire, she instructed nurses to save the records first.[35]

Breckinridge's concern with record keeping reflected the Progressive Era emphasis on rationality. By the early twentieth century, benevolence had grown systematized and highly organized, with professional social workers replacing unpaid "friendly visitors." "Sentimentality and religious zeal" became an insufficient motive for reform work; instead, "dispassionate analysis and business sense" were expected.[36] Breckinridge recognized that to attract donors' support, she must convincingly demonstrate the professional, "scientific" nature of her enterprise. Only by providing airtight statistics could she prove the effectiveness of her demonstration.[37]

Although nurses joined the service with the intention of delivering babies, they spent more of their time in the committee's first three years doing public health work and disease prevention than midwifery.[38] By 1925, trachoma, previously deemed the "scourge of the mountains," had practically disappeared in eastern Kentucky as a result of the efforts of the Kentucky Society for the Prevention of Blindness, which Linda Neville had organized in 1910. But Breckinridge's nurses still had to treat a variety of afflictions. Modern science offered antidotes to many of the health problems facing rural Americans, such as communicable diseases, infected tonsils, and intestinal parasites. In keeping with their mission, committee nurses attempted not only to treat the symptoms of these illnesses but also to prevent future occurrences through education.[39] Prevention was the service's primary objective. The nurses regularly visited all their patients, not just those who were sick. Ideally, each nurse tried to examine every infant (less than one year old) twice a month. She visited preschools (children between one and six years) once a month. Schoolchildren were seen every three months and adults twice a year.[40]

Breckinridge's nurses sought every possible opportunity to spread the "gospel of health." Again using serum provided by the state, they held vaccination clinics throughout Leslie County to protect patients against the typhoid, smallpox, and diphtheria epidemics that had so frequently plagued the area.[41] Nurses also set up booths at local fairs to demonstrate proper infant care. Service employees shared with mothers the "correct" way to feed, dress, and bathe babies while showing fathers how to build sanitary toilets and explaining how to keep disease-carrying flies and mosquitoes out of homes by screening windows and cribs.[42]

In addition to teaching patients new, more healthful ways of living, Breckinridge's nurses also paid special attention to what she saw as mountain children's greatest nemesis, intestinal parasites. More than one-third of the area's children had hookworms, and nine out of ten were afflicted with roundworms.[43] Poor sanitation and mountain children's tendency to go barefoot in the summer made them susceptible to these parasites, which left them malnourished and emaciated. Playing up the devastation caused by these "Minotaurs," Breckinridge evoked potential supporters' sympathy.[44] Armed with stereopticon slides of worms that committee nurses had removed from hapless patients, Breckinridge attempted to make every American "worm-conscious."[45]

The committee's work required nurses to have not only strong stomachs but also sturdy backs and a sense of fearlessness. Freda Caffin noted that spending days in the saddle "on roads, which when they were not in the rocky river beds, were apt to climb an almost perpendicular mountain," physically exhausted nurses unused to riding.[46] Riding to and from cases in the dark in inclement weather through areas where it seemed "the last person there was Daniel Boone" could undermine the resolve of even the most committed professional.[47] The danger was not imagined—swinging bridges, icy trails, floods, snakes, and skittish horses posed very real threats. One of Breckinridge's early nurses, Elizabeth Stevenson, described her first night call: "I think it will always remain in my mind that first fording of a river, the horse picking his way over rock, the swirling water underneath, and the intense dark." Stevenson praised the skill of her horse, Snip, who led her safely home without the benefit of even a flashlight.[48]

AFTER NURSES arrived at an emergency call, they had to be prepared for any situation. Creating an aseptic field in homes where often even basic items such as bowls were not available required nurses to carry a wide variety of instruments and medications. At all time, nurses kept two sets of saddlebags packed, one for general calls and one for midwifery cases. The midwifery bag alone weighed forty-eight pounds and contained, among other things, a rubber apron, an operating gown, soap, a scrub brush, gloves, a thermometer, scissors, basins, and pharmaceuticals.[49]

The most important item committee nurses carried, however, was the *Medical Routine*. This twenty-page booklet, which they referred to as their Bible, detailed what to do in case of gunshot wounds, snakebites, coughs, hookworms, and a myriad of other general and midwifery conditions. Because doctors and well-equipped hospitals were not easily accessible, committee nurses often had to perform procedures that fell beyond the scope of their training. The *Routine*, written by physicians and surgeons who belonged to the organization's Medical Advisory Committee, acted as a stand-in when nurses could not secure orders directly from a doctor. The document allowed nurses to "meet emergencies and carry on until physicians [could] be had." The publication included instructions for suturing "when necessary," setting fractures "if obliged," and prescribing narcotics such as morphine and codeine in cases when such medications were warranted.[50]

Practically speaking, the Kentucky Committee's *Medical Routine* existed to make the work of its nurse-midwives easier and more effective, but Breckinridge also used the document to stave off critics' suggestions that her nurses were illegally practicing medicine. The *Routine*'s authors were careful to protect the prerogative of their colleagues practicing in eastern Kentucky. The Medical Advisory Committee emphasized that "it is the nurse's duty, as well as privilege to sell the idea of this [state licensed] practitioner to her patient."[51] In other words, because they encouraged patients to seek professional medical treatment, committee nurses were not competing with area doctors but were helping them to increase their clientele.

Breckinridge publicly stressed that her nurses deferred to doctors in all situations, but in reality, their remote location often forced them to handle procedures that doctors would have been expected to perform if available. The organization carefully avoided publicizing that its nurses sutured wounds, gave anesthesia, and set bones. "We don't like to stress this side of our work on account of the Medical Profession," Freda Caffin explained. "We want them with us and not against us."[52] Describing her new organization in the *American Journal of Obstetrics and Gynecology* in 1928, Breckinridge recognized that she might encounter some resistance from obstetricians who saw her nurses as a threat and consequently emphasized, "We are not substituting one method for another." Instead, she stressed, the mothers her nurses served "have no other trained assistance at near hand."[53]

Breckinridge understood the importance of remaining within local physicians' good graces to enable her organization to survive and prosper. Early-twentieth-century doctors were concerned with shoring up their professional status. Medical education was being upgraded and standardized, and physicians throughout the country, under the auspices of the American Medical Association and local medical societies, were pushing state legislatures for tougher licensing laws that excluded irregular practitioners. In the 1920s, physicians directed their attention primarily against chiropractors, but anyone practicing outside the bounds of "regular" medicine became a target of physicians' concern. Kentucky doctors shared the fear voiced by their colleagues across the nation that alternative practitioners provided dangerous competition. Addressing the Owensboro meeting of the Kentucky State Medical Association in 1926, Dr. William Pusey warned against "the Europeanizing of medical practice . . . the turning over of childbirth of a majority of the people to midwives, [and] the use of the visiting nurse in place of the family doctor." Though there is no reason to believe he was speaking directly against Breckinridge, his words reveal the latent hostility directed toward those who operated outside the bounds of traditional medicine. Breckinridge realized that nurse-midwifery was an innovative concept understood by few, even physicians, and she therefore took every opportunity possible to reassure doctors of their supremacy.[54]

In large part because of Breckinridge's careful diplomacy, the Kentucky Committee encountered little early resistance from doctors. In fact, many physicians wholeheartedly supported the committee's work and became important allies. Doctors across the nation endorsed her plan, including such notable figures as prominent New York obstetrician Dr. Ralph W. Lobenstine; Dr. William H. Welch, who established the Johns Hopkins University School of Medicine; and Dr. George W. Kosmak, editor of the *American Journal of Obstetrics and Gynecology*.[55] Practitioners from Lexington, Louisville, and Cincinnati enthusiastically participated in Breckinridge's Medical Advisory Committee and consulted on her patients' cases at no charge, either in their own offices or at tonsil, gynecological, eye, and dental clinics held locally.[56] Even doctors in nearby Hazard applauded her project. Dr. H. C. Capps, a surgeon from Perry County, supported Breckinridge, agreeing to care for the organization's abnormal cases in exchange for the services of a committee nurse who dealt with his routine cases.[57]

Historian Sandra Barney contends that physicians "tolerated, and often encouraged" Breckinridge for several reasons. Her social position combined with her decision to work in a very remote, rural region helped win physicians' support. Barney contends that Breckinridge would not have received the same welcome had she chosen to establish her organization in an urban center. Just as importantly, she maintained doctors' cooperation because she honored and upheld a physician-centered model of medical delivery. She did not question doctors' control of medicine. She argued that in a perfect world, every person would have access to a physician's services. When this was not possible, however, she saw nurses, trained to deal with normal situations and able to distinguish abnormal cases and to request assistance, as an appropriate alternative. Doctors appreciated Breckinridge's willingness to defer to them.[58] Then too, in some cases, doctors may have supported the committee out of guilt. Unwilling to practice in poor rural areas because of the limited financial rewards and the lack of access to new technology, some doctors saw Breckinridge's model as a practical solution to the misdistribution of health care.[59]

Doctors from New York, Lexington, and even Hazard supported Breckinridge's work because they did not compete with her nurses for patients. Three physicians moved into Leslie County soon after Breckinridge began work, however, and they were more critical of her methods. Local doctors first voiced complaints in 1928, after Breckinridge announced that the committee was planning to build a hospital. Several months before the facility was to open, a physician identified only as Dr. Keith attacked the organization, accusing its nurses of overstepping their boundaries. Breckinridge saw through his hostility, attributing his complaints to greed. "A state licensed doctor . . . of low professional and moral character," he wanted sole permission to practice surgery in the new hospital, which she was unwilling to give, and he feared that the nurses' preventative measures would interfere with his fledgling business.[60]

Breckinridge dismissed Keith's charges as nothing but "virulent hot air" and asserted that there was not "the smallest shadow of any question of illegality" in the services her nurses were providing.[61] She was prepared to respond to the disgruntled physician in the press if need be, seeing the dispute as an opportunity to explain to "large audiences" the role of the Kentucky Committee and its relationship to the medical community.[62] Instead, she wrote to Keith privately, stressing that she wanted to build "harmonious and amicable" relationships on every front. She added, however, that her committee was fully backed by legal and medical experts who agreed that his charges were groundless.[63] For further support, she asked Dr. Josephine Hunt, a member of the Medical Advisory Committee (and her cousin), to write to reassure Keith and other area physicians. Hunt noted that the organization's nurses were "giving such medicines as they have instructions to do under my direction." Just like nurses working under physicians in urban hospitals, the service's nurses were following doctors' orders and were not making clinical decisions on their own, Hunt promised.[64]

Keith's animosity toward Breckinridge's enterprise and his fear for his economic well-being were warranted. Not long before Keith challenged the Kentucky Committee, the Perry County Medical Society had met to address the problem of nonpayment by patients. In June 1926, the doctors agreed to identify delinquent patients who were capable of paying their fees and to share this list with their colleagues. The physicians resolved not to attend to patients who failed to show proper appreciation for services provided.[65] But in the case of the Kentucky Committee, the problem went beyond the failure of those who could pay to do so. Local practitioners recognized that they were competing against a heavily subsidized organization that charged patients only a fraction of services' worth on the open market. Doctors had typically dealt with indigent patients by setting standard fees and then reducing them according to patients' need. Physicians preferred to continue with this approach because it reinforced medical care's status as a commodity, and they feared that organizations such as Breckinridge's would pauperize medical practitioners.

Breckinridge shared physicians' concern that patients would begin to take medical care for granted and would become dependent on charity. Believing that it was important "not to lessen the native pioneer independence of the patients," the Kentucky Committee charged every family, no matter how destitute, a flat yearly one-dollar fee for general care. Mothers expecting babies were required to pay a separate five-dollar fee, which covered prenatal care, delivery, ten days of postpartum care, and a layette set.[66] Strapped for cash, patients rarely paid even these modest fees. In 1929, Breckinridge discovered that only 283 of the 942 families that received care from committee nurses had paid their annual fees. Those that did pay off their debt usually did so not in cash but, as Breckinridge explained in her best mountain dialect, with goods such as "quilted 'kivers,' skins of 'varmits,' [or] split-bottomed chairs." Men in the community often worked off the cost of their families' medical care by helping to build new outpost centers or barns. Children also contributed. Breckinridge proudly reported that several young girls earned their toxin-antitoxin injections by emptying the dispensary slop buckets.[67] Unlike local doctors, who needed their fees to support themselves, Breckinridge from the start looked outside the mountains to keep her organization solvent, and doctors such as Keith understandably feared that they could not compete in an area where medical care was available at such low cost.

BRECKINRIDGE OBTAINED the money to run her nursing service outside the mountains, and fund-raising placed a heavy burden on her shoulders. Her constant travels in and out of the mountains strained her physically and emotionally. While she developed bonds with her employees, she continued to lean on old friends outside of Kentucky for moral support. Her old friend Lucille "Pansy" Turner and her British spiritual advisers, Maud and Adeline Cashmore, provided needed reassurance that Breckinridge's efforts were worthwhile. These women not only praised her for improving the health of "her mountaineers" but, more important, reminded her that she was performing "God's work" through her organization.[68] Adeline Cashmore argued that although committee statisticians would measure success in terms of "human life," the number of "human souls quickened" truly revealed Breckinridge's contribution.[69]

Breckinridge was a product of the nineteenth century, and her close relationships with female friends throughout her life reflected the values of the era in which she was raised. The "Victorian emotional ethos" encouraged intense "romantic friendships" among women and even sanctioned physical contact between same-sex friends.[70] Although Breckinridge married twice and embraced the twentieth-century ideal of companionate marriage, which encouraged close emotional ties between men and women, she continued to seek sustenance from female friends, particularly after the dissolution of her second marriage.[71] Breckinridge corresponded frequently with the Cashmores and Turner throughout the 1920s, exchanging affectionate letters. The comforting words of her international support network buoyed Breckinridge and allowed her to suppress lingering worries that her venture might fail.

With an eye to the donors she was attempting so vigorously to court,

Breckinridge announced in 1927 that the Kentucky Committee for Mothers and Babies would change its name to the Frontier Nursing Service (FNS). According to Breckinridge, two factors influenced her decision to rename the organization. First, because the conditions her nurses were attempting to improve constituted a problem of national rather than just statewide scope, a name with broader implications made more sense; second, a significant portion of the organization's support came from donors outside of the Bluegrass State, and she wanted to recognize these contributions.[72]

Breckinridge's decision certainly had deeper significance, however. Using the word "frontier" in her organization's name allowed her to evoke important symbolic imagery. Suggesting adventure and infinite possibilities as well as old-fashioned values such as independence, thrift, and hospitality, the new name aided Breckinridge in generating enthusiasm among potential employees and patrons. The new name also revealed that the organization's goals had changed. Breckinridge was no longer devoted solely to helping mothers and babies. As she grew more familiar with her clients' needs, she developed a more sophisticated understanding of community health care. She realized that to improve the quality of life for Appalachia's inhabitants, her nurses would have to do more than ensure the safe delivery of the next generation. They had an obligation to treat the diseases prevalent among the mothers, fathers, and siblings of the children being brought into the world. By adopting a new name for her organization, Breckinridge conveyed a more extensive model of health care.

FROM THE start, Breckinridge planned to build a hospital in Leslie County as soon as money became available. The twelve-bed facility she envisioned would provide a center of operations for a full-time resident physician, who would consult on the nurse-midwives' irregular cases. To pay for a hospital, she first looked not to her growing network of individual donors but to corporations with ties to the region. Arguing that these enterprises had a "public spirited duty" to give back, she leaned on them to pay for the hospital. She compiled a list of coal companies that owned land in Leslie County and in the spring of 1926 met with their representatives to explain her plan and to "coax" them into financially supporting her endeavor.[73]

Though Breckinridge insisted that she was not motivated by a sense of noblesse oblige and rejected any suggestion that in her service to Appalachia she was acting as lady bountiful, she sincerely believed that elites had a duty to give back to the less fortunate.[74] Breckinridge had faith that these companies would see the value in her plan and would be willing to do their share. She previously had convinced coal companies to contribute land and supplies to her venture. In 1925, the Kentucky River Coal Corporation indefinitely loaned the Kentucky Committee two houses that would become outpost centers. The following year, the Kentucky Union Company, a coal operation that owned twenty-five hundred acres in Leslie County, agreed to donate half of its holdings to Breckinridge. Soon thereafter, however, the FNS deeded the land back to the Kentucky Union Company, an act that suggested that the land was already ravaged and that the continuing tax burden would have outweighed any advantage the service, like the company, would have gained from owning the property.[75]

Using tactics similar to those she used to develop fund-raising networks in the Northeast, Breckinridge attempted to win over coal representatives by entertaining them at Wendover, where they could view her work firsthand, and by asking industrialists with whom she was familiar to provide her letters of introduction to others she did not know.[76] As she began her hospital campaign, however, Breckinridge was disappointed to find that these companies refused the opportunity to improve the health of the community in which they operated. Only the L & N Railroad, which had representatives on the FNS's executive board, offered to help by providing a 50 percent rebate on the freight costs of shipping building materials to the new hospital site. Other companies rebuffed her requests for assistance, leading her to admit that "perhaps corporations have no souls."[77]

Breckinridge's relationships with the coal companies that owned land in Leslie County challenges historian David Whisnant's scathing critique of female mountain reformers in *All That Is Native and Fine: The Politics of Change in an American Region*. According to Whisnant, instead of attacking the true problems facing the region—industrial exploitation, political corruption, and cultural erosion—female reformers at best failed to understand the true situation and at worst consciously sold out to the corporate sponsors who provided funding. It is true that Breckinridge rarely criticized coal companies publicly, and she may have too quickly abandoned her campaign to raise financial support from Leslie County investors. She deserves credit, however, for attempting to hold industrialists accountable for their actions. These investors had profited from the region, often at the expense of its residents. She confronted them with the implications of their actions, erroneously believing that they would embrace the opportunity to assist their neighbors. Breckinridge idealistically assumed that her powers of persuasion, combined with industrialists' internalized sense of duty, would naturally culminate in a new hospital for the county. She was mistaken. Still, Whisnant gives too little credit to reformers such as Breckinridge who wanted to challenge (if not remake) the industrial order and soften its impact on the area. He views these women as operating within a set of limitless options instead of taking into account the constraints they faced and the concessions they had to make to raise funds and attract supporters.

When her plan to secure corporate support fell through, Breckinridge turned to individual sponsors both within and outside Leslie County. Northern donors provided the bulk of the funds, with FNS patients contributing in ways they could with gifts of supplies, such as stone and timber, and labor. The local committee, Breckinridge proudly reported, pledged to raise one thousand dollars toward the cost of the hospital and ultimately exceeded that amount.[78]

Breckinridge expected that when the costs of building the hospital were worked out, the hard part would be over. She did not foresee the numerous challenges that would delay construction. A Lexington architectural firm drew up the blueprints at no cost. However, the firm did not send representatives to visit the land that the FNS had purchased and consequently failed to assess adequately the terrain of the site, perched high on Thousandsticks Mountain overlooking Hyden.[79] The service was plagued with other problems that did not affect builders of urban hospitals. The new facility could not hook into existing electrical lines and sewage systems; the FNS had to bring in expert consultants, run lines, and find creative solutions.[80]

The FNS finally dedicated Hyden Hospital on June 26, 1928.[81] Believing that it would be appropriate to have an authentic "Scottish Highlander" and a respected "Anglo-Saxon" medical pioneer present at such an important event, Breckinridge invited Sir Leslie MacKenzie, the director of the Scottish Highlands and Islands Medical Service, to serve as the keynote speaker at the dedication.[82] She also invited more than two thousand members of the community and FNS supporters to enjoy fireworks and musical entertainment.[83]

In the days leading up to the ceremony, Breckinridge and her staff busily prepared for the arrival of the dignitaries. They sought to make the difficult twenty-mile trek from the rail station to the hospital site as easy as possible. Steady rain the day before the dedication made the journey to Hyden more difficult, but, Breckinridge recalled, no one complained. The guests' "sporting qualities never failed," even when they had to climb mountains and creep along ledges.[84] One guest, Dr. J. A. Stucky, declared that the sacrifice was "well worth while because it [was] for . . . genuine Anglo-Saxon people."[85] When the rising river detained the wagon carrying the luggage, the guests went barefoot and changed into the "odds and ends" their hosts could gather. Breckinridge remembered having to "put some of the men in skirts," but "it was a gay party." She later remarked, "I had far rather handle a crowd of well bred people than any other."[86]

The festivities kicked off the following day when a twenty-piece band made up of miners from Hazard struck up "My Old Kentucky Home." Following the invocation, given by Berea College president William Hutchins, MacKenzie delivered a "splendid" dedication speech. According to Breckinridge, "He abandoned all of the learned things he had expected to say . . . and spoke from his heart, almost in tears." "The beacon lighted here today," he proclaimed, "will find an answering flame wherever human hearts are touched with the same divine pity." In the future, he predicted, "men and women, generation after generation, will rise to bless the name of the Frontier Nursing Service."[87] Following MacKenzie's address, the band broke into "Hieland Laddie." A fireworks display, "the first that the mountaineers had ever seen," enchanted the crowd that remained into the evening. Reporting on the festivities several days later, Breckinridge remarked that they were "exceptional," coming off "without a flaw."[88]

HYDEN HOSPITAL, with its electric lights, General Electric refrigerator, and state-of-the-art sterilizers, became the heart of Breckinridge's medical system.[89] It served as a hub, linking the organization's growing network of outpost nursing centers. By 1929, FNS nurse-midwives staffed six clinics, and two more were under construction. The scope of its operations now extended from Leslie County into Clay, Perry, and Harlan Counties. More than ten thousand people over a seven-hundred-square-mile area relied on the FNS for health care, more than half the twelve hundred square miles Breckinridge sought to cover. She looked forward to extending her experiment to the Ozarks, the Alleghenies, the Rockies, and other rural American communities. Soon, she hoped, the FNS would leave "no territory uncovered, and no people uncared for."[90]

A s the Frontier Nursing Service (FNS) expanded during the 1920s and the costs of operation swelled, Mary Breckinridge's need to find a steady source of funds became pressing. She looked toward philanthropic agencies to provide the funding necessary to continue and to expand her demonstration, with the idea that after she had proven the value of her system, the government would eventually pick up the tab, leading to public health care at the very least for women and children but ideally for all Americans. However, Breckinridge ultimately funded her organization not through foundations or through government support but by creating a network of wealthy individual donors who, attracted by her charisma and the organization's romantic appeal, gave generously. This decision to tap individual donors resulted largely from expediency, but it profoundly affected the scope of Breckinridge's work and inadvertently limited her organization's ability to transform American health care in the way that she intended.

MANY PRIVATE philanthropic boards concerned themselves with health projects during the early 1920s, and Breckinridge hoped that she could convince one of these organizations to underwrite the entire cost of her operation, thereby freeing her from the worries of fund-raising. Breckinridge's first attempt at securing foundation support ended unsuccessfully in 1924 when she withdrew her proposal from the American Child Health Association after her falling out with Dr. Annie S. Veech. In 1926, Breckinridge tried again, this time approaching the Laura Spelman Rockefeller Foundation.[1] Armed with statistics from the Kentucky Committee for Mothers and Babies's first few months of work, Breckinridge confidently mailed off a proposal for funding, sure that others would see the value and potential of her ideas.

By 1919, at least twenty-six U.S. charitable organizations were supporting medical research. Foundations understandably sought the most bang for their buck and consequently favored projects with broad, national implications, such as prestigious northern medical schools.[2] Rarely did local charities receive funding. Major philanthropies commended mountain settlement schools, community centers, and medical providers such as the FNS for fixing immediate needs but hesitated to support these groups because they failed to address the root of Appalachia's problems.[3] Breckinridge stressed that rather than just serving one locale, her organization was engaged in a demonstration that would eventually spread to other rural areas. This argument, however, did not sway the Rockefeller board. Breckinridge was frustrated to learn that her organization did not fulfill the Rockefeller Foundation's larger goals.

The rejection disappointed Breckinridge, not only because she had hoped for the money but also because such an endorsement would have brought the FNS credibility. The announcement that she had won the Harmon Foundation Quarterly Award for her article, "An Adventure in Midwifery: The Nurse-on-Horseback Gets a 'Soon Start,'" published in *Survey Graphic* later that year, raised her confidence, but the $250 cash prize that came with it did little to advance the organization's financial fortunes.[4] The FNS received $150 a month from the Kentucky State Board of Health beginning in 1927, but this amount covered only the salary of one nurse.[5]

Breckinridge's hopes for the FNS appeared within reach when she approached the Commonwealth Fund for support in 1928. With its mission of addressing the challenges facing vulnerable populations and of helping the United States create an efficient and innovative health care system, the fund's interests meshed nicely with those of Breckinridge.[6] She requested twenty-five thousand dollars yearly for five years, an amount that would allow her to extend her organization's work into new areas. In return, Breckinridge promised to raise matching funds and to launch an endowment campaign designed to raise three million dollars before the end of the five years.[7]

In what must have been a humiliating blow to Breckinridge's pride, the Commonwealth Fund rejected her proposal for funding, dismissing her nurses' work as unscientific and misguided. The fund's records noted that an investigation into Breckinridge's organization revealed "a group of nurses doing individually as good a piece of work as a group untrained in the fundamentals of sound public health could be expected to do." The report went on to criticize the service's misplaced goals. "Good roads and the ability to reach economic independence" would really benefit the community, the report noted. The fund's directors advised that rather than attempt to alleviate the area's problems "through the guise of a nursing service which operates without a scientific basis and has no clear definition of function," subsidies to state health departments, funding for workshops for local lay midwives, and "even subsidies to individual physicians to practice in the county, would produce more effective and lasting results." In a direct assault on the director's ego, the report concluded, "Without Mrs. Breckinridge's intensely personal concern and her standing in her own community, it is to be doubted whether the enterprise would have gained any foot-hold whatsoever."[8]

After it became clear that she would not receive the endorsement and financial backing of a national organization, Breckinridge convinced herself that remaining autonomous would be the best thing for the FNS. Her words almost became a rallying cry: "Co-operation every turn with every agency is our policy; but incorporation with none." Breckinridge did not view dismissal by foundation boards or government officials such as Veech as a reflection of the value of the project. Instead, Breckinridge saw these rejections as testament to the inventive nature of her plan. She fashioned herself as a maverick challenging a rigid system that prevented new ideas from being implemented. Writing to her publicity secretary in 1926, she confided that she was relieved that she had parted ways with Veech's Bureau of Maternal and Child Health. Had they allied with the state agency, the FNS's nurses would have been "hampered with red tape at every turn." Remaining independent gave Breckinridge the freedom to try new things and to avoid the bureaucracy that often stymied innovation.[9]

This freedom, however, brought financial uncertainty and the stress of constant fund-raising. In the late 1920s, Breckinridge threw herself into campaigning for the service outside of the Bluegrass State. She specifically targeted northeastern cities, relying on family and friends there to introduce her to other wealthy, philanthropic-minded individuals.[10] She worked tirelessly to spread the word about the important work her nurses were doing, penning more than two thousand letters each year to donors and traveling in and out of the mountains on average every ten days in 1926.[11] In correspondence with her nurses, she frequently expressed her desire to return to Wendover, but she often put her homecoming on hold as she attempted to "squeeze" as much "gold" as possible out of another city.[12]

The American economy was booming in the late 1920s. Manufacturing output rose 23.5 percent between 1923 and 1929, and real per person income increased nearly 13 percent during the same period.[13] Breckinridge's organization reaped the benefits of this prosperity. Northern elites responded enthusiastically to her appeals. During fiscal year 1926–27 alone, donations to the organization increased by more than 400 percent from the preceding year.[14] David Whisnant notes that Americans looked at Appalachian residents in one of two ways in the early twentieth century, either as " 'backward,' unhealthy, unchurched, ignorant, violent, and morally degenerate social misfits who were a national liability" or as "pure, uncorrupted 100 percent American, picturesque, and photogenic pre-moderns who were a great untapped national treasure."[15] Breckinridge and her supporters clearly fell into this second group. The romantic reputation of the FNS's work attracted many contributors. Fans were enamored with nurses' uniforms and saddlebags and especially intrigued by their use of horses at a time when cars were becoming the preferred mode of transportation for most Americans. Supporters shared Breckinridge's concern that a new urban, industrial society threatened to supplant America's traditional rural, agrarian ways of life. In addition, the FNS's backers were reassured by her promise that Appalachian residents possessed pure blood and with assistance could provide an antidote to the forecasted weakening of American stock.

Breckinridge relied on personal charisma and her extensive contacts with prominent individuals throughout the country to build a fund-raising network from the ground up. One of the first steps she took once she decided that government or foundation support was not a possibility was to hire a public relations coordinator to develop a system of city committees. With Jessie "Kit" Carson's assistance, Breckinridge scoured the country in search of individuals sympathetic to her cause. The city committees allowed Breckinridge to create a strong following for her organization and helped its treasury to "run . . . into the thousands" in just a few years.[16] By the end of the decade, Breckinridge was raising more than $130,000 annually.[17]

Breckinridge carefully selected where and when to solicit support, seeking the most fertile ground in which to sow her seed. She set her sights on such large cities as New York, Chicago, and Boston not only because they were home to some of the wealthiest Americans but because they had successful visiting nurses' services. She assumed that she would have a better chance of winning residents over to the value of her plan in areas where public health was already a priority. An area's reputation for generously supporting other mountain projects also figured into her choice of fund-raising territory.

After identifying the areas she wanted to target, Breckinridge sent Carson ahead to lay the groundwork. As with her state and local committees, Breckinridge attempted to recruit the "leading citizens" of each location, believing that if she could get them on board, others would follow. Carson conducted careful research to identify each city's most respected residents. She searched the local society registers and rosters of charitable organizations for names. She also scanned newspapers for leads. In Chicago, she clipped columns listing those who held box seats at the opera and naming those who served as honorary pallbearers at a wealthy citizen's funeral.[18] After Carson compiled a list of possible committee members, she wrote to each individual, requesting an opportunity to explain in person the FNS's purpose. After Carson generated initial enthusiasm for the project, Breckinridge then made a sweep, speaking to as many groups and personally calling on as many individuals as possible. Organizations she often targeted included the Rotary Club, the Optimists, Junior Leagues, the General Federation of Women's Clubs, the Daughters of the American Revolution, and the Colonial Dames.[19]

Those not immediately attracted by written descriptions of Breckinridge's project often found themselves drawn in by the director's charm and energy. When asked to describe Mary Breckinridge, friends and patrons nearly always emphasized her talent for public speaking.[20] Her presentations left audiences inspired and emotionally moved. Like her famous male ancestors, who had won acclaim for their stump speaking abilities, Mary never failed to impress listeners with her "spellbinding stories."[21] She used microphones only when necessary and never relied on notes. She once commented, "If I should get the ideas out of my head on paper I could never get them back in my head again."[22] She was not known for brevity, often speaking for an hour and a half; according to one supporter, however, audiences always "wanted to hear more."[23]

During her long presentations, Breckinridge used graphic pictures of tapeworms and vermin removed from young patients to hold listeners' attention. At one particular engagement, when she noticed several older ladies nodding off, she launched into her discussion of parasites. According to Breckinridge's niece, Marvin Breckinridge Patterson, "The dozing ladies woke up with a start, horrified, and listened attentively thereafter."[24] One former FNS volunteer, Patsy Lawrence, recalled that the normally prim and proper women to whom Breckinridge spoke loved to hear "the gory details" of the "newest worming methods." They would "sit up on the edge of their seats" to catch her every word. Lawrence observed, "It was really as if these women were seeing a pornographic movie or something."[25]

A reporter for Rhode Island's *Providence Evening Bulletin* praised Breckinridge's speaking ability, noting that "she had a great stage presence, an electric personality, and a magnificent rhythm."[26] Likewise, a nurse in one of Breckinridge's audiences recalled that hearing her was like watching a "maestro" who had the listeners "in the palm of her hand."[27] In testament to her skill, she won praise from some accomplished public speakers. Kentucky governor Albert B. "Happy" Chandler commended her oratorical abilities, claiming that she could "charm the birds off the trees."[28] Congressman Thruston Morton praised Breckinridge's ability to inspire her audiences, noting that he longed for similar skills.[29]

Breckinridge's physical appearance certainly did not captivate audiences. Her haunting blue eyes—inherited from her grandfather, John C. Breckinridge—were her only distinctive feature. She was about five feet, two inches tall, on the plump side, and later in life had a slight hunchback. She had short "bristly" gray hair, which she wore "clipped like a boy's." The "cow man" at Wendover usually cut her hair. Fashion meant little to her, much to her co-workers' dismay. Her clothes were always neat and clean but never fancy. Although Patterson urged her to "dress smartly" when speaking to city committees of chic women as a way of proving that "she belonged to their group," she paid no heed. She appeared at every annual meeting in the same black dress and black suede shoes, hand-me-downs from her sister-in-law. "She had no vanity," Patterson recalled. "She thought her work, her kinfolk, her friends, and books were far more important than her looks."[30]

Breckinridge and her associates claimed that she never directly asked for donations from those who attended her presentations.[31] Her policy was simply to share her enthusiasm for the FNS's work without pressuring those in attendance to give immediately. Several days after each speaking engagement, she sent a follow-up appeal, thereby allowing audience members to consider what she had said and willingly send contributions. Breckinridge contended that this policy inspired donors to give larger sums than they would have if immediately solicited at the end of her presentations. When a fellow reformer asked for advice on raising money, Breckinridge responded, "All I try to do is to get them to love [the service] as I love it." She noted that this approach best suited her. This way, "money that comes is from people who are glad to give it, I am glad to get it, and that is a nice state of gladness all around."[32]

The value of Breckinridge's plan, combined with her calculated approach to fund-raising and the passion with which she delivered her appeal, helped her to win favor from what one historian has dubbed America's "charity trust."[33] As she had hoped, some of the country's most recognizable names graced the list of FNS supporters. Contributors included William Cooper Proctor, founder of Cincinnati-based Proctor and Gamble; Gustavus Swift, a successful meat packer; and J. S. Pillsbury, a wealthy flour merchant. The *Louisville Courier-Journal* reported that no other charity had ever "attracted so influential a following in New York."[34] Although the bulk of her support came from elites such as these, who could "by the stroke of the pen provide all or a large part of the amount necessary," many supporters of more moderate means sent only a few dollars each.[35] Everyone who heard Breckinridge's impassioned speeches in the 1920s seemed to want to do their part to further the service's work.

BY 1930, most Americans, whether or not they had attended one of Breckinridge's presentations, were aware of her quest to save mountain mothers and babies. Romantic tales of the FNS's work had appeared frequently in mass-circulation magazines in the latter part of the preceding decade. Journalists praised the nurse's willingness to "leap into her saddle at a moment's notice and ride wherever duty calls," traveling "over mountain paths that hardly deserve the name even in the best of seasons." Once there, the nurse "safely usher[ed] a new being into the world" with no more than the light of an open fire and her lantern. Likened to soldiers and to Royal Mounted Police, frontier nurses became "angels on horseback" and "heroines of the highlands."[36]

Breckinridge recognized that her nurses' exciting exploits attracted many supporters, and she capitalized on the fascination. She frequently described the thrills and challenges of their work in the *Frontier Nursing Service Quarterly Bulletin*. In 1926, for example, she reported in vivid detail a night call made by Edna Rockstroh during which the dedicated nurse-midwife did not let freezing rain keep her from reaching a patient in need. She willingly offered her services in spite of the potential danger and discomfort. After bringing a new baby into the world, the exhausted nurse returned home in the middle of the night frozen into her clothes and onto her saddle. Two men had to hoist her from her horse and then lift her poncho, "stiff as a board," over her head. "So, loosed from her bonds," Breckinridge recounted, "she emerged every inch a nurse."[37] Another nurse, nicknamed Harry, had "bits of shrapnel left inside" from her service during World War I. After beginning work with the FNS, she was thrown from her horse and fractured her skull, but she never let her pain stand in her way of serving her patients.[38]

Breckinridge stressed that FNS nurses were prepared to save mothers and babies at any cost, including that of the nurses' own lives. In 1931, Nancy O'Driscoll became the first FNS nurse to die "in service," reinforcing Breckinridge's claim. The *Lexington Herald* printed a tribute to O'Driscoll, praising the "Irish heroine" for ignoring her pain to tend to the needs of others. Even after her appendix ruptured, she refused to return to headquarters because she had not yet completed her rounds. The article concluded, "No soldier in the field of battle, no pioneer carrying the flag of civilization, ever died a more heroic death in a nobler cause than did . . . O'Driscoll."[39] O'Driscoll continued to serve the FNS long after her death: she became a mythic hero in Breckinridge's fund-raising appeals, illustrating her nurses' bravery and commitment.

The prevailing theme in Breckinridge's early fund-raising literature was that the people of Appalachia were proud and noble. Through no fault of their own but simply as a consequence of isolation, they lacked access to modern ideas and conveniences. The *Quarterly Bulletin* became one of the FNS's most important fund-raising tools, giving patrons frequent glimpses into how nurses' efforts were making a difference in the lives of their deserving mountain patients. Early issues of the *Bulletin* used both words and images to communicate in romantic terms the hardships Leslie County residents faced. Birth became a mystical experience, as the account of one delivery that took place on a cold night in 1926 reflected. A special fund-raising appeal told the story. Following a "cold stumbling ride," a nurse arrives at a "ramshackle" cabin to find a sixteen-year-old wife in labor. As she lies moaning "on the home-made bed," "smoke eddies out of the chimney and fills the room with weird mistiness." Pale dawn begins to shine through the cracks in the walls, and as it does, "the moaning ceases suddenly, and the faint small wail of a new-born infant reaches waiting ears."[40] In service literature, a simple birth—albeit one occurring under difficult circumstances—becomes heroic, mysterious, and idealized. Service supporters found such images, very skillfully and eloquently penned by Breckinridge, compelling and responded by giving generously.

The language with which she described FNS patients helped emphasize the distance that separated Leslie County from donors in other parts of the nation. Breckinridge claimed that "mountain people, like lowlanders, are just people," but she clearly saw them as different and exotic. In keeping with the portrait painted by local color writers, she referred to "the Leslians" as though they were a distinct species.[41] Distinguishing them in such a way connoted a degree of respect for their unique culture, but by emphasizing their differences from other Americans and by celebrating their hardiness, Breckinridge oversimplified the problems faced by residents of the area's "vast primeval forests."[42]

More than anything, FNS publicity stressed that its patients were worthy of the help they were receiving. A courier described a case in which a nurse-midwife delivered the baby of a mother who was sick with pneumonia. This care, she claimed, had inspired the oldest child, Susie, to improve the house. Each day when the nurse visited, she noticed some little change in the cabin. After just a few weeks, she noted, "I hardly recognized that room. Everything was clean and neat."[43] In another case, Breckinridge used the story of Sally to illustrate the difference the service was making. Relying on her district nurse as a resource, this local mother had gone to great lengths to create a clean, safe environment for her family. Her neighbors considered her "the sewinest an' workinest woman on the creek."[44] Unwilling to accept charity, she had "knocked at the clinic door with five pennies saved from her egg money" to purchase old copies of the *American Journal of Nursing* and the *Public Health Nurse*. She used the journals to paper the walls of her remote cabin, shutting out the cold while simultaneously improving the cabin's appearance. The people of Leslie County needed the FNS, according to Breckinridge. Without the nurses' help, not only would residents' health suffer, but they would continue to live in squalid conditions without the opportunity to improve their surroundings that the nurses and their discarded journals provided.[45]

ROMANTIC DEPICTIONS of the FNS's work alone, however, only partly explain why Breckinridge raised so much money during the late 1920s. Her plan to make maternity safer for the women of Appalachia succeeded in large part because she capitalized on the nation's paranoia that the white race was in danger. For those who feared that immigrants would overtake America's old stock, Appalachia, with its population of "pure Anglo-Saxons," appeared to provide a haven from the forces threatening the country. Glamorous images helped to attract patrons, but only a deeper affinity with the service, an agreement with the philosophies and goals it espoused, inspired people to continue opening their wallets.

The turn of the twentieth century was an uneasy time for Americans, particularly white, middle-class American men, who felt threatened from within and without by the rapid technological and social changes that accompanied industrialization. Although confident they were members of the world's most advanced civilization, American men feared that their privileged position was in jeopardy. Many believed that the new conveniences that industrialization brought would make them "soft" and unable to compete in the human struggle to be most "fit." Experts pointed to neurasthenia and the increased visibility of homosexuals as proof that the United States was becoming "overcivilized." Concurrently, other groups appeared to be gaining in power. Women's push to expand their sphere by obtaining the right to vote and by pursuing careers contributed to the growing fear that traditional power structures had come under attack. Likewise, the perception that African American men were regressing toward their "natural" state now that they were no longer held in check by slavery challenged prevailing hierarchies, leading American men to fear that white women and ostensibly the white race were in danger.[46]

Although these fears may today appear irrational, they were rooted in tangible threats to middle-class power and authority. Historian Gail Bederman argues that during this time, social mobility contracted, and it became more difficult to become a self-made man after 1900. Fewer middle-class men were self-employed. In addition, frequent economic depressions undermined Americans' sense of security. Small entrepreneurs particularly felt threatened as they encountered increasing difficulty in competing with powerful conglomerates such as Standard Oil and U.S. Steel.[47]

Instead of blaming industrialists and capitalist structures, many Americans identified the immigrants flooding the cities as the enemy. Nativism, the hatred of all things foreign, first emerged in the United States in the 1840s and 1850s and continued to ebb and flow throughout the remainder of the nineteenth century. As World War I approached, Americans began to argue that new blood from other races would not improve the nation's stock, as experts had previously predicted, but instead would dilute older Americans' superior heritage. Experts now stressed that foreign germs and foreign ideas, particularly autocratic political theories, threatened democracy.[48] Following the war, nativist sentiment exploded. One hundred percent Americanism, invoked during the conflict to unify the country, later became the rallying cry of anti-immigrationists. The 1920s brought a rejuvenation of the Ku Klux Klan, the Red Scare, and stricter immigration policies, culminating in passage of the 1924 National Origins Act.[49]

While decay introduced from without was a concern, fear of weakening from within also abounded during the early twentieth century. The field of eugenics, developed in the late nineteenth century by Sir Francis Galton, became popular among many leading Americans, including Mary Breckinridge. Supporters of the eugenics movement applied the concept of survival of the fittest to human reproduction. Just as selective breeding had improved horses and dogs, so too could it improve humans, eugenics supporters argued.[50] They warned that if unworthy parents were allowed to breed unchecked, they would pass along to their offspring such acquired characteristics as degeneracy, alcoholism, crime, and mental illness.[51] Critics viewed "defectives" as a threat to the nation's health. Comparing the nation to a body, eugenics supporters warned that inferior individuals would "infect" the country, causing it to sicken and die.[52]

Madison Grant, an upper-crust New Yorker and author of a popular book, *The Passing of the Great Race* (1916), helped draw attention to the urgency of the eugenics cause. He called for improvement of the population in "quality rather than quantity." The melting pot, he stressed, should not be "allowed to boil without control." Otherwise, he cautioned, "the type of native American of Colonial descent [would] become as extinct as the Athenian of the age of Pericles, and the Viking of the days of Rollo."[53] He urged concerned Americans to "completely repudiate the proud boast of our fathers that they acknowledged no distinction in 'race, creed, or color,' " else they soon "turn the page of history and write: 'FINIS AMERICAE.' "[54]

Eugenics supporters varied in their approach to addressing the crisis they saw developing. Some saw forced sterilization as a crucial way to fight degeneration. Indiana passed the first sterilization law in 1907, and by 1931, thirty-one states had followed suit. California led the way in limiting reproduction of the unfit; between 1909 and 1929, more than sixty-two hundred of its residents were involuntarily sterilized. These laws were constitutionally sanctioned by the U.S. Supreme Court, and even liberal reformers supported the measures.[55] At the same time, many eugenics supporters focused less on the unfit and more on the nation's best citizens, whom they encouraged to have more children. Leaders such as President Theodore Roosevelt warned that the Anglo-Saxon descendants of America's Founding Fathers were not producing large enough families. He issued a national challenge, cautioning that unless white birthrates increased, "race suicide" would result. He criticized white women who chose to remain childless as "criminal against the race." According to Roosevelt, an ideal, upper-class family should have six children. Any fewer than four, he argued, contributed to the nation's genetic degradation.[56] His warning received wide press. Between 1905 and 1909, popular magazines published more than thirty-five articles on the subject of race suicide.[57]

In this climate of fear, hostility, and uncertainty, Americans found Breckinridge's descriptions of her pure white Appalachian patients very compelling. She was not the first to argue that Appalachia would provide a cure for the nation's ills. For more than two decades, William Goodell Frost, president of Berea College, had been publicizing the value of the mountains and their people. According to Frost, Appalachia would save the country from race suicide. "The American families in eastern cities have few children and are dying out," he explained, "but a mountain household always numbers a good 'baker's dozen.' "[58] Contrasting eastern Kentucky with America's urban areas, Breckinridge claimed that the mountains were "a feeder for the city . . . a nursery for the finest flower of the old American stock."[59]

Appalachian birthrates indeed remained high, even as other areas of the nation experienced a steady decline during the nineteenth century.[60] Not only did Appalachian families have many children, they had what anxious Americans viewed as the "right kind" of children. Writing in 1901, geographer Ellen Churchill Semple noted that the people of the mountains "bear about them in their speech and ideas the marks of their ancestry as plainly as if they had disembarked from their eighteenth-century vessel yesterday." She stressed that the residents of the region, though poor, were America's best. Their "gentle, gracious, and unembarrassed" manners made one forget "their bare feet, ragged clothes, and crass ignorance" and led one to bow "anew to the inextinguishable excellence of the Anglo-Saxon race." Like Frost, Semple credited isolation with keeping the mountain stock "free from the tide of foreign immigrants which has been pouring in recent years into the States." Not only were "foreign elements" scarce, blacks reportedly were absent: according to Semple, Appalachia was "as free from them as northern Vermont."[61]

Mary Breckinridge shared the prevailing fear that the American race was in jeopardy, and she believed strongly that mountain residents would strengthen the nation against foreign threats. Breckinridge was well-read and was familiar with eugenics experts' arguments. She was concerned about immigration and served on the Americanization Committee of the Colonial Dames.[62] Breckinridge viewed race in strict hierarchical terms. She described African Americans as naturally inferior and supported the system of segregation that had developed in the South, seeing it as beneficial to both races. Even among whites, she drew sharp distinctions. Nordic races, she claimed, possessed the finest blood and the strongest leadership ability, while inferior stocks, such as the Italians and Slavs, were naturally subordinate. She reserved her highest praise for Anglo-Saxons, who possessed both superior blood and an impressive cultural history as the creators of democracy.[63]

In the early years of the FNS, Breckinridge's fund-raising literature consistently stressed the racial identity of her organization's patients. She inaccurately praised Kentucky mountaineers for being "all of British descent, with here and there a sprinkling of Huguenot and Pennsylvania Dutch."[64] According to the census, Leslie County had more than ten thousand residents, only two of them foreign-born. In all her travels throughout the county, however, she insisted that she never found either of them.[65] She used the intelligence tests she commissioned in 1923 to reinforce her claims that the county had a superior population that deserved assistance to reach its full potential.

Breckinridge recognized that some observers might question why the people of eastern Kentucky needed outside help if they belonged to such a noble race. In response, she stressed that her patients were "handicapped by geographical conditions and not by native ability." She described eastern Kentucky as "a land of few good roads, where an eighteenth century civilization continues to exist . . . in the heart of America."[66] The territory her organization covered was so rough "that a golf course, or even a croquet set, could scarcely be laid out within its borders," she explained.[67] Although she did not go as far as one of her contemporaries, who likened mountain residents to modern-day "Robinson Crusoes" "marooned in the mountains," Breckinridge firmly believed that their remote location accounted for their economic distress and for their lack of progress in medicine and education.[68]

Although Breckinridge blamed isolation for many of the problems plaguing Appalachia, she argued that isolation had benefits as well. The region's insularity, she claimed, had protected traditional American values at a time when the nation was in transition. Breckinridge stressed that her patients were "unadulterated by foreign infusions, untouched by the jazz-mad world all about them." She praised the mountain people for "holding still to the convictions and beliefs of their forefathers" and for "speaking a language which [clung] to the idioms and phrases current at the time when Jamestown and Plymouth were settled."[69] In a rapidly changing world, Breckinridge and her nurses looked to the mountaineers, who "continued to live their lives and think their thoughts in much the way their forebears had done for the last hundred and fifty years"—that is, to preserve the ideals of past generations.[70]

Breckinridge specifically asked contributors, "What responsibility do you feel for these American citizens?"[71] The overwhelming response her appeals generated shows that the images she painted of FNS patients resonated with her supporters. Patrons and volunteers, like Breckinridge, appreciated the "pure" blood of the region's residents and admired their traditional values. FNS accountant W. A. Hifner Jr. described the satisfaction he received from working with the organization. He rejoiced that the service was endowing those who "by reason of a natural heritage" had "better bodies" with "better minds and hearts."[72] The members of the executive committee similarly revealed their pride in contributing to Breckinridge's "worthy experiment." Summing up their first year of work in 1926, they wrote, "We challenge any section to show finer babies than these wee Leslians of ours—and here and now we pay a tribute of respect to the intelligent and eager cooperation of their mothers. This is the old stock, with modern care and teaching—America's own. Hasn't the year been worth while?"[73]

BRECKINRIDGE EXPERIENCED a great deal of fund-raising success during the late 1920s because the wealthy, white Americans who comprised the bulk of her supporters shared her racist views. Some, like Elizabeth Perkins, explicitly expressed their motivation for donating. Perkins deeply admired all Breckinridge was doing for her "sturdy, upright God fearing" patients.[74] After faithfully supporting the FNS throughout her lifetime, she bequeathed the service $150,000 in 1952. She did so, her will confirmed, to further the FNS's efforts to save mothers and babies, "preferably those of the Anglo-Saxon race."[75] Anne Morgan, daughter of wealthy financier J. P. Morgan, echoed Perkins's concern with protecting white Americans, explaining, "I am particularly interested in this movement of Mrs. Breckinridge's . . . because I feel that it means so much towards the survival of our oldest American stock."[76]

Others, including automaker Henry Ford, did not explicitly state their reasons for giving to the FNS. However, Ford's well-publicized racial prejudices suggest that he was similarly motivated to contribute. Ford was one of the most famous and most generous supporters that Breckinridge recruited to her cause. His wife, Clara, became a particularly loyal donor. In January 1926, she heard Breckinridge speak at the Girls' Protective League of Detroit, was deeply moved, and sent the organization a check for seven thousand dollars with instructions to "build and furnish a health center at once."[77] A long relationship between the service and the Ford family was thus established. Beginning in 1927, Clara Ford faithfully donated one thousand dollars every year until her death in 1950. She contributed an additional fifty dollars annually to the organization's Christmas party fund. Beginning in 1928, the Fords' only son, Edsel, followed his parents' lead by pledging one thousand dollars annually.[78]

At first glance, the Ford family, Leslie County's largest landholder, might seem to have had ulterior motives for donating to the FNS, but the evidence does not support this contention.[79] The Fords only reluctantly publicized their contributions. When Breckinridge first announced that a supporter had pledged to build a nursing center at Red Bird, she listed the gift as coming from an anonymous donor. Only later did she reveal that Clara Ford had provided the funds.[80] The Fordson Coal Company, a subsidiary of Ford Motor, donated land on several occasions, and its engineers often advised the organization on building projects, but the *Bulletin* never recognized these gifts. If the Fords had been interested in Breckinridge's work because they desired to improve their image in the region, they surely would have made their contributions known. The Fords may have sought to downplay their extensive holdings in the region and therefore shied away from Breckinridge's spotlight, but that still does not explain their interest in her cause.

Like Breckinridge, the Fords saw Appalachia as the hope of a nation inundated by immigrants. History well remembers Henry Ford's anti-Semitic views. As an ardent proponent of racial purity, he feared race suicide and sought to preserve the values of Anglo-Saxon America. Writing in 1923, he praised the mountain people, calling them "the real Americans." He appreciated that "fellows" in Appalachia "talk American . . . act like Americans . . . are simple in their living habits [and] work hard." "Precious little" American stock remained, but as he saw it, the mountains, in their isolation, were preserving the true American values.[81] The Fords became loyal contributors not only to the FNS but also to other Appalachian reform projects, including the Berry schools, Lincoln Memorial University, Berea College, and the Hindman Settlement School.[82]

In donors' minds, the racial purity associated with the mountains went hand in hand with the preservation of traditional values. At the turn of the century, as industrialization transformed the nation, Americans nostalgically looked to the mountains, where older ways of life persisted. This nostalgia manifested itself in a fascination with Appalachian folk crafts and a mad rush to collect and preserve old ballads still sung in the region. In her book, *Selling Tradition: Appalachia and the Construction of an American Folk, 1930–1940* (1998), Jane Becker investigates the use of tradition as a "symbolic construction." She contends that Americans' early-twentieth-century preoccupation with folk culture stemmed from a desire to invoke "a distant past that was vague and conflict-free, untroubled by class, racial, or ethnic divisions."[83] Scholars convincingly have argued that this picture of a mountain area frozen in time was inaccurate; in fact, as Dwight Billings explains, "Half of the coal-mining workforce in the central Appalachian coalfields of southern West Virginia were European immigrants and one-fourth were African American at the very moment in time when folk song collectors were searching for traditional British ballads in the region's most remote areas."[84] By 1929, quaint ballads were being superseded by "hillbilly records" broadcast across the nation's radio waves.[85] But in spite of the changes, Americans continued to see Appalachia as representing a key repository of traditional values that were dying out elsewhere.

Mountain folk, Americans believed, were hardworking, independent, and virtuous and behaved as true men and women should. According to one contributor to the serial *Mountain Life and Work*, the mountains offered "a constant stream of vigorous native manhood and charming, simple womanhood, fresh, unspoiled and in the deepest sense American."[86] This picture contrasted starkly with the cities, where gender roles were in flux. J. A. Stucky, a physician active in mountain health projects, appreciatively noted that the Appalachian people were not "laborers, operatives, or salaried folk, but soil-owners and home-makers." Not only did his mountaineers embody the Jeffersonian ideal on which the nation had been built, but he admired the fact that each person understood his or her proper gender role.[87] Breckinridge reinforced this reassuring image, stressing that Appalachian men retained "the utmost chivalry for women" while mothers remained "the heart of the household."[88] Separate spheres may have been breaking down in urban regions, but in Appalachia, men still knew how to be men and women still acted like women.

The rugged terrain of the mountains combined with its perceived isolation, observers noted, to allow Appalachian residents to continue to experience life in its truest form. Just as America's frontier history was closing, with the nation settled from shore to shore and its great wilderness conquered, Appalachia appeared to be a new "pioneer" region where men could continue to test their "wits."[89] Americans were striving to become "civilized," but at the same time, they feared that they would become too civilized, thus losing the toughness and strength necessary to keep civilization on its forward path. Convinced that comfortable living and working conditions were making city residents "soft," critics applauded the rugged mountain lifestyle for allowing people to remain vigorous and hardy.[90]

Americans sought opportunities to reconnect with nature in hopes of testing their vitality and experiencing the primitive. Most Americans embraced progress, but they recognized that while they were gaining comforts, they lost a way of life that they could never recover. The desire to experience the primal (and to prove his masculinity) led Theodore Roosevelt to travel through Africa after he left office in 1909.[91] Wealthy industrialists such as J. P. Morgan bought camps in the Adirondack Mountains where they could "play at roughing it" in a sort of "rustic fantasy," while servants—often as many as three to each "pioneer"—ensured comfort.[92] Similarly, many people flocked to Appalachia to find adventure and a simpler way of life. In *The Land of Saddle-Bags: A Study of the Mountain People of Appalachia* (1924), Berea College professor James Watt Raine encouraged such pilgrimages to the mountains: "Have you ever thought, when rummaging in an attic, how delightful it would be . . . to visit the home that your great-great-grandfather built after he left his Elizabethan England and came to America?" According to Raine, traveling to Appalachia, like boarding a time machine, would allow one to do so.[93]

Intrigued by the struggles Appalachian people faced and curious to see how their grandparents had lived, FNS supporters traveled to eastern Kentucky to witness firsthand Breckinridge's work. One newly married bride and groom even chose to spend their honeymoon making the rounds of FNS nursing centers.[94] Visitors described their trips as life-changing experiences. Julia Henning, a vice chair of the Kentucky Committee for Mothers and Babies, using language rich with symbolism, described her 1925 trip "into the heart of the mountains." "A spiritual experience," the journey was filled with new undertakings—sleeping on a corn shuck mattress, mistakenly taking a swig from the slop bucket, and hearing testimony in "a perfectly good murder trial." Being able to "lodge . . . with a native," Henning recalled, was one of the highlights of her journey. She described the mountain residents she encountered with a mixture of curiosity and appreciation, commenting on their intelligence, industriousness, and respectability. One of her hostesses "smoked a pipe with the air of a Duchess." Conditions in this "wild country" were rough, but, according to Henning, she and her companion managed to maintain their dignity. After arriving at the "primitive . . . abode" where the two women stayed, her companion "rescued her Roger-Gallet soap, her Cody perfume, her Bonwit Teller costume, [and] her pearls."[95] In her report of their trip, Henning sharply contrasted her civilized way of life, complete with its many luxuries, with other Americans' "primitive" lifestyles. Doing so allowed her to rejoice in the nation's progress while mourning the loss of a simpler time.

Breckinridge played on her supporters' oversimplified images of the area. Even those who could not visit in person could share in the excitement of the service's work by reading dramatic accounts of nurses' rounds and anecdotes that starkly contrasted life in the mountains against the way of life to which most Americans at the time were accustomed. The material that filled the organization's *Quarterly Bulletin* resonated with FNS supporters such as Virginia McKee, who later recalled how she loved reading the "little quaint old poems . . . and little stories about [the Appalachian] people, . . . you know, farmers and simple people."[96]

WHEN MARY Breckinridge established the Kentucky Committee for Mothers and Babies in 1925, she was unsure how she would raise the money needed to pay for nurses, supplies, and horses. She forged ahead anyway. Inspired by the image she painted of the region's "pure Anglo-Saxons" and her predictions concerning their ability to contribute to the nation, patrons gave generously to her project. Breckinridge's constant traveling and extensive correspondence paid handsome dividends. In the five years following the launch of her demonstration, she raised more than $336,000 in contributions.[97] By 1930, strong committees were in place in twelve cities, and one donor had promised $50,000 to start an endowment fund.[98]

Supporters were good to Mary Breckinridge and her organization, but in the long run, her decision to pursue private funding undermined her original goal of revolutionizing American health care. Breckinridge arrived in Leslie County convinced that she had the answers to the problems that plagued the area. Lay midwives were dangerous; trained nurse-midwives could provide an efficient alternative not only in eastern Kentucky but throughout the nation wherever physicians were scarce. When state health officials and charitable board administrators criticized her plan as impractical and misguided, her resolve only strengthened.

Breckinridge later emphasized that she loved the mountain people and had nothing but their best interests at heart, but the oversimplified view of the region's culture that she initially brought to her work caused her to ignore the deeper structural changes occurring in Appalachia in the early twentieth century. She romanticized her patients and in so doing made the problems they faced appear less a national issue that required true reform of the system and more an isolated instance of cultural dissonance. Breckinridge did not publicly critique the industrialists who were transforming the mountains and exploiting the region's resources for private gain. She did not condemn the American capitalist system that had led to such glaring disparities of wealth. Instead, she celebrated an area that had been left behind and provided Americans with quaint stories of admirable folk and a way to assuage their consciences by supporting the work of her brave nurses.[99]

Breckinridge arrived with good intentions and certainly plenty of enthusiasm, but her confidence that she had all the answers and her romanticized impression of mountain life drawn from media representations instead of true interaction with the area's people initially blinded her to the challenges they faced. Breckinridge expected patients to welcome her nurses with open arms. In reality, FNS nurses struggled for nearly a decade to sell their project to the residents of Leslie County.

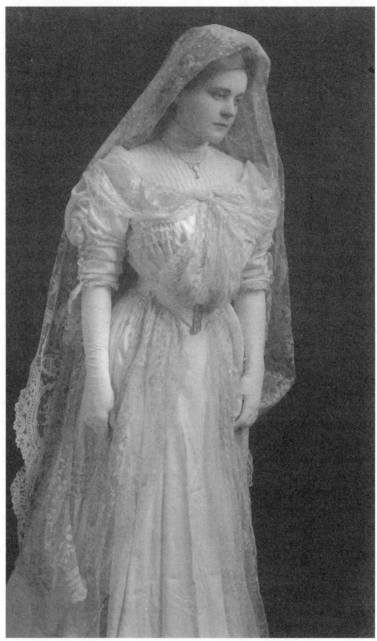

Mary Breckinridge as a young bride, 1904. Breckinridge claimed that when she married Henry Ruffner Morrison, she renounced all of her own ambitions to devote herself to home and family.
(Courtesy of the Audio-Visual Archives, Special Collections and Digital Programs, University of Kentucky Libraries, Lexington)

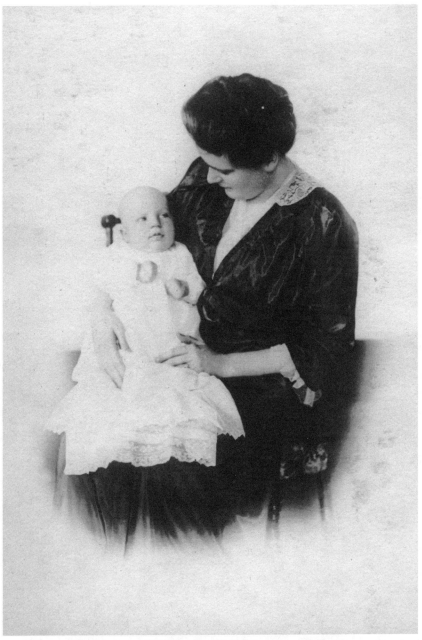

Mary Breckinridge with her son, Breckie, Eureka Springs, Arkansas, 1914.
For the rest of her life, Breckinridge would make women and children the focus of her
reform efforts, using her position as a mother to justify her public involvement.
(Courtesy of the Audio-Visual Archives, Special Collections
and Digital Programs, University of Kentucky Libraries, Lexington)

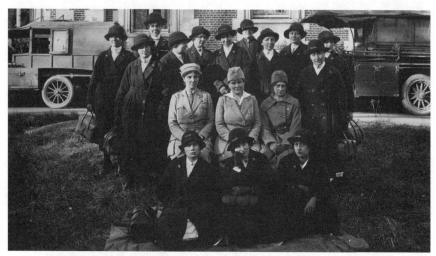

Mary Breckinridge (second row, center) with her colleagues from the Comité Américain pour les Régions Dévastées de la France, Soissons, February 1921.
(Courtesy of the Audio–Visual Archives, Special Collections and Digital Programs, University of Kentucky Libraries, Lexington)

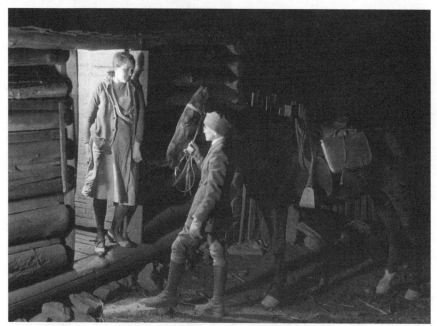

FNS assistant director Mary B. Willeford making a late–night home visit, ca. 1929. Nurses kept two sets of saddlebags packed at all times, one for general calls and one for midwifery calls. In the service's early years, horses provided the only form of transportation.
(Courtesy of the Audio–Visual Archives, Special Collections and Digital Programs, University of Kentucky Libraries, Lexington)

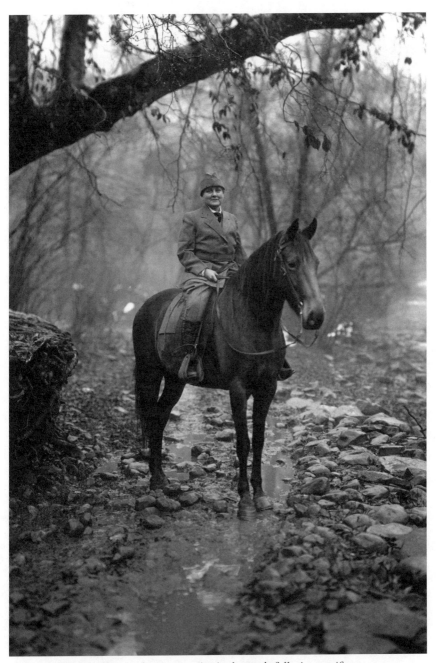

Mary Breckinridge standing at attention in the FNS's full winter uniform, ca. 1931. She designed the uniform, which closely resembled the one she wore in France, to command respect and to reinforce comparisons between her nurses and soldiers.
(Courtesy of the Audio-Visual Archives, Special Collections and Digital Programs, University of Kentucky Libraries, Lexington)

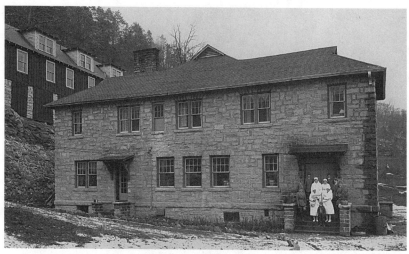

Hyden Hospital, ca. 1940. This twelve-bed facility, built in 1928, served FNS patients until the Mary Breckinridge Hospital opened in 1975.
(Courtesy of the Audio-Visual Archives, Special Collections and Digital Programs, University of Kentucky Libraries, Lexington)

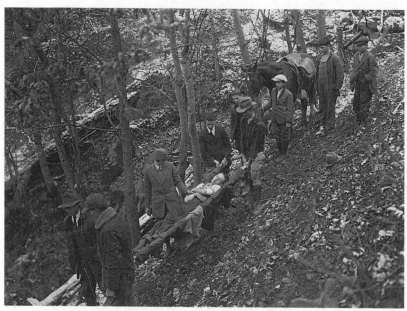

With assistance from local men, FNS nurse-midwife Betty Lester transports a gunshot victim to the hospital by stretcher, 1931. The stretcher consists of two poles run through the arms of coats and shirts. Patients often had to be carried this way for several miles over rough terrain.
(Courtesy of the Audio-Visual Archives, Special Collections and Digital Programs, University of Kentucky Libraries, Lexington)

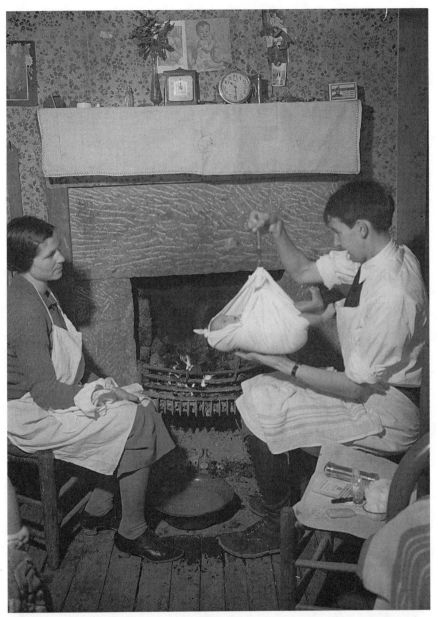

Nurse–midwife Dorothy Buck weighs a newborn during a postpartum checkup as the mother looks on, ca. late 1930s. The service provided thorough care both before and after delivery.
(Courtesy of the Audio-Visual Archives, Special Collections and Digital Programs, University of Kentucky Libraries, Lexington)

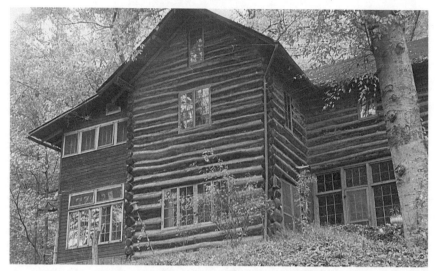

Wendover, Mary Breckinridge's home and the FNS's headquarters, ca. 1980.
(Courtesy of the Audio-Visual Archives, Special Collections and Digital
Programs, University of Kentucky Libraries, Lexington)

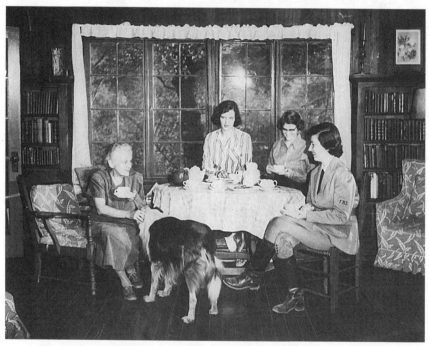

*All action at Wendover stopped each afternoon at four o'clock for tea time. Here,
Breckinridge sits with several unidentified couriers and a nurse-midwife, ca. 1940s.*
(Courtesy of the Audio-Visual Archives, Special Collections and Digital Programs,
University of Kentucky Libraries, Lexington)

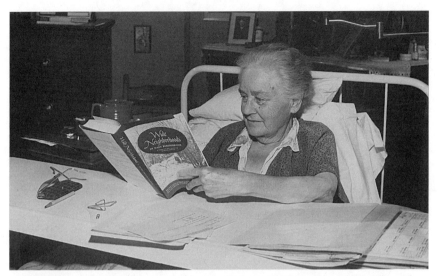

Breckinridge reads from her autobiography, Wide Neighborhoods, *published in 1952. Because of a riding injury, Breckinridge often worked propped up in bed.*
(Courtesy of the Audio-Visual Archives, Special Collections and Digital Programs, University of Kentucky Libraries, Lexington)

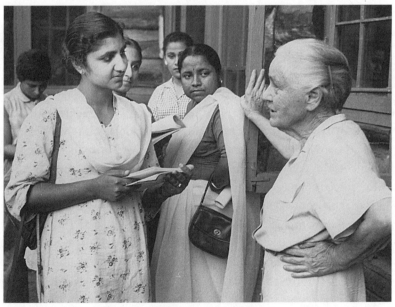

Breckinridge meets with representatives from the International Farm Youth Exchange, 1955. Visitors from around the world came to Wendover to study the FNS's rural health care methods.
(Courtesy of the Audio-Visual Archives, Special Collections and Digital Programs, University of Kentucky Libraries, Lexington)

The early years of the Frontier Nursing Service (FNS) appear an unqualified success by the measures of its swelling treasury, its growing staff, and its expanding territory. Yet while the organization's literature painted a glowing picture of its work and the warm welcome nurses received, the relationship between FNS workers and local residents in reality proved adversarial at first. Breckinridge expected her patients gladly to abandon traditional health care methods in favor of the new standards of care the FNS introduced, but mountain residents did not immediately or unquestioningly do so. Patients did not trust the foreign nurses whom Breckinridge recruited but instead remained wedded to the folk medicine on which they had always relied and continued to depend on the lay midwives who were their neighbors and friends. The relationship between Breckinridge's organization and her clients was one of both give and take, with patients and staff initially struggling to understand one another's alien cultures. Breckinridge's nurses eventually won the confidence of Leslie County residents, but the process was long and was plagued by misunderstandings on both sides.

WHEN MARY Breckinridge made her home in eastern Kentucky in 1925, she arrived with a clear mental picture of how her project would unfold. She expected to assimilate easily into her adopted community. She believed her family's Kentucky roots, combined with her years spent living in the Ozarks and in the Swiss Alps, would provide her with a natural bond with Leslie County residents. "There is a kinship between mountains and mountaineers the world over," she noted. "I am at heart a mountaineer."[1] Appalachia was renowned for its hospitality, and Breckinridge assumed that she and her nurses would receive a hearty welcome.

Breckinridge looked forward to creating a new life in Leslie County. She planned to build a "Lodge" for herself, with a "Cabin" to house a family of Swiss servants that she had recruited to join her.[2] She expected that Appalachia would provide her a safe haven, a place to escape the pain of her divorce and the deaths of her children, just as the Swiss Alps had allowed her to escape the loneliness of her childhood. Long before she built Wendover, Breckinridge had a detailed vision for her home and the grounds. The rustic structure would be surrounded by terraced hillsides and vegetable gardens, and at the foot of the hill would be "the most ideal of fishing holes for her father."[3] Breckinridge imagined that she would spend her days nestled in her lodge with her servants close at hand, while her father, relaxed and happy, passed his time fishing and gardening. Her neighbors would embrace her project, receiving her as a savior and hero who brought needed medical care as well as access to the comforts of modern life.

According to Breckinridge, conditions were so bad in Leslie County substantial improvement would require but little effort. Privately describing to a friend the area that she found in the spring of 1925, she noted that the county "has many moonshiners and much bootlegging and much pistoling—and the babies are born and die and their mothers are maimed or die and the children are untended and hardly learn to read and write." All that was needed to make a difference, she believed, was "clean hands and a sure-footed horse."[4] The stereotypical accounts of the area that so frequently circulated in the media colored her impressions of what she would find. She celebrated the basic accommodations mountain cabins offered, marveling over relics such as hand-pieced quilts, spinning wheels, and dulcimers.[5] The area, according to Breckinridge, was locked in time, simply waiting for outsiders such as her organization to introduce improvements.

As a consequence of the rugged climate and the lack of trained doctors, Breckinridge assumed that medicine in the mountains was of a poorer quality than that found elsewhere. She believed that midwives practicing in the area were dirty and ignorant, and to illustrate the need for her service, she sought proof that they posed a threat to the women they served. The director conducted thorough studies before the FNS began operation to assess the true state of health care in the area. Although Breckinridge and her team of investigators visited every home in the county to uncover unreported births and deaths, and although she interviewed all the area's lay midwives, she never released the mortality figures she calculated before the FNS began work. She loved data and firmly believed that accurate numbers would provide her with credibility, and she did not hesitate to give exact figures to show her nurses' success rates, but she appears to have covered up the data about conditions before she arrived.[6]

Responding to a reporter's question in 1941, Breckinridge explained, "There is no way of knowing what the maternal death rate was in here before we began our work." She vaguely estimated that a "high maternal death rate" plagued the region, explaining, "We infer a high maternal death rate because we have known of so many maternal deaths in similar areas. . . . There are no accurate figures, however, to cover this territory prior to the time we began our work in it."[7] In early publicity, Breckinridge simply noted that the FNS was starting in the Kentucky mountains because the problem was "in its most acute form there."[8]

Breckinridge consistently claimed that infant and maternal death rates in the mountains were much higher than the national averages when the FNS began work, but the opposite may in fact have been true. In his landmark study of Appalachia, *The Southern Highlander and His Homeland* (1921), John C. Campbell acknowledged the poor state of medicine there; however, he claimed that the death rate among women in childbirth was lower in the mountains than in other rural areas.[9] Similarly, in a 1929 *Harper's Monthly Magazine* report, journalist Dorothy Dunbar Bromley suggested that rural areas had lower maternal mortality rates from septic causes than urban areas. According to Bromley, lay midwives achieved better outcomes because they tended to intervene less than doctors and thus were less likely to spread infection.[10] More specifically, Breckinridge's rival, Dr. Annie Veech, head of the Kentucky Bureau of Maternal and Child Health, challenged Breckinridge's claim that mothers in Appalachia faced greater risk than their counterparts elsewhere. Veech calculated the death rate in one unnamed eastern Kentucky county that might well have been Leslie County to be 4.4 per 100,000, much lower than the 6.6 per 100,000 rate found in the rest of the state. Similarly, the infant mortality rate in this county was considerably lower than state and national averages. Veech's statistics reinforced her argument that Kentucky's "midwife problem" could be remedied by training and supervising lay midwives.[11]

Breckinridge disagreed, however. Her need to prove that conditions were dire in Leslie County, that lay midwives could not effectively be trained, and that her nurses were the answer to the problem influenced the way she framed her questions and interpreted the data she collected through her preliminary studies. When lay midwives' answers to her questions did not match what she expected to hear, she assumed that they were lying. For example, she was skeptical when interviewees would "admit to no knowledge of old customs."[12] She doubted the claims of three midwives who said they could read. Several of the midwives she interviewed reported having attended classes offered by the state bureau of hygiene and noted that they had changed their methods as a result, but Breckinridge's follow-up interviews with local mothers, doctors, county judges, and teachers led her to conclude that "their unhygienic practices of many year's standing had not been supplanted by a few hours' instruction." Lay midwives often assured her that they had never lost a mother, but she noted, "Rarely ever did I feel that the statements given me regarding maternal deaths and stillbirths were accurate." She placed more weight on indictments midwives offered of their colleagues, highlighting claims such as, "I never lost a woman but Aunt Nora has lost three." Breckinridge cited several cases in which midwives' daughters and daughters-in-law had died in childbirth to reinforce the threat mountain midwives posed.[13]

Breckinridge took the midwives' answers to her questions into account when formulating her conclusions but based her assessment of her subjects' competence as much on her impressions of their appearances, attitudes, and living conditions as on the information they provided. She complemented one midwife from Owsley County for being an "exquisite looking old woman." She described another as "clean and fairly tidy, although she chews and spits [and has] bare [feet]." Others she dismissed as "slovenly" and "ignorant looking." When midwives did not provide her their full cooperation, she attributed their resistance not to the fact that they might feel threatened by her condescending attitude but to flaws in their character. Under the heading "Personal Appearance," she described one midwife as "reticent and sour" and another as "difficult to question." She displayed no recognition that these women might have resented her probing and her disdainful attitude.[14]

While Breckinridge challenged the veracity of local midwives' answers, she provided little evidence to support her supposition that they had underestimated complications. She quickly dismissed as undocumented midwives' claims concerning their personal records of success, but she was quite willing to accept hearsay that other women had lost babies or had high rates of complications. In the summary of her midwife study, she supplied no specific statistics concerning maternal and infant death rates, though she and her colleagues had visited every home in the county to compile these data.[15] She simply wrote off lay midwives as well-meaning but dangerous and above all untrainable.

Breckinridge did not feel guilty about criticizing local midwives because she believed they had not chosen their role; rather, "it was thrust upon them" out of sheer necessity.[16] Although her interviews revealed that some women had taken up midwifery in search of income, her report downplayed economic motivations, instead stressing their desire to do their neighborly duty. She predicted that lay midwives would welcome the arrival of qualified replacements. Soon after the service began operation, she noted that "the old, native midwives [were] willing to pass the torch" to the FNS because they were "tired and rheumatic."[17] By emphasizing that midwives practiced only reluctantly and that they were glad to see professional nurses enter the area, Breckinridge portrayed her service as a worthwhile endeavor and showed the people it served in a favorable light. FNS nurses came across as heroes rather than intruders, while she depicted local residents as charitable and self-sufficient when necessary but also forward thinking and worthy of available assistance.

More than providing a portrait of the type of medical care available before the FNS arrived, Breckinridge's detailed midwifery study, built on casework methods popular at the time, allows an assessment of the preconceived notions and foundational assumptions she brought to her work.[18] In recent years, historians have used case records of social workers and public health officials to shed light on the relationships that developed between reformers and their clients. Scholars warn that case records, while intended to provide an in-depth assessment of conditions facing the poor and downtrodden, actually say more about their authors' class biases. Linda Alcoff reminds us that rather than "a simple act of discovery," representation is the product of construction, mediation, and interpretation. In a similar vein, historian Emily Abel cautions that scholars must carefully consider case records, with an understanding that they serve as "texts of the dominant."[19] Breckinridge felt certain that she understood the medical challenges Appalachia faced and the solutions that were needed; rather than revealing the true situation, her studies of the region highlight her firm belief that she had the answers to the area's problems.

BRECKINRIDGE ASSUMED that the superior blood coursing through local mothers' veins would allow them to recognize the value of her ideas and make them willing participants in her plan. Though poor, her patients retained great promise. Sick children's unkempt clothes, worn shoes, and uncombed hair, she declared, could not conceal the "intelligence and eager yearning" that shone in their eyes.[20] Leslie County residents had suffered from isolation, which had prevented their exposure to modern ideas. FNS nurses could remedy this problem by bringing improved medical care along with information on house-keeping, farming, and child care.

Breckinridge viewed her clients as raw material, waiting to be transformed, and not just in a medical sense. She charged FNS nurses with modeling middle-class values such as cleanliness, order, and thrift even as they extolled the value of scientific medicine. Public health nurses trained at the turn of the century learned to see patients as empty vessels to be filled. The nurse bore respon-sibility for gaining patients' confidence: clients would heed advice only if they had faith that the nurses' ways were superior. In her classic text, *Notes for Visiting Nurses* (1893), Rosalind Gillette Shawe instructed caregivers to "find [their] way to patients' hearts" and to convey lessons "in simple form easily understood."[21] Nurses served as "missionar[ies] of health," bringing physical well-being in place of spiritual salvation.[22] They could not wait for patients to come to them but had to actively recruit followers to their cause. The best nurses had "the natural gift of personality," which, combined with a talent for teaching, allowed them to convert even the most resistant individuals to healthier ways.[23] While she often reminded her nurses to respect their patients' free will, Breckinridge, reflecting her training in public health, insisted that patients were blank slates, knowing "nothing but such confidence and under-standing as the nurse can inspire."[24]

The line separating health and hygiene from moral and social uplift often blurred. Like public health nurses serving elsewhere, FNS staff members brought a "message with their medicine."[25] Breckinridge often claimed to be simply another member of the mountain community, but in reality, her im-pression of Wendover's function signifies more accurately the top-down rela-tionship she expected to have with her neighbors. Breckinridge believed that simply inviting local residents into her home would inculcate in them a new respect for progressive, modern ways of living. In 1925, as one of the first events sponsored by the Kentucky Committee for Mothers and Babies, she, in cooperation with the area's "leading citizens," hosted a Christmas party at Wendover, inviting the ten thousand residents of the organization's service area. She used the occasion to weigh and measure the children in attendance and to dedicate her home in memory of her own deceased children. The party also allowed visitors a chance to taste the good life that her service could bring—what she described as "a radiance of joy beyond [their] power to dream." The five hundred guests who attended the "splendiferous" event feasted on ham, puddings, cake, and hot cocoa. Children left with gifts and bags of candy. Many, she noted, admired their first Christmas tree.[26]

Breckinridge saw Wendover as providing an important model of middle-class domesticity, which she hoped her neighbors would replicate. She often referred to her home as "the Big House," suggesting that it, like a master's plantation home, stood out as a beacon of civilization in comparison to the tiny, "ramshackle cabins" found nearby. She expected that her home, outfitted with modern plumbing, an extensive library, and a well-equipped kitchen, would provide an example for those "living in the hoot owl hollows" who hoped to improve their own dwellings. With Clifton Rodes Breckinridge demonstrating fishing and farming techniques, her home had the male figure needed to present a traditional model family.[27]

But in addition to serving as an example to neighbors, Wendover also provided a refuge for its residents, allowing Breckinridge and her colleagues to escape the "heart of Leslie."[28] Breckinridge's home looked rustic, with its massive stone fireplace dominating the living room and stuffed wildlife decorating the walls, but in reality the structure was comfortably equipped. More than once she pointed out that her home accounted for two of Leslie County's five bathtubs.[29] In her study of mountain reformers' "built environments," Karen Hudson argues that although Wendover's "mountainside setting and native log and stone skeleton might have suggested that it was the home of a pioneer, the interior provided a sense of middle-class 'culture' and modernity."[30]

Breckinridge often asserted that all mountain residents "have the same social status" and that her nurses were working "through" rather than "for" their patients; however, in spite of her claims, she did not believe that her employees' relationship with their new neighbors represented an equal partnership.[31] An FNS bookkeeper, commenting on the matriarchal way service employees treated patients, questioned, "Why is it that we always call them by their first names and they use our Miss or Mrs. titles?"[32] Coming from the outside, FNS employees brought modern information that not only included health advice but also extended to methods of cooking, farming techniques, and even the proper way to celebrate Christmas. Breckinridge expected that her nurses would improve the area in multiple, needed ways while always taking care to help residents preserve the values and traditions that made Appalachia appealing.

REPORTS FOUND in the FNS's *Quarterly Bulletin* and Breckinridge's correspondence with supporters give the impression that her nurses were indeed blessed with the "natural gift of personality" and that they quickly won their patients' trust. In August 1925, the director insisted that the service received a warm welcome and that "*everywhere*, each section [was] begging for the first centers and longing to help!"[33] "They came crowding around with their sickly babies," she claimed, "so many it fairly broke my heart."[34] After the work was under way, she again reported that the organization enjoyed an "immediate and handsome" response from the people in the area.[35] "The Leslians" were so "progressive in claiming health protection" that nurses could not keep up with requests for inoculations, Breckinridge noted.[36]

Despite the glowing reports in the *Quarterly Bulletin*, tension plagued the Kentucky Committee's relationship with Leslie County residents during its earliest years. Winning local support proved much more difficult than Breckinridge had anticipated. Based on the number of deliveries annually performed by local midwives as revealed in her 1923 study, the director predicted that her nurses would deliver at least one hundred babies in their inaugural year.[37] Indeed, the service registered twenty maternity cases during its first month of operation, reinforcing Breckinridge's assumption that women of the area were excited to have trained care available. However, FNS nurses became discouraged as the women they enrolled called local midwives when it came time to give birth. In their first year, Breckinridge's nurses delivered only thirty babies.[38]

After the arrival of FNS nurses, Leslie County mothers continued to turn to their neighbors to attend their deliveries because they knew and trusted these women and valued the assistance they provided. In her study of Wisconsin midwives, Charlotte Borst shows that women's choice of childbirth attendants was typically guided by a shared geographical and cultural background; even when these Wisconsin women began to turn to doctors in the early twentieth century, they continued to seek out caregivers who lived in their ethnically segregated neighborhoods. In short, they preferred birth attendants who shared their worldviews.[39]

Appalachian women similarly privileged cultural ties over professional credentials. As Leslie County native and local historian Sadie Stidham explains, "The Granny was not too well educated," but the lack of formal training mattered little to the women she served. "Baby girls were often named after the Granny, Creeks and branches were also named for her."[40] The nicknames given to local lay midwives—"Aunt Nancy," "Aunt Jane," "Aunt Tildy," and so forth—suggest their esteemed status.[41] Local residents' affectionate descriptions of individual lay midwives appear in stark contrast to Breckinridge's detached reports. For example, both Stidham and Breckinridge profiled "Aunt Sarah" Morgan. While Stidham admits that this granny midwife had no formal training and could not read her "doctor book" (others read it to her) and that later in her career she had trouble mounting a horse, Aunt Sarah still provided high-quality, personalized care. She traveled to families, her wagon filled with clothes and food so she could stay "as long as she was needed." Stidham adds, "She never lost a baby and folks always loved and respected her."[42] Breckinridge, in contrast, simply notes that Morgan, age fifty-seven and born in Bell County, was "fairly neat and clean, crippled from a broken hip 5 years ago, which does not interfere with her practice [and] does not read or write."[43]

Local midwives' techniques diverged significantly from those of FNS representatives. In some cases, Breckinridge's criticism of lay midwives seems justified in light of modern theories concerning asepsis. She rightfully disapproved of local midwives' practice of applying hog grease to their hands and performing frequent vaginal examinations during labor "to see if the baby is comin' straight." The common tradition of cutting the umbilical cord with unboiled scissors, tying it with string, greasing the navel, and then putting a scorched rag over it likewise legitimately troubled Breckinridge.[44]

Other techniques employed by granny midwives, however, posed less of a true threat and simply contradicted the modern conventions Breckinridge and her nurses had learned as part of their professional training. For example, Breckinridge questioned lay midwives' practice of delivering women in an upright position. Lay midwives instructed a laboring woman either to sit on her husband's knees or to stand and, as the phrase suggests, truly did "cotch" babies. The FNS, by comparison, endorsed the newer method of laboring while lying in bed, following the theory that doing so lessened a woman's risk of perineal tearing.[45] Breckinridge claimed that her updated methods provided a better outcome, but continuing debate on such issues today suggests that her recommendations reflected passing trends rather than patent scientific advancement.[46]

Local women trusted the lay midwives who had always served them and were reluctant to turn to newcomers, regardless of their promises or credentials. In 1926, FNS nurse-midwives Gladys Peacock and Mary Willeford expressed dismay at repeatedly seeing parturient women turn to granny midwives instead of calling the service. Frustrated, Peacock and Willeford appealed to Breckinridge, who advised them to "sell their personalities." Finally, three months and nineteen days after the establishment of the Beech Fork clinic, the first mother registered. The nurses' excitement quickly dissipated, however. "Emily" gave birth before her next scheduled visit, assisted by a local midwife. More than seven months passed before the Beech Fork nurses delivered their first baby in

May 1927.[47] As late as July 1929, nurses continued to complain that women in their districts rejected attempts to provide care.[48]

Expectant women who called lay midwives after they had registered with the Kentucky Committee were not the only ones who shunned the nurses' methods. Local residents rebuffed nurses' efforts at general health promotion as well. On one occasion, two nurses ready to inoculate a long line of children against typhoid almost found themselves thwarted by a teacher who warned children that the injections would be painful and were unnecessary. In response, according to a report in the *Quarterly Bulletin*, the nurses told the teacher, "It is our personality against yours." They then proceeded to speak for thirty minutes with "glowing fervor" on the benefits the shot would bring. As the nurses later recounted, a nine-year-old boy "of good stock," inspired by their remarks, shyly stepped forward to announce that he would go second if someone else would be first. Another child's father volunteered to be first, and the young boy, "gallantly true to his word," went second. That day, the nurses proudly reported, they inoculated more than one hundred students and parents.[49]

In this case, the nurses seemingly managed to sell their methods. They did not always succeed, but of course they did not advertise their failures. After the service went to great lengths to arrange for "special" cases to travel to Louisville or Cincinnati for treatment, patients often changed their minds and refused to go.[50] They may have believed the rumor circulating that the nurses were "trying to do all the harm [they] could to the County." One mother heard this rumor and assumed that the organization had kidnapped her daughter, who had not returned quickly from Louisville. When asked about the girl's whereabouts, nurse-midwife Freda Caffin reassured the mother that no one would take her child from her. After all, Caffin condescendingly pointed out in a private letter to a colleague, "With her sickness no one would want Mallie."[51]

Dorothy Buck, a nurse-midwife who eventually became the service's assistant director, later conceded that she was not surprised that Leslie County residents reluctantly accepted the FNS. "It was no wonder. The people were not used to professional assistance and many were the tales that passed from mouth to mouth." Some feared that "the 'doctor women'" would turn baby boys into bears. Others suggested that the nurses "were there to sit by the women and give them something to kill them." Still others warned that the FNS performed circumcisions on newborns in an attempt to "fix 'em so when they married they couldn't raise children." "Is it any wonder," Buck concluded, "that mothers hesitated to entrust themselves to such monsters?"[52]

Patients found FNS practices unfamiliar and intimidating. One expectant mother was so scared of all the organization's "paraphernalia" that she "beat it to the hills" before the nurse-midwife arrived. Fear left patients as "wild as deers," one nurse observed.[53] Lay midwives criticized the different methods used by FNS nurses.[54] Older women frequently asked FNS nurses when they were going to "hive" new babies to assure clear skin and health.[55] Nurses and local women also disagreed about how soon to bathe infants. FNS nurses advised that they be washed on the second day, but this recommendation alarmed older local women, who argued that it was "sure death" to bathe a newborn baby.[56] FNS methods did not accord with the folk remedies on which its Appalachian patients had long relied, and rather than embrace newcomers who offered to inject children with vials of strange liquid and to send them hundreds of miles away for treatment in the name of progress, mountain residents understandably remained skeptical and hesitant.

INSTEAD OF downplaying the gulf that separated FNS nurses from their patients to allow the service to assimilate more smoothly into the community, Breckinridge in many ways exacerbated the cultural differences that distinguished her staff members from their neighbors. FNS employees certainly stood out in the homogenous community they came to serve. Most of the organization's nurses were new not only to the region but to the United States. Breckinridge recognized the impossibility of recruiting American nurse-midwives since no schools in the country offered such training. She could send interested American nurses to Britain for specialized instruction, but this approach proved costly and time-consuming. Instead, until she could create a FNS-run school, she recruited foreign women already trained as nurse-midwives. By 1930, fourteen of the organization's twenty-one nurses hailed from Britain, Scotland, or New Zealand.[57]

Breckinridge did not consider the nationality of her nurses a problem; in fact, she saw British nurses as fitting caregivers for Appalachian patients. She dismissed the idea that cultural differences could separate patients and her nurses because, in keeping with the theories of the day, Leslie County's Anglo-Saxon residents were "descendants of [the nurses'] ancestors."[58] Discussing the ethnicity of Breckinridge's staff, a journalist agreed that "British nurses [had] a dramatic appropriateness" in Appalachia because they shared the same heritage and culture as their patients.[59]

Breckinridge assumed that the organization's patients would feel comfortable with British nurses, but in fact, the relationship proved uneasy. Ott Bowling, a resident of Leslie County, recalled that in the early years, he and his neighbors "didn't like none of 'em." Bowling attributed the community's reluctance to trust the nurses to their foreign roots: the region's residents "could 'bout understand Italian as good as [they] could" the nurses. In addition to the language barrier, he claimed, the British nurses "didn't understand these mountain people, they didn't understand they was poor."[60] Local residents immediately assumed that FNS representatives did not comprehend the difficulties they faced. When she visited homes around the county to compile data, researcher Bertram Ireland was surprised to be greeted with such questions as, "Did you ever have to hoe corn? I'll bet you never carried wood on your back." Ireland chafed at these assumptions and responded privately, "Yes, we carried wood, drew water from the well, saddled and groomed our horses and took stones from their shoes, all under the critical eyes of the practiced mountaineer, but never quite up to his way of thinking, I imagine!"[61]

FNS nurses' marital status further marked them as strange and to some extent threatening. Ireland also noted that the questions and comments directed at her often focused on her personal life: "Where do you stay? You don't look like you were married?"[62] Children, who were unused to seeing professional, single women, were especially curious. One nurse told the story of a little boy she encountered playing along a creek. She could tell he was eager to know who she was and why she was there. He waited until she passed and then he could not hold back any longer, asking, "Are you'ns married?" She replied, "No. . . . Why do you ask?" "Well," he replied, "then you'ns must be a narse."[63]

Along with their strange accents and unmarried status, nurses were further distinguished by the FNS attire. By the 1920s, many visiting nurses rejected uniforms, anxious to blend in rather than stand out when arriving at homes for fear of stigmatizing patients.[64] Breckinridge, conversely, argued that uniforms brought her nurses recognition and inspired patients' confidence. Uniforms marked them as professionals and gave them a needed air of authority. Breckinridge demanded that nurses wear their full uniforms any time they went out on the districts.[65] Nurse-midwife Betty Lester recalled, "We were . . . told in no uncertain terms that . . . we did not go out in uniform unless it was absolutely perfect." The service's director contended that only through careful attention to their uniforms could nurses convince patients of the need for respect and of the soundness of the FNS's methods.[66]

To her credit, Breckinridge considered the region's norms when advising the first nurses on what to wear. Because area residents were not used to seeing women in pants, the director instructed nurses to cover their riding breeches with walking skirts whenever they dismounted.[67] Ultimately, however, nurses' rather than patients' needs won out. Breckinridge recognized that the physically demanding nature of the work required that the nurses wear "simple and sensible" clothing; she therefore abandoned split skirts when designing the

FNS's official winter and summer uniforms in 1928.[68] She patterned the FNS's winter riding uniform after the one she had worn during her years with Comité Américain pour les Régions Dévastées de la France. It consisted of a blue-gray hip-length coat with the FNS logo embroidered on the shoulder, breeches, a self-fabric belt, white riding shirt, tie, cap, and knee-high boots. She styled the summer uniform after women's sportswear fashions popular at the time. Nurses wore loose-fitting, sleeveless jackets, knickers, cotton hose, panama hats, and oxford shoes.[69] The uniforms were practical and designed for comfort and durability and above all emphasized the distance that separated nurses from their patients.

LESLIE COUNTY residents hesitated to trust Breckinridge's nurses for a variety of understandable reasons, and the media attention she directed toward the area undermined what little confidence existed in the organization. In the beginning, the director attempted to limit newspaper coverage of her cause. She refused to admit reporters to the Kentucky Committee's first annual meeting because she feared they would "get things twisted."[70] She claimed that she wanted to protect the people of Appalachia, but she was probably also trying to guard her reputation in case her venture failed.[71] Despite—or perhaps in part because of—her initial refusal to speak with reporters, newspapers printed degrading stories about the nurses' work. "It is discouraging to think that in closing the doors to reporters one does not always effectually bar out the newspaper world," she complained.[72]

After Breckinridge resigned herself to the fact that she would have to rely on a network of individual donors to fund her work, she began to seek out print publicity, but she still retained tight control over the stories printed. Coverage in newspapers and mass circulation magazines allowed her to communicate the value of her plan to a much larger audience than she could hope to reach through speaking engagements. As the 1920s drew to a close, accounts of the service's work began to appear more frequently in national publications.

As the service's work gained increased publicity, so did Breckinridge's need to do damage control. Following the appearance of an unflattering article in January 1926, she immediately wrote to Kentucky health commissioner Arthur McCormack to apologize: in spite of her refusal to speak with reporters, "at least one vulgarly worded and inaccurate description has found its way in the Press." Reiterating her recognition of "the immense value of silence," she repeated her promise to "not wittingly say or do anything which might embarrass you or us."[73] She also wrote to Ethel DeLong Zande, from Pine Mountain Settlement School, to defend herself, warning, "If you read an inaccurate and stupid description of our Committee in one of the New York papers, please bear in mind that it does not come from me!" She blamed the article on "leakages," which unfortunately sometimes occurred "through friends."[74]

Leslie County residents protested pieces that they saw as unfair and demeaning, further emphasizing in Breckinridge's mind the dangers of publicity. In late 1926, a review of *On the Trail of a Pioneer*, a cutting-edge "MOTION picture" documenting the work of Breckinridge's nurses, appeared in the *New York Times*.[75] The organization's director, with the consent of the local committee, had authorized the production of this film as a way of "bringing [the] cause before the public." When Elizabeth Perkins, a friend from Breckinridge's days in Europe, approached her and offered to assume all financial risks and costs in exchange for 35 percent of the film's profits, Breckinridge agreed but stipulated that her executive committee must have final say over the captions that accompanied the silent picture.[76]

Few Leslie County residents saw the film, but many read the *Times* review. The degrading article, reprinted in the *Lexington Herald* and the Hyden newspaper *Thousandsticks*, painted a positive image of Breckinridge's nurses but ridiculed the area and its people. The piece blamed mountain residents for the high infant mortality rate, claiming that they had not known how to take care of their children before Breckinridge's service arrived. The article further engendered resentment by describing Hazard, the nearest city, as "no more than a few stores and a group of miner's shacks."[77]

Several Leslie County residents protested the way the *New York Times* article portrayed their community. In a letter to the editor of the local paper, Hyden resident M. C. Roarke politely endorsed the work of the Kentucky Committee but argued that the people of Leslie County should not have to sacrifice their dignity to receive care.[78] Another local resident wrote directly to Breckinridge to express his displeasure with the article. He declared his appreciation for the "wonderful work" that the committee was doing but concluded, "We would rather not have the work done at all than have false impressions deliberately scattered to the four corners of the earth."[79]

There is no recorded response from Breckinridge addressing these complaints; however, in a rejoinder printed in *Thousandsticks*, Perkins apologized for "any hard feelings" the article created. In a backhanded attempt to placate Leslie County residents, Perkins suggested that "the writer . . . was trying to pay a compliment to Kentucky by giving space in a Metropolitan paper." She blamed the reporter for twisting her words, claiming that she had never meant any harm. "We pure blooded Americans must stand solidly together," she argued, "for we Americans are the inheritors of this wonderful country and we are very distinct from the foreign-born element which is overpowering us in the great cities."[80] In keeping with the nativist atmosphere of the early twentieth century, Perkins apologized to a group she admired by denigrating another group that most of her audience saw as undesirable.

Although neither Breckinridge nor anyone connected with her organization penned the *New York Times* article, unhappy residents rightfully blamed her for turning the spotlight on them. Area residents who were already highly sensitive to stereotypical images of their region criticized Breckinridge for adding to the "wornout, half baked, exaggerated falsehoods" that authors typically had written about Appalachia.[81] The people from Leslie County did not care whether service representatives had written the article; they held Breckinridge accountable for attracting outsiders' attention to the region.

Breckinridge promised that she would never do anything to degrade her clients, but she ultimately faced the same challenge that other reformers who publicized their work to generate funds confronted. In 1928, Mary Swain Routzhan, a representative of the Russell Sage Foundation, described the common mistakes mountain workers made when presenting their work to the public. Routzhan criticized those who focused on stories of the poorest individuals and who used images of log cabins and bedraggled children to build support. According to Routzhan, these tactics led readers to view exceptional cases as normal. She warned against the temptation to romanticize Appalachian poverty, suggesting that "perhaps in real life Lizzie Ann is no longer barefooted." However, she recognized the dilemma reformers faced. If they began to display Lizzie Ann wearing shoes and stockings, Routzhan admitted, "It is doubtful whether she will appeal so greatly to the hearts of those on whose gifts the work depends."[82]

As chief fund-raiser, Breckinridge faced a significant burden every year as she attempted to raise enough money to fund the work of her nurses. This necessity forced her to spotlight the problems plaguing the region, and she quickly found that tugging on donors' heartstrings helped increase the size of donations. Local residents, however, resented the attention, and the publicity further drove a wedge between the organization and its patients in these early years.

LIKE BRECKINRIDGE, FNS nurses came to eastern Kentucky with a missionary zeal and a romanticized impression of the welcome they would receive. When they did not find doors and arms open to them as they expected, they quickly became frustrated. As one of the first two nurse-midwives Breckinridge hired, Freda Caffin was caught off guard by the hostility directed at her during her time with the FNS. Caffin was a native New Yorker and the daughter of a well-known *New York Post* art critic. She worked with the Henry Street Settlement and New York's Maternity Center Association before taking a pay cut to come to Kentucky in 1925.[83] Caffin was surprised when patients did not follow the cultural script that she expected. She assumed that they would bow to her professional expertise and embrace her promises of progress, but she instead watched as patients rejected her services, and she became increasingly suspicious of her neighbors.

In December 1926, Caffin publicly praised the area's residents for their "enthusiasm for the prevention of disease . . . and their eager acceptance of the newest ideas."[84] Simultaneously, however, her private correspondence expressed a sense of alienation from her patients: "We live a very shut in form of existence and all who are not born in Leslie County are Foreigners."[85] Rather than seeing FNS staff and their neighbors as allies, she viewed her patients as adversaries, out to get as much as they could from the service. Her suspicion of local residents was apparent in 1927 when a dispute developed over a manure pile. According to Caffin, their landlord had given the nurses permission to keep a manure pile on the property, but then he began "taking it without leave" and refused to provide compensation, threatening to "turn [them] out if [they] try and do anything." She emphasized that she was concerned not with the actual value of the manure but with "the principle." "So many of the people here," she complained, "are trying to block the work by over charging for everything they do or sell." She suggested that the situation might improve if residents understood that they would have to pay for the administration of "the work" after a certain number of years. She admitted that "one can't all together blame them for wanting all they can get." According to Caffin, all they saw was "a steady stream of money pouring in from outside."[86]

Though she had no fund-raising responsibilities, Caffin apparently worried constantly regarding the service's finances. When a thirteen-year-old boy wrote to request a pass to Richmond, Kentucky, to seek treatment for trachoma, Caffin responded harshly to the young man's petition, explaining that it was against the FNS's policy to "send any child away who we haven't seen." Instead of praising him for recognizing the value of scientific care, she admonished him, stressing, "You do not seem to realize that it is a very expensive business sending people away [and] a great privelege." She advised that he come to a weekly clinic to be examined, and then she would consider his request.[87] In response to a local man who needed hospital care, Caffin adopted a similarly callous tone, explaining that the service could not spend its "hard earned money" on men when its mission was helping mothers and babies.[88]

A visitor to the service in 1926 was struck by Caffin's hostile relationship with her patients and brought the issue to Breckinridge's attention. Elizabeth Bruce, a nurse from Louisville and a member of the organization's founding committee, spent almost a month in Leslie County to view for herself the service's work. She felt she had a duty to visit, she explained, as "it was not fair to act on a board that is to endorse work, that I . . . do not know at first hand."[89] What she saw troubled her greatly. The lack of harmony between nurses concerned her, but her largest worry centered on the condescending attitude displayed by nurses in general and Caffin in particular as well as the nurses' failure to integrate themselves into the community. Bruce suggested that "unless a complete reversal of attitude results, the work had better stop at once before harm is done."[90] She accused Breckinridge's nurses of having "an imperfect understanding of the mountain people" and concluded that other organizations doing similar work had dealt with their clients "with a truer grace."[91]

Breckinridge responded crisply to Bruce, defending the nurses. Breckinridge was surprised by Bruce's charges, aware only of "good will" between the nurses and the local population. She emphasized that the clinics run by Caffin and Edna Rockstroh were "thronged" and praised local residents for raising nearly eight hundred dollars in money, labor, and supplies to build a new nursing center. She did not deny that the mountaineers were sometimes the subject of jokes among the nurses after a hard day of work but claimed that these jokes were not a product of mean-spiritedness but instead provided a way of coping with the "isolation . . . hardship and tragedy" of the situation. Breckinridge emphatically argued that "fun among ourselves is *not* ridicule among the people." Breckinridge, who was older than Bruce, reminded her of the difference in their ages and questioned her "hastily formed and harshly worded judgments," suggesting that perhaps the younger woman did not understand people.[92]

Breckinridge's explanations failed to reassure Bruce, who remained convinced that an "atmosphere of ridicule" existed within the service.[93] After several exchanges of letters between the two women, Bruce threatened to resign from the board. They never reached a compromise, and Bruce's name disappeared from the roster of the board of directors less than a year later.[94] Breckinridge immediately dismissed Bruce's accusations, apparently without seeking to confirm them. As before, when faced with criticism, she remained convinced that her plan was sound and that her approach was justified. She failed to acknowledge that her nurses truly might not understand the challenges their patients faced and that the jokes they made, whether spoken privately or publicly, revealed hostility rather than compassion.

CAFFIN RESIGNED from the service in 1927, leaving Breckinridge and the remaining nurses to win their patients' confidence.[95] Throughout the 1920s, nurses frequently expressed their frustration to Breckinridge as they watched maternity patients turn to local midwives. While Breckinridge shared her nurses' concerns, she encouraged them to remain steadfast in their efforts to sell their ideas. FNS nurses must never give up on patients. Noncooperation was not a valid reason for closing cases.[96] Breckinridge urged nurses to get to know their patients on a personal level. She reminded the nurses that they might have to make "several friendly visits" before patients would begin to trust them and recognize the worth of their suggestions.[97]

Breckinridge remained confident that with a little encouragement, most patients would soon recognize the value of the care FNS nurses had to offer; still, she instructed her nurses that they must always respect the free will of their clients. When a woman refused to seek desperately needed care outside the mountains, Breckinridge stressed to the staff that they must not "adopt a paternalistic attitude in which we say that our decisions must be met." Instead, she just as paternalistically insisted that the nurses' ideas were right and that the nurses must use their superior knowledge to convince their misguided clients. She recommended explaining clearly and concisely the "probable results" of failing to follow their advice. Then, she noted, they "must stand by the patient no matter what the outcome. . . . [I]t is her life and she has the right to make the decision herself."[98] Breckinridge insisted that local women had the "liberty of choice," and if they wanted lay midwives, they had the right to do so, but, she stressed, they "cannot have both the native midwife and the F.N.S."[99]

Breckinridge felt sure that with time, as the number of babies and young children her nurses saved from needless death increased, the service would naturally win the hearts and minds of the women of the community. Healing a sick child, Breckinridge contended, would allow the nurses to prove the superiority of their methods. "When we have restored a baby," she insisted, "we hold its mother forever after in the hollow of our hands."[100] The service, however, directed much of its attention at young girls, who would be more pliable and receptive to new ideas, rather than older women, who were more wedded to folk medicine. Hoping to reach as many future mothers as possible, the FNS offered homemaking and child-rearing classes in the local grade and high schools.[101]

Though Breckinridge wished to convert Leslie County's young residents to the gospel of good health that her nurses offered, she could not bring herself to see her patients as equal partners. Critics have charged that the FNS never sought to train local women as nurse-midwives.[102] In a few cases, FNS officials selected particularly bright children and paid their tuition to attend schools outside the mountains, but no large-scale effort was ever made to equip Appalachian residents to become caregivers. Breckinridge's desire to carve out a space for herself in an era when the public realm afforded women few options led her to guard carefully the role she created for herself and her nurses. Though no evidence suggests that she coined the phrase "angel on horseback," she clearly relished being perceived in that light. She could not move beyond the impulse to be the lady benevolent, coming in to uplift the area. Her failure to recognize that her patients were not blank slates or empty vessels waiting to be filled blinded her to the reality of life in the mountains and ensured that the early relationship between FNS nurses and local residents would prove contentious.

DAVID WHISNANT harshly criticizes "fotched-on women" such as Breckinridge who came to Appalachia in the early twentieth century, arguing that they viewed the area's culture in simplistic terms and attempted to remake it in a way that fit their tastes and values. Whisnant emphasizes that "interveners" typically misjudged the existing culture. Rather, they built their cultural vision on "a *selection*, an *arrangement*, an *accommodation* to preconceptions."[103] The female reformers who came to the mountains, according to Whisnant, viewed themselves as "rescuers." Coming with a mission to protect and enshrine an outdated "sanitized" culture, these women displayed a "rather shallow liberal commitment." As Whisnant explains, they took the "cheapest and safest" route, avoiding confrontation with vested interests and requiring only minimal sacrifice from supporters.[104]

As Whisnant points out, Appalachian reformers' efforts were invariably colored by the culture in which they were raised, for it was their "most available touchstone."[105] Mary Breckinridge was no exception. Nearing middle age when she created the FNS, she brought to her work in Appalachia years of assumptions concerning society and her place in it. As the well-connected daughter of a prominent family, she believed in a natural aristocracy. She also believed that God had given particular advantages to certain "leading citizens," who then had a responsibility to share their resources and superior ideas with the less fortunate. Breckinridge often claimed that all mountain residents "have the same social status," but she clearly distinguished the "best" mountaineers from their less cooperative neighbors.[106] Breckinridge's definition of "worthiness" largely hinged on who was most willing to accept her ideas.

Breckinridge firmly believed she had the answer to Appalachia's problems, but while she tried to replace folk medicine with scientific theories and to discredit lay midwives, she consciously avoided trying to remake the local culture in some of the more visible ways that reformers who had come before her had. For example, Hindman Settlement School founders expressed a goal of "liv[ing] among people in a model home, to show them by example the advantages of cleanness, neatness and order, and to inspire them to use pure language and to lead pure, Christian lives . . . thereby to elevate and uplift them."[107] While Breckinridge shared these broad goals of elevating and inspiring her patients, FNS nurses were told that they must never discuss politics or religion. They were there to convert patients to the gospel of modern medicine, but the organization did not proselytize in the traditional sense. Many female reformers working in the mountains had been strong temperance advocates and had often helped to uncover stills in the area.[108] But Breckinridge explicitly instructed her nurses to turn their heads if they came across moonshine operations.[109] As the director explained, "We keep strictly neutral. . . . Our business is nursing." The FNS also avoided becoming involved in feuds. "When a man is shot in a fight and we are called, we do all we can," Breckinridge noted. "The fight behind it is not our concern."[110]

Instead of criticizing these behaviors that troubled critics, Breckinridge defended them and attempted to place them in historical perspective. Rather than seeing moonshining and feuding as products of moral weakness, she described these practices as manifestations of a unique pioneer code of honor and an understandable outcome of isolation. Moonshining was a practical economic response to the harsh conditions under which mountaineers lived. Like past generations, Leslie County residents distilled corn into alcohol because doing so provided a practical way to transport and market a surplus commodity. Similarly, she rationalized that the violence characterizing the region represented a throwback to an earlier time when, in the absence of the law, individuals took matters into their own hands.[111] However, Breckinridge pinned most of the blame for the violence on federal revenue agents, who earned fifty dollars each time they enforced Prohibition laws. She explained that unlike the cities, where people had money to bribe agents, "the poor little mountaineer ha[d] to face the music."[112] One nurse-midwife defended her patients' production of "mountain dew": "The folks that ran a still had screens at their windows, better house and food."[113] Instead of levying moral judgments against the moonshiners, this FNS employee praised them for providing safer living conditions for their families, reinforcing Breckinridge's claim that nursing was the service's sole concern.

WHILE IT may be tempting to dwell on the patriarchal nature of the FNS's relationship with its patients and to emphasize nurses' attempts to force their ideas on their patients, the relationship between local residents and organization staff ultimately was a negotiation. Instead of adopting wholesale the new modern methods FNS nurses taught, patients carefully selected from the services offered.[114] In his study of Appalachian folk medicine, Anthony Cavender argues that families were "inventive and adaptive," melding traditional folk remedies with new methods introduced by practitioners of biomedicine. Even when scientific medicine became available, mountain residents continued to rely on a wide range of healers, depending on the ailment—wart doctors, burn doctors, goiter rubbers, and herb doctors, among others.[115] FNS patients likewise continued to rely on folk medicine when it served their needs and sought the organization's services when they believed its nurses could provide better care.

In some cases, the benefits of scientific medicine were obvious. For example, physicians working with the U.S. Public Health Service could offer patients suffering from trachoma pharmaceuticals that provided immediate, almost miraculous results. Breckinridge, however, found it more difficult to convince her patients that professional nurse-midwives could provide better results than lay midwives could. In many cases, local women sought prenatal advice from service nurses, since the local midwives did not offer this kind of care, but continued to rely on their neighbors to attend deliveries, as had previously been the case. FNS nurse-midwives offered postnatal care, which surely attracted some patients but, unlike lay midwives, did not help with household chores. Mothers weighed the costs and benefits of both types of care and made decisions based on very practical criteria.[116]

DESPITE HER claims to the contrary, Mary Breckinridge had a simplistic understanding of her patients' ways of life and little sense of the depth of Appalachia's problems when she began her work in Leslie County in 1925. She arrived in the mountains idealistic and naive. She shared the romantic view of the mountains that was popular at the time, emphasizing the isolated, picturesque nature of Appalachian life. She assumed that the community would greet her enthusiastically and would recognize at once the value of her plan, embracing the "progress" she brought. She confidently predicted that the medical care her organization provided would allow those it served, individuals possessing some of the nation's best blood, to fulfill their promise. The FNS's arrival would transform puny, wan children into "rosy-cheeked boys and girls, dressed in overalls and gay ginghams."[117]

Over time, however, Breckinridge developed a more realistic understanding of the region's culture and the roots of its economic problems. Her impressions of Appalachia and its residents grew more nuanced and sophisticated as the decades passed.[118] The 1930s precipitated an economic crisis that would force her to acknowledge the deeper, structural roots of inequality. Instead of seeing her patients as stock, cardboard characters who had chosen a life of poverty, she grew to understand that prosperity elsewhere was strategically connected to economic suffering in the mountains.

Breckinridge steadily became more aware of the challenges that Leslie County residents faced, and as she did so, their trust in the organization deepened. As their familiarity with the region increased, nurses learned that they could not rush in and out of patients' homes but instead must sit and visit a while before getting down to business.[119] Though "shy of 'em" at first, FNS patients gradually came to recognize that its nurses had their patients' best interests at heart.[120] While the service struggled to register maternity patients in its earliest years, it averaged more than one delivery per day by 1934.[121]

seven Praying for Better Times Ahead

By 1932, Mary Breckinridge could proudly announce that her nurses had made "great headway against disease."[1] They had introduced prenatal care and according to Frontier Nursing Service (FNS) publicity had made childbirth safer; they had provided thousands of inoculations against the epidemic illnesses that previously had taken so many lives; and they were well on their way toward eradicating the parasites that stunted mountain children's growth. Dr. Louis Dublin, vice president and statistician for the Metropolitan Life Insurance Company and president of the American Public Health Association, in his expert evaluation of the service's first one thousand maternity cases, had enthusiastically endorsed the value of Breckinridge's plan, concluding that ten thousand fewer mothers would die and thirty thousand more babies would survive each year in the United States if all women had access to the type of care the FNS offered.[2] The Committee on the Costs of Medical Care, made up of some of the nation's leading economists, physicians, and public health specialists, likewise praised the value of Breckinridge's service, noting its potential as an "economical and efficient" answer to America's rural health care crisis.[3] In spite of these accolades, Breckinridge stressed that the FNS's work was far from complete. "We've still to attack their poverty," she explained to readers of *Good Housekeeping* magazine.[4]

Much had changed since 1925, when Breckinridge had chosen to name her organization the Kentucky Committee for Mothers and Babies. The renamed Frontier Nursing Service no longer limited itself to serving women and children. The director recognized that to improve the lives of these most vulnerable members of society, she must make the whole family her concern. A firm believer that women should remain at home and that men should be the sole breadwinners, she noted that it was essential for her organization to care for the men of the community. No good could come of saving a baby who was doomed to starvation because there was no father to earn a living for the family, she contended.[5] In rural work, Breckinridge noted, no detail could go unnoticed. "If the mule is sick, we do our best to help doctor it and share the drugs that the veterinarians have sent us. We even vaccinate the family dog against rabies."[6]

As her ties to the Leslie County community strengthened, Breckinridge came to see health care as only one part of a complicated equation. While treating physical ailments was important, she could not hope to improve patients' situations unless she addressed their emotional and financial needs as well. Breckinridge became an advocate for FNS patients both locally and nationally during the 1930s, fiercely championing causes that would improve the quality of their lives, and as she did so, local residents' faith in her organization grew.

AS THE FNS entered its second decade of existence, Breckinridge's thoughts turned to expansion. From the start, she had planned to share her "saddlebag-and-cabin-technique" and to eventually cover the "length and breadth, heighth and depth" of America's mountain ranges.[7] In 1930, a year earlier than her original plan had specified, Breckinridge announced that the FNS would soon begin limited operation in the Ozark Mountains.[8] The developing economic crisis, however, forced her to place on hold all thoughts of expansion. Throughout the next decade, Breckinridge's dream of creating a network of rural health organizations across the United States faded as she struggled "just to keep a toehold" in Leslie County.[9]

During the 1920s, subscriptions to the FNS had increased every year, and the FNS experienced several budget surpluses. But following the stock market crash and the deepening depression it ushered in, service contributors began to lower their donations.[10] Subscriptions that normally would have ranged from twenty-five to one hundred dollars fell to five and ten dollars on average. In September 1930, the FNS experienced its first budget shortfall. The following summer, Breckinridge found that again she had no choice but to borrow money to balance the books. In May 1931, the director recommended that the executive committee increase the service's debt limit from twenty-five thousand to one hundred thousand dollars.[11]

With her financial concerns growing daily, Breckinridge began to look for new, creative ways to raise money. The Northeast had always been profitable fund-raising territory for the service, and to tap more fully into the area's resources, the director established publicity offices in New York and Boston in 1931. Breckinridge hired a full-time public relations specialist for each office, placing them in charge of coordinating fund-raising events and gaining media attention for the service.[12]

A key part of the FNS's strategy of building support in the Northeast centered on young upper-class women. In the early 1930s, the organization began recruiting girls from "social register type families" to serve in an auxiliary role as couriers. Breckinridge realized that by allowing these volunteers to participate in the organization's work for just a short time, she could foster lifelong allegiances, and, indeed, many couriers went on to serve as FNS trustees and donors.[13] Breckinridge patterned her courier service after the chauffeur system that she had observed during her time in France. She enlisted the aid of four couriers at a time. These young women, all of whom who were at least nineteen years of age, lived at Wendover for an average of six to eight weeks. Couriers performed a variety of odd jobs, thereby freeing nurses to concentrate on health care. They carried messages between centers, tended the nurses' horses, and made tea for the nurses each afternoon, among other tasks.[14]

Being selected a FNS courier became a badge of honor among the nation's elite. Girls seeking the opportunity endured a rigorous application process. The FNS required candidates to submit three letters of recommendation attesting to their horsemanship and personality. Breckinridge selected only girls from the "best" families. In 1932, the Associated Press reported that the social registers of Chicago and other cities had come to view selection as an FNS courier as "a special mark of distinction." By the 1950s, a waiting list of girls who wanted to work with the organization existed. Former couriers registered their daughters with the service at birth, hoping that they too could one day work with the organization.[15]

Breckinridge further tapped into northeastern social circles by hosting elaborate benefits with the hope of compensating for declining revenues. Always a perceptive fund-raiser, Breckinridge recognized that although many wealthy Americans cut their philanthropic budgets in the wake of the financial crisis, most continued to spend money on leisure activities. Tennis matches, ice pageants, and Easter balls became yearly events for the service during the depression years, offering upper-class supporters the opportunity to relax and to mingle with other elites.[16] But Breckinridge set her sights on cruises as a way to "float [their] budget by means of floating a ship."[17] Wealthy Americans enjoyed annual vacations to exotic locations as a way to leave behind the "ugliness of the urban melting pot" and to circulate with other "solid Yankees" while demonstrating their wealth and status. Breckinridge hoped to capitalize on this tradition.[18]

In both 1932 and 1933, the FNS chartered ships to carry FNS patrons to the Caribbean. The service agreed to publicize the excursion and to sell tickets in exchange for 25 percent of the profits.[19] Breckinridge's publicity secretaries went to great lengths to advertise the "mountain cruise" as the social event of the season, carefully sending their brochures to the "right people." Breckinridge recruited special cruise committees, consisting of men "of outstanding financial positions," to sell tickets. Flyers were posted in "the most fashionable" hair salons for the "rich and swell to gaze at while being manicured." The FNS assured supporters that the cruise was being booked privately and that the passenger list was being "hand picked."[20] In an attempt to attract wealthy debutantes, Breckinridge recruited handsome young men from Ivy League schools to serve as "assistant cruise directors." Their main duty was to organize shore excursions, but as Breckinridge pointed out, "naturally they liked to dance in the evenings with the girls."[21]

Breckinridge held high hopes that these cruises would become a yearly event, allowing her to raise a large part of the organization's budget in one shot. However, both of these ventures ended in failure. In 1932, only three weeks before the first cruise was to set sail, the Boston Committee reported that it had not sold a single ticket.[22] In the end, the FNS grossed only four thousand dollars for its share of the receipts.[23] In 1933, Breckinridge looked forward to the cruise "going over the top with a bang" and was pleased with initial ticket sales.[24] But when banks across the nation began to fold just days before the cruise was to sail, many prospective passengers canceled their reservations. The cruise went on as scheduled, allowing the service to pay off its obligation to the shipping company, but the FNS made no profit.[25]

EXACERBATING HER financial woes, Breckinridge suffered a riding accident in the fall of 1931 that left her in pain for the rest of her life. After traveling for several months publicizing the FNS's work, she had returned to Leslie County for Thanksgiving, spending an enjoyable holiday with her father and her coworkers. She left Wendover on a new mount to catch a train back to New

York. She had received the horse as a gift from her colleagues a few days earlier, naming it Traveller in honor of her hero Robert E. Lee's horse. She knew the horse was not familiar with the mountain landscape and was jumpy, but as an experienced rider, she felt confident that she could control him despite the rainy weather. Breckinridge and her two companions had not gone far when her flapping raincoat spooked Traveller, and he took off with a jolt. "He seemed to skim through the air," Breckinridge recalled. After horse and rider sped across three miles of mountainous territory in less than fifteen minutes, she decided that she would not be able to outlast Traveller and planned her fall. Reaching a clearing, she rolled to the right. As soon as she hit the ground, she knew "there would be the devil to pay."[26]

Local men transported the injured director several miles by stretcher to Hyden Hospital. Although she was in blinding pain, Breckinridge in characteristic fashion joked with the stretcher bearers that she would have dieted if she had known they were going to have to carry her. Recognizing that her injuries were serious, local doctors sent her to Lexington. X-rays revealed that she had crushed a vertebra in her back. Doctors informed her that she would have to remain immobile for eight weeks and then would have to wear a brace for several more months. She was relieved to know that she would make a complete recovery, but the question of how she would raise money in the meantime troubled her.[27]

Immediately after receiving the diagnosis, Breckinridge had her secretary cable her close friends, Lucille "Pansy" Turner and Adeline and Maud Cashmore, to request their prayers. Adeline quickly wired back, "Indeed I am with you, little one, may he hold you in his healing hands." Breckinridge later recalled that as soon as she turned to Adeline, she "began to come out of [her] slump, which was just as well because [she] had a lot of work to do." Adeline reassured Breckinridge that she did not need to worry about raising money because God would provide. Pansy and Maud likewise wrote to assure Breckinridge that God would never place burdens on her that she could not handle.[28] Breckinridge accepted her friends' advice, declaring several days after the accident that she had placed her concerns "absolutely in God's hands."[29] Still, she remained legitimately concerned that unless donations increased, she would be forced to close some of the nursing centers.

The FNS trustees capitalized on the director's accident by issuing a special appeal to "Friends of the Service." In a dramatic letter, they praised their "stricken leader's" bravery. They stressed that after Breckinridge fell from her horse, she "insisted on continuing her journey," but doctors forbade her from doing so. According to the appeal, Breckinridge bravely "asked whether it would not be possible for the specialist to furnish her with braces which would enable her to meet her Detroit engagement." She valiantly declared that she would "be willing to run the risks and suffer the future consequences if only she could now carry on her work." The trustees urged patrons to take the load "from her overburdened shoulders" and donate to the service, stressing that such generosity would hasten her recovery.[30]

Doctors allowed Breckinridge to travel from Lexington to Hyden on December 20, 1931, just in time to spend Christmas with her staff at Wendover. She spent the next month recuperating, "living chiefly on soda water, whiskey, morphine and mentholated cigarettes."[31] In mid-February, her doctors permitted her to travel to New York. For the rest of her life, however, Breckinridge would suffer nearly constant pain. She compared her discomfort to "a great dental drill gnawing through [her] back day after day and hour after hour."[32] In an attempt to strengthen her "patched-up bargain-counter back," she underwent several operations, wore a steel brace, and periodically visited spas, but these treatments provided only temporary relief.[33] Breckinridge acknowledged that the pain did "cramp one's style," but she did not dwell on her misfortune.[34] Instead, she found ways to compensate. For example, when she traveled she always arranged for her host to place a board under her mattress. To alleviate her pain, she did most of her work from bed, propped up on pillows. She found it difficult to ride on horseback for prolonged periods after her accident, but she continued her yearly rounds of the outpost centers.

Though supporters rallied around the FNS's "stricken leader," the organization continued to struggle financially. FNS executive committee members had loaned the organization fifty thousand dollars after Breckinridge announced that she would have to close several outpost centers.[35] These loans temporarily allowed the service to maintain its full level of care, but in May 1932, Breckinridge decided that she had no choice but to cut nurses' salaries if the organization was to survive.[36]

When she gave the twenty-three nurses on her staff the option of taking a pay cut or of temporarily resigning, only three chose to leave; the others agreed to accept severe salary reductions.[37] Most employees gallantly informed the director that they were happy to take a drop in pay if it meant alleviating her worries even slightly. Sybil Johnson felt honored to be "asked to do a little to help in this depressed time." Dorothy Buck assured Breckinridge, "We have plenty of money so don't worry about us. We can go for a while on our hoarded wealth." Edith Batten likewise agreed to stay on at reduced wages: "I could no more dream of giving up the FNS than I could expect to fly by flapping my arms." Besides, she remarked, "If we didn't have a few trials it wouldn't be any fun at all."[38]

Although most employees were willing to work for reduced salaries, Breckinridge still had to "release" seven nurses and three members of the administrative staff to balance the budget. She also disposed of several old horses that could no longer earn their keep. To compensate for the reductions, Breckinridge staffed each center with one nurse instead of two and temporarily reduced the territory of each center from five miles to three. When explaining the changes to the Boston secretary, she remarked, "Of course, it is like cutting out my heart and giving it to the dogs to do this, but it is the only way in which we can make our budget balance."[39]

Following the failure of the second cruise, Breckinridge admitted that her new fund-raising methods were not working. She would have to return to the tactics that had brought results in the past, although doing so required a monumental effort on her part. The director reluctantly closed the service's northern publicity offices in the spring of 1933. They were expensive to run and had raised few additional funds. Until the economy improved, she decided that the organization should focus on spending as little as possible on development, allowing all donations to count as pure profit. She believed that patrons would appreciate the FNS's thriftiness and hence more enthusiastically support its work.[40] Instead of relying on glitzy benefits and cruises, Breckinridge returned to raising money through direct mail appeals and personal appearances.[41] She continued to emphasize many of the same issues that had won the organization financial support in the 1920s. She kept as her main themes the purity of the mountain stock, the region's isolation, and the value of the FNS's methods.

Early in the depression, Breckinridge targeted her appeals at wealthy Americans, but as the crisis worsened, she began to encourage smaller contributions from anyone who could afford to give. In 1932, she reminded the Boston contact secretary to send the "Saddlebag Appeal" to as many people as possible: "Remember that we don't want them sent only to the elite, but to many less well known people who could make small contributions."[42] In the *Quarterly Bulletin*, Breckinridge pointed out that those who had only five or ten cents to give could still help. She advised that handkerchiefs made a good gift because they would be given to the "thousands of children" to whom they were attempting "to teach good health habits." She assured potential donors that although the FNS attracted many wealthy patrons, "no one need feel on that account that his small gift will not be as useful as it is welcome."[43]

The FNS's financial situation continued to decline, with contributions finally bottoming out during the 1934–35 fiscal year. Although revenue plummeted, the number of donors increased yearly. The receipts generated during this difficult period represented a 50 percent decline from those collected just five years before.[44] The organization's debt continued to grow, with no end in sight. The service's financial position grew so desperate that Breckinridge chose to auction six pieces of rare Russian china that her mother had purchased during her father's tenure as ambassador. Though she estimated the collection's value at five thousand dollars, it sold for just eighteen hundred dollars, but she realized that even this small addition to the organization's coffers was better than nothing.[45]

As her organization suffered financially, Breckinridge's personal finances took a similar hit. She had devoted much of her savings to the organization during the 1920s. She relied on her investments with Arkansas Valley Trust, a venture that her father had originally helped finance, to pay her living expenses, refusing to accept a salary from the FNS. However, her dividend checks dwindled steadily as the depression wore on. Funds were so tight that Breckinridge resorted to cutting her cigarettes in half to save money. Without one hundred dollars sent by her brother before the service's 1933 cruise sailed, she "couldn't have even had one glass of beer," she reported.[46]

Unable to afford upkeep on Wendover any longer, Breckinridge deeded the property to the FNS in July 1936. She apologized to the executive committee for placing the burden of the facility's operating costs on the service. The committee, however, praised her generosity, describing her contribution as "additional evidence of the consecration and devotion of their leader." They went on to declare that her material gifts, "as generous as they [were], could not compare with the gift of her genius, enthusiasm, and constant and untiring efforts throughout the years."[47]

WHILE THE early 1930s brought great struggles for Breckinridge and her organization, she optimistically noted that the FNS's poverty "endeared" it to its neighbors, who were suffering as well, and as a result the relationship between nurses and patients improved during this decade.[48] From the start, Breckinridge and her nurses recognized that poverty was pervasive in the mountains. In fact, to a certain extent, she had capitalized on the challenges patients faced to advance her fund-raising efforts. In FNS literature, mountain residents appeared proud, hospitable, and above all content. Their trials had forced them to develop a "dogged determination to survive" that Breckinridge greatly admired.[49] Breckinridge celebrated the work ethic of the region's residents and their ability to make do, but in the early history of the service, she placed little priority on improving the economic situation of her patients. Her tendency to romanticize the area and its people, reflecting media stereotypes so prevalent at the time, led her to overlook the day-to-day hardships Appalachia's residents faced. Now, challenged by trials of their own, Breckinridge and her staff began to appreciate that life in the mountains was not exotic and romantic, as media representations suggested; rather, it was taxing and often tragic.

At first, the depression had little noticeable effect on the people of eastern Kentucky, for whom poverty was a familiar state. While the 1920s brought a heady period of economic growth for much of the United States, eastern Kentucky struggled, dependent on three of the nation's four "sick industries" —agriculture, timber, and coal. "Public work" had become available throughout much of Appalachia at the turn of the century as the region shifted from an agricultural to an extractive, industrial economy. But while Leslie County lagged behind in this process, the mainstay of its economy, subsistence farming, was becoming increasingly unworkable.[50] A system that had previously provided a decent standard of living now resulted in dire poverty for many. As Harry Caudill later explained, "The stork outran the grubbing hoe and plow," leaving families destitute.[51] Many Leslie County residents became tenants, living on land owned by the Ford Motor Company.[52] Others were forced to relocate. But with the financial downturn sweeping the country, those who had left Leslie County seeking economic opportunity began to return home, stretching already meager resources even thinner. The land could not support the existing population, let alone those streaming back in.[53]

When a severe drought hit a portion of the nation's midsection from Arkansas to West Virginia in 1930, residents faced unprecedented devastation. The drought was one of the worst in U.S. history. From June to August of that year, Kentucky received only 43 percent of its normal rainfall. To make matters worse, temperatures topped one hundred degrees and remained there for weeks in July. Experts declared the potato and hay crops a complete loss and reported 75 percent of farmers' corn destroyed. Rural Kentuckians helplessly watched their crops wither and wondered how they would survive the upcoming winter.[54]

The hot, dry summer ended, and the fall brought no relief. Breckinridge reported that in Leslie County, four out of five wells had gone dry and pastures were "parched to brown ruin." Mountain residents floated logs down the river each spring to earn a little extra cash, but the lack of rainfall hampered these plans as well. The service's director predicted that unless the county's unemployed residents found work soon, starvation would ensue.[55] Recognizing that its patients were "headed for famine," the FNS began to provide food and jobs in addition to medical care, straining its budget ever further.[56]

BRECKINRIDGE HAD long admired Appalachian communities' tradition of self-help. Mountain residents did not seek charity in times of crisis; instead, neighbors willingly stepped forward to do their part. If a man's barn burned, the community worked together to rebuild. Friends and relatives took in orphaned children, no matter how crowded their own households. Those who had a surplus at harvest time shared their bounty, ensuring that no one went hungry. Breckinridge wished Americans throughout the nation would emulate her patients' willingness to care for one another.

The drought that ravaged the eastern Kentucky countryside in the summer and fall of 1930, however, brought into sharp focus the limitations of the informal community safety nets Breckinridge so admired and forced the director and her nurses to consider more seriously the causes of the region's poverty. Nearly all crops were destroyed, leaving few, no matter how willing, with surpluses to share. The depth of the devastation challenged the assumption held by so many Americans that hard work constituted a sure path to success. Their neighbors were not just facing temporary hardship. They had been poor during the 1920s, when most Americans' fortunes were on the rise, and they would continue to suffer after the national economy recovered.

In the fall of 1930, the FNS conducted a study to assess how long area families' food supplies would last. Breckinridge hired a local man to make an exact count of the number of bushels of corn each family had stored. His findings were grim. He estimated that by the following January, 17 percent of Leslie County families would be without food; by June, the number would rise to 70 percent. He predicted that unless conditions improved by the next harvest, 92 percent of county residents would face starvation.[57]

With conditions reaching a crisis point that fall, Breckinridge resolved that her organization needed to look beyond its medical mission to begin addressing patients' pressing material needs. The need for immediate stopgap measures led the FNS to establish the Social Service Department in 1931. Alpha Omicron Pi sorority voted to make the FNS its national service project and provided funds to pay the salary of a trained social worker and to cover the new office's operating costs. In the days before county welfare agencies existed, the Social Service Department gave FNS nurses a place to refer patients whose emotional and financial troubles interfered with their medical healing. The Social Service Department stepped in to provide aid in various forms. Director Bland Morrow held educational workshops on topics such as canning and sewing. She arranged for local children to attend school and paid their tuition. Most importantly, the Social Service Department helped feed and clothe patients by distributing secondhand clothing donated by FNS supporters as well as cod liver oil and canned milk to sustain malnourished parturient mothers and children. Emergency gifts of seed, fodder, shoes, eyeglasses, and "store teeth" were common.[58]

Breckinridge committed her organization's scarce resources to provide material assistance to the community through the Social Service Department, but she quickly recognized that the FNS could not begin to solve a crisis of this magnitude on its own, especially as donations steadily declined. Outside assistance would be necessary. Armed with data from the survey of area families' food supplies, she began corresponding in the fall of 1930 with the American Red Cross, which Congress had chartered in 1905 to administer relief in such times of national crisis. She urged the Red Cross to begin providing assistance as soon as possible.[59]

Although Leslie County Red Cross agents "show[ed] great and kind interest," Breckinridge quickly grew frustrated by their conservative response.[60] She deemed the monthly food allotment of $2.00 per person the agency reluctantly began issuing in January insufficient and questioned the restriction that no family, no matter how large, could draw more than twenty dollars each month. At Breckinridge's urging, the Red Cross increased allotments slightly to $2.50 per person, but many of the area's fundamental needs still remained unmet. Thousands of families had no cows and therefore no milk to supply growing children. Red Cross aid did not cover seed for the following year's crop or fodder for mules. Residents might escape immediate starvation, but families would lack the basic tools to ensure their future subsistence.[61]

Breckinridge did not blame the Red Cross for the inadequacy of the assistance it was providing. She praised the agency for doing splendid work with limited resources. Instead, she urged the government to increase the funding it provided the cash-strapped organization. She wrote to Kentucky's U.S. senator, Alben Barkley, in January 1931 to draw his attention to the dire conditions his constituents were facing. Describing the suffering as worse than that she had witnessed in France after the Great War, she implored him to use his influence to funnel additional funds to the Red Cross.[62] The following month, Breckinridge traveled to Washington, D.C., to attend a conference on drought relief sponsored by the Red Cross and attended by several sympathetic U.S. senators, including Barkley.[63]

Breckinridge was happy to hear that in the days following this conference,

Congress passed a $20 million measure that would supplement earlier legislation offering "feed and seed" loans to devastated farmers for "purposes incident to crop production."[64] The government stipulated, however, that only specific commercial crops such as cotton and corn could be used as collateral, assuring that eastern Kentucky would be almost completely left out of the federal crop loan program. After the U.S. Department of Agriculture denied her request that it consider timber, the area's only cash crop, as security for loans, Breckinridge again contacted Barkley for assistance in February 1931, urging him to act quickly, before Congress adjourned.[65] Much to her dismay, however, timber failed to qualify as a collateral crop. Very few area farmers remained eligible for the government loans, leaving many of the hardest hit to scrape by on their Red Cross allotments.

Breckinridge stepped in when the federal farm loan program failed to adequately serve her region. She again intervened on area farmers' behalf when the federal government began collecting on these ten-month loans in the fall of 1932. Having before found Senator Barkley a sympathetic ally, she encouraged him to introduce legislation that would delay the collection of federal farm loans. Data compiled by her staff revealed that the organization's patients who had qualified for the loans, like many other borrowers across the country, would suffer extreme hardship if required to repay them according to the original terms. Mountain residents were more than willing to pay their debts; they simply needed an extra year to get back on their feet. Though still bedridden following her recent riding accident, Breckinridge offered to "use [her] first strength" to address Congress on behalf of loan relief legislation.[66]

While she waited for Congress to act, she contacted the federal agent in charge of collecting the loans. Following a bedside conference with the FNS's director and, according to Breckinridge, having fallen victim to her charm, the loan officer pledged to do everything in his power to avoid forcing payment. After seeing the devastation in Leslie County, he regretted that he could not cancel the loans altogether. In the meantime, the fight in Washington continued. Breckinridge encouraged FNS supporters to contact their local congressional representatives in favor of a loan moratorium that the nation's farmers so desperately needed. Still, Breckinridge took comfort in knowing that her organization had played an instrumental role in convincing the Department of Agriculture to adopt a more lenient policy concerning farm loans in her territory.[67]

After more than a year of drought and famine, the rains finally came in April 1931. Creeks and rivers began to rise, replenishing wells and allowing local families to send their stockpiled timber to market. The people of Leslie

County welcomed the roaring, muddy "tides." Journalist Ernest Poole offered a dramatic account of the scene. Children ran to the river to watch, people cheered, "women dropped their hoes in the fields and men at their ploughs stood waving their hats. For the Great Drought had come to an end."[68] Families returned to work, clearing land, repairing fences, and planting gardens. The immediate crisis had ended, but poverty would remain a constant companion for eastern Kentucky's residents.

ALTHOUGH THE Social Service Department had initially sought to provide day-to-day emergency assistance during the drought, Morrow led the agency to become a vehicle through which to "reconstruct . . . the economy of the region." Morrow came to the FNS after completing two years of postbaccalaureate work at the New York School of Social Work and brought a macro-level perspective to her work. She believed that the "mountain problem" could be solved through study, and she thoughtfully considered how Appalachia's economy could be retooled to move beyond subsistence farming. Unlike Breckinridge, Morrow did not hesitate to point out that by limiting renters' ability to make full use of the land, outside investors, who claimed title to more than half of the county's territory, held its residents hostage. She recognized that the harsh mountain environment as well as absentee ownership posed problems for residents, and she looked both within the region and outside it to find new economic opportunities.[69]

Morrow in large part attributed the mountain problem to the fatalistic attitude of the people living there, which, she noted, was to be expected after "generations of helplessly watching the ravages of typhoid, dysentery, tuberculosis, diphtheria, seeing over and over again women dying in childbirth without means to prevent it, [and] seeing the crippled and deaf and blind doomed to useless lives."[70] Community development became a central part of the service's mission to deliver health care in the 1930s.[71] The nursing stations offered more than simply a place to receive medical treatment; they offered an opportunity to socialize with neighbors and to learn new skills such as patching and darning, baking, and home beautification, and they empowered local residents to improve their economic situations.[72] These outreach efforts resembled the work urban settlements such as Hull House were doing at the time and foreshadowed the work rural extension agents would later do.

Possum Bend, run by nurse-midwife Nora Kelly, was perhaps the most active outpost center. Kelly sponsored a literary and debating society that met weekly to discuss current local and national issues. Leslie County's newspaper, *Thousandsticks*, reported that meetings often filled the room to capacity, with participants spilling out onto the porch. Besides providing a forum for lively debate on topics such as arms reduction and the merits of single versus married life, the gatherings provided a venue in which neighbors could read poetry and display musical talent.[73]

Similarly, Wendover became a popular meeting place. Neighbors came to take part in organized activities such as the singing classes offered every Saturday afternoon or to check books out of its circulating library. A study of Leslie County conducted in the 1950s observed that Wendover provided a "hangout" for neighbors, who visited regularly to retrieve their mail, gossip, or pitch horseshoes. Young men wrangling for dates especially liked to congregate there and socialize with the girls the service employed as maids.[74]

As Breckinridge and her colleagues developed close personal relationships with their neighbors, their understanding of the region's problems grew more sophisticated. Although the terminology would not come into vogue until many decades later, Breckinridge, with Morrow's help, began to realize that Appalachia suffered from "underdevelopment."[75] The region was rich in resources but had profited little from this generous endowment. In later years, those who criticized the kind of development that occurred in the mountains focused on the coal industry, which made absentee developers wealthy while leaving area residents to face environmental destruction. At this point, however, Breckinridge was most concerned with the exploitation of the region's manpower. She resented that urban industries had "drawn the labor out and used it," only to "cast it back upon the mountain country" when the economy turned sour. In this way, Breckinridge reasoned, urban areas grew wealthy at the expense of the rural hinterlands. The capricious nature of the modern, industrial state, she concluded, bore primary blame for Appalachia's poverty.[76]

RED CROSS aid and loan extensions would help FNS patients in the here and now, but as the depression wore on, Breckinridge set her sights on providing more far-reaching economic uplift. She recognized that even after depression conditions lifted elsewhere, the Appalachian economy still would fail to support the area's population. She believed, however, that with careful planning, this "frontier" region could move from being one of the poorest sections of the country to one of the most prosperous. She envisioned "self-sustaining" communities where residents would earn their livings by combining environmentally friendly farming techniques with light industry such as woodworking shops that would not destroy the region's natural beauty or unique culture. Tourism seemed an obvious way to bring new revenue to the area, and she predicted that her organization's efforts to combat typhoid would help transform Appalachia into "the safest playground in America."[77] Improved roads, of course, were also necessary for economic development to occur. To this end, Breckinridge lobbied the state highway commission in support of a new road connecting Hyden to Manchester in 1932.[78]

More than anything, however, Breckinridge believed that selective forestry would be key to Leslie County's transformation. In 1931, the FNS commissioned a study of the timber industry in Clay and Leslie Counties. The director invited two representatives from the Yale School of Forestry to devise a plan "whereby [the area's] forests could be developed in perpetuity as an economic outlet." The report of their findings, which she reprinted in the *Quarterly Bulletin*, blamed "the stagnation of the region and the misery and poverty of the people" on the misuse and mismanagement of its forests. The Yale scholars advised that the region could preserve its natural resources and establish a steady source of income by implementing a plan for selective timbering. This plan would include new transportation networks, the construction of local mills to process lumber, and the development of national markets to sell the finished products.[79] After hearing the experts' findings, which supported her vision, Breckinridge immediately sent the results to the U.S. Forest Service.

In the 1930s, the federal government was in the process of establishing a system of forest stations, and Breckinridge hoped her area would be included. The Forest Service first proposed setting aside land for conservation in eastern Kentucky in 1911, after the passage of the Weeks Act. Lack of money put the plan on perpetual hold. However, interest in the plan, particularly among those who had cutover acres they wished to unload, continued to build for the next twenty years. Finally, when Franklin Delano Roosevelt took office in 1933, he made money available to fund the project.[80]

In July 1933, Breckinridge submitted a report to the U.S. Forest Service, citing the Yale study and her "intimate knowledge" of the area and detailing her recommendations for the proposed Cumberland Purchase Unit. She urged the Forest Service to include the counties her organization served in the area set aside for conservation. Clay, Perry, and Leslie Counties were particularly important, she argued, because they were home to some of the last stands of virgin timber in the area. Moreover, the strategic location of these counties would allow for better protection of the Kentucky and Cumberland River watersheds. Of course, she had other motivations as well. Becoming part of the national forest area not only would protect the environment, which was facing rapid destruction, but also would boost the local economy, providing an outlet through tourism to absorb jobless individuals who had returned home to the mountains at the start of the depression.[81]

To convince Forest Service representatives that her ideas were sound, she encouraged them to visit Leslie County to study conditions in the area for themselves. She promised them cooperation as well as "hospitality and horses." She cautioned that they would need to allow at least two weeks to make a thorough study of the rugged area, but she reassured them that they would be comfortable during their stay. FNS nursing outposts were equipped with bathtubs and running water, so an inspector could expect a "fresh bath after his day's ride."[82] The Forest Service took Breckinridge up on her offer and in August sent W. P. Kramer, a regional forester, to tour the three counties.

Breckinridge was impressed with Kramer's "sound knowledge and . . . approach to local situations" and felt comfortable that his recommendations would follow her own. In a preliminary report of his visit, Kramer agreed that the FNS's territory offered certain advantages, but he stressed that the reluctance of the area's large absentee landholders to sell lands at a reasonable price would make it difficult to acquire the selected areas.[83] Still, the Forest Service promised to conduct a more thorough investigation of the area as soon as possible. While waiting for forest officials to make a return visit, however, Breckinridge was disappointed to learn that the government had purchased land in Laurel, McCreary, Pulaski, Rockcastle, and Whitley Counties to form the Cumberland Purchase Unit.[84]

Over the next two years, Breckinridge went to great lengths to convince Forest Service officials to extend the Cumberland National Forest to include her counties. She personally visited the chair of the National Forest Reservation Commission and the chief of the Forest Service. She kept up a steady correspondence with these men, frequently resorting to flattery.[85] In a letter to the chief of the Forest Service, she offered her utmost compliment to his men. "Nothing in private life," she noted, "begins to approach [them] in efficiency, economy, integrity and splendid achievement." In a subsequent letter, she again praised the Forest Service employees: "All of your Foresters impress us as the most outstanding single group of men with which we come in contact."[86] Considering her high regard for mountain men, whom she praised for respecting a "pioneer code of honor," this was indeed a compliment.[87] Based on the Forest Service's original reasons for rejecting Clay, Leslie, and Perry Counties, she also contacted the Ford family, members of whom were not only the largest landholders in the area but also her close personal friends, to urge their cooperation.[88]

Breckinridge's efforts at persuasion came to an end when a Forest Service representative wrote in June 1935 to inform her that "the time [did] not seem ripe to extend the Cumberland Forest eastward." The Forest Service rejected this proposition because "the majority of the landowners [were] not now willing to dispose of their holding at prices which the Government would consider equitable." The cost was too high and funds too limited. Nothing more could be done until "the attitude of the owners changes."[89]

Breckinridge dashed off a letter protesting the Forest Service's decision. She declared that she did not see why lack of funds would be an issue at a time when the government was spending vast sums on public works projects. In a final attempt to have Leslie County included, Breckinridge offered to speak with the person responsible for rejecting the plan. "If you would let me know confidentially where the hitch in the matter of funds comes in and would be willing for me to do something about it, I would be glad to act." In case her influence was in doubt, she added that she knew Franklin and Eleanor Roosevelt "very well."[90] She did not offer to attempt to persuade the Fords to accept a lower price but instead viewed the federal government's thriftiness as the problem.

Years later, Robert F. Collins, a retired representative of the U.S. Forest Service, praised Breckinridge's vision. In his *History of the Daniel Boone National Forest* (1975), Collins contended that had the Forest Service followed her advice and acquired the areas she suggested, strip mining might not have had such a disastrous impact on the watersheds of the Kentucky and Cumberland Rivers.[91] Breckinridge had identified an important opportunity for the region to protect its environment, but her unwillingness to challenge the industrialists who owned so much of Leslie County's land contributed to the area's later destruction. She advocated a retooling of the Appalachian economy, but her vision for the area largely followed the conservative approach endorsed by the reformers who preceded her. Though she recognized that mountain poverty was connected to prosperity elsewhere, she failed to hold industrialists' feet to the fire and failed to suggest innovative strategies for moving the area forward economically. Her desire to preserve the quaintness of the area limited her ability to look beyond folk crafts and small-scale industry.

BRECKINRIDGE BECAME an active booster for Leslie County in the 1930s. She believed that her experience living and working in eastern Kentucky gave her the intimate knowledge needed to implement a plan for economic uplift. Although many others were working to solve the "mountain problem," the FNS never worked closely with other reformers. In the beginning, the director promised "cooperation with any existing agencies of whatever character," and very early in the FNS's history it sent representatives to the Southern Mountain Workers conference and contributed frequently to *Mountain Life and Work*, a publication that allowed those working in the area to share ideas.[92] But by the 1930s, Breckinridge had little interaction with other projects located in the mountains. In part, Breckinridge distanced herself from evangelical agencies such as the Presbyterian Settlement at Wooten because she preferred a nondenominational approach that emphasized detached professionalism.[93] The fact that these mountain reform organizations were competing for funding certainly discouraged cooperation as well. But Breckinridge's belief that she understood the mountain people best and had the answers to the problems that stifled development in the region particularly inhibited her ability to work cooperatively with fellow reformers.

Breckinridge preferred to work autonomously, but she recognized that to enact her sweeping vision, she must tap into government resources.[94] During the 1930s, the United States entered a period of massive federal spending, and although Breckinridge was a vocal proponent of the value of private voluntarism, she hoped to draw some of those federal dollars her way. As it did for many individuals, the Great Depression and FDR's groundbreaking New Deal forced Breckinridge to reconsider the relationship of individuals to the federal government. Breckinridge had long grappled with the state's proper role in welfare work. She believed firmly in the principles of social justice and in every individual's right to a basic standard of living. In particular, she saw Americans as having a collective responsibility to ensure the well-being of women and children, and she supported federal efforts on behalf of these dependent groups. She worked briefly as an agent for the Children's Bureau, and she endorsed the Sheppard-Towner legislation, which funneled federal money toward improving the health of mothers and babies. Like many maternalists, Breckinridge saw women and children as naturally deserving of state aid, but she shared many Americans' pervasive fear that a comprehensive welfare system would lead men to lose their will to work and would result in corruption.[95]

When Breckinridge first laid out her plan for a rural health care demonstration in 1923, she suggested that while private initiative would lead the way, only through "national recognition and support" could it extend into other areas of the country. She expected that federal funds eventually would cover the costs of running the service. Her project assumed "that the bearing and rearing of children is not a local, or even a state, but a national function."[96] For the cost of one battleship, the government could furnish an endowment sufficient to fund a nursing service that could serve millions of mountain residents.

As she saw it, the federal government was committing funds to much less important pork barrel projects such as river widening. Instead, she believed, legislators should commit dollars to the preservation of human lives. Mothers and infants, she insisted, should not "be sacrificed to the resources of the community where they chance to be living."[97]

In 1923, Breckinridge clearly viewed an alliance with government as having positive implications for her organization. A falling out with the head of the Kentucky Bureau of Maternal and Child Health, Dr. Annie Veech, however, made Breckinridge briefly reconsider the role public funding would play in her enterprise. Stung by Veech's criticisms of her proposal, Breckinridge smugly noted that the most innovative programs always began under the auspices of private agencies. Still, Breckinridge did not rule out the possibility that tax dollars would one day underwrite her organization's budget. She remained convinced that public monies would be necessary to carry out her project on the scale she envisioned. Public endorsement would bring needed funds as well as recognition and respect.

By the early 1930s, however, Breckinridge had become an enthusiastic advocate of the value of private aid. She often claimed that she resisted government interference because she believed that private organizations were a better judge of local conditions and could respond more flexibly to need.[98] Considering that she initially had argued in favor of public reform projects, her desire to exert her authority and to act independently surely influenced her celebration of voluntarism. She liked the autonomy that came with running a private agency and hesitated to accept the bureaucratic restrictions typically tied to government funding. She praised the British system, in which hospitals received government funds to cover their deficits but "were left to the control of their own boards of governors."[99] As the primary decision maker within her organization, she had no interest in sharing her authority with Uncle Sam.

The generous financial support Breckinridge received from donors strengthened her faith that voluntarism could meet America's economic and social needs. She firmly believed that the country's wealthy urban dwellers had an obligation to subsidize the costs of rural medical care, and she felt sure that individuals could be trusted to act in socially responsible ways if given the opportunity.[100] Writing in 1929, however, she expressed concern that the increasing availability of state aid would undermine Americans' sense of responsibility for the less fortunate, especially those hidden from view. She pointed out the irony that within the United States, the wealthiest nation in the world, such extreme poverty existed. Using the body as a metaphor, she challenged supporters: "Is anyone whole while there is sickness in one part?" The responsibility of caring for others, she emphasized, belonged not to the federal government but "to each one of us."[101] She chastised wealthy individuals who did not take seriously their duty and chose instead to gorge themselves on rich foods while others went hungry. She warned that "corruption and crime and disorder" would result if the upper class failed to live up to its responsibilities. Conversely, she offered nothing but praise for FNS patrons who demonstrated their social maturity through their donations.[102]

Breckinridge recognized that during times of economic crisis, generous Americans could not maintain their charitable giving. Unfortunately, these drops in donations came at the precise moment that agencies found their resources most strained. Breckinridge acknowledged that during troubled economic times, such as those America was facing in the 1930s, government had no choice but to commit resources to welfare work. She recommended, however, that federal authorities provide grants-in-aid to private groups rather than attempting to oversee relief themselves. The Hoover administration established such a relationship with the American Red Cross in the early days of the depression, an arrangement that Breckinridge praised.[103]

In many ways, Breckinridge's views matched those of President Herbert Hoover. Hoover upheld the nineteenth-century liberal philosophy that valued self-help and private charity, and he argued that government assistance must at all costs be avoided. Historians have roundly criticized Hoover for reacting so cautiously to the depression. The president viewed the stock market crash as a natural economic downturn that would soon correct itself, and he hesitated to make long-term structural changes to government. Public aid would "pauperize" individuals, he argued, undermining their will to work and making them forever wards of the federal government. Instead, voluntary agencies should remain responsible for providing assistance. "Progress will march," Hoover stressed, "if we hold an abiding faith in the intelligence, the initiative, the character, the courage, and the divine touch in the individual."[104]

Breckinridge shared Hoover's concern that aid given too freely would ruin its recipients. One of the qualities she most admired in the Appalachian people was their unwillingness to accept charity. In fund-raising material, she stressed that even the service's most destitute patients refused "hand outs," insisting that they be allowed to pay their debts by "whitewashing barns, mending drains and so on."[105] Despite her claims to the contrary, however, the possibility that mountain residents might become a burden on society seemed very real. In a February 1931 letter to FNS staff, the director urged nurses to remind their patients that the milk and food the organization supplied were "not charity." She instructed nurses to stress that they were providing supplies "due to an act of God." As soon as the drought ended, so too would the distribution of food.[106]

Breckinridge took her stand against public welfare programs at the exact moment that her goal of providing affordable health care to all Americans perhaps had the best chance of becoming reality. Government traditionally had taken a hands-off approach when it came to medical issues. State and federal governments usually limited their public health efforts to the control of infectious diseases that threatened the population at large. Starting in the 1920s with the passage of the Sheppard-Towner Act, the federal reach extended to health prevention work, but only among women and children. Medical doctors were a powerful lobbying group, and politicians hesitated to infringe on their territory.[107]

The New Deal, however, stood to change the government's role in health care. Created in 1935 to rehabilitate farm families by attacking sources of rural poverty and promoting economic self-sufficiency, the Farm Security Administration deemed lack of access to medical care a significant problem and responded by developing a network of health cooperatives. Established throughout the country, these cooperatives bore a marked similarity to the system Breckinridge administered. The cooperatives sought to ensure that illness would not interfere with borrowers' ability to pay back their Farm Security Administration loans. The cooperatives took disease prevention very seriously. Although the specifics varied from area to area, these cooperatives typically resembled prepaid insurance plans, a concept with which few rural Americans were familiar. Patients paid yearly dues, usually in the range of fifteen to thirty dollars, in exchange for unlimited doctor's visits. With risk distributed among a wide number of individuals, costs were affordable. In cases of extreme hardship, such as in migrant communities, the government absorbed some of the operating expenses. At the program's peak, Farm Security Administration health cooperatives served more than 650,000 clients, and many people viewed them as a step toward national health care.[108]

While the New Deal promised to address many of the inequalities Breckinridge had long viewed as a problem, including lack of access to health care, her desire to protect her power and autonomy prevented her from publicly endorsing Roosevelt's program. Though a staunch Democrat, she rejected the ideas of big government on which FDR's plan for economic recovery rested.[109] For the rest of her life, she insisted that welfare efforts were best left in the hands of private individuals—preferably her hands.

BRECKINRIDGE WAS skeptical of the New Deal because she feared massive government spending. She worried that government would become paternalistic, undermining its citizens' initiative in its attempt to provide relief. While she acknowledged the danger that the FNS too might erode patients' independence, she felt sure that her knowledge and experience left her better equipped to address her neighbors' problems. She criticized the format of the New Deal yet agreed with the goals of its key programs, and she adopted some of its basic ideas when crafting her organization's response to the depression. In one sense, Breckinridge rejected FDR's New Deal in favor of her own.

By the 1930s, Breckinridge saw few issues as falling outside her realm of authority. Like other maternalists, she emphasized woman's natural role as caregiver to justify her incursion into realms traditionally considered off limits to members of her sex.[110] She used the license provided by her position as a trained health care provider to step well beyond the roles she had been taught to view as appropriate for women.

Although Breckinridge clearly enjoyed the power her position afforded her, she was careful not to appear too self-serving. She lived in a region where women often held a great deal of power within their own families but rarely publicly displayed their authority. As John C. Campbell documents, a rigid patriarchal system existed in the mountains, with men controlling politics, religion, and domestic relationships. "From babyhood," he notes, "the boy is the favored lord of all he surveys."[111] Girls were rarely educated, for their greatest aspiration was to marry and start families of their own. Mountain gender norms corresponded well to Breckinridge's own upbringing, which stressed that motherhood was a woman's highest calling and the domestic sphere her proper place.

Breckinridge carefully couched in feminine terms projects that others might view as crossing into the male domain, thereby making her actions appear less threatening. For example, when she wanted roads built or a particular candidate elected, she did not work directly toward those ends but instead led "whispering campaigns." For those who might see her efforts on behalf of highways, no matter how quietly communicated, as inappropriate, she claimed to be concerned about the danger primitive roads posed to public health. It only took "one streptococcal throat spittle out of a coal truck cab" on a dusty road to infect everyone living or traveling on it, she warned.[112]

Impressed by her leadership skills and practical solutions to complex problems, supporters more than once urged Breckinridge to perpetuate her family's political legacy by running for public office.[113] She declined, however, convinced that her work with the FNS allowed her to have a greater impact than she could possibly have by serving in Congress. Though she did not practice politics in the traditional sense, her actions had significant political implications, and by staying above the fracas of politics, Breckinridge avoided the fate faced by other reformers such as literacy crusader Cora Wilson Stewart. Stewart became heavily involved in state and national affairs, only to find her methods shunned and her cause co-opted by bureaucrats who rejected grassroots, voluntary efforts in favor of standardized, state-supported, and university-trained leadership.[114] Breckinridge carefully avoided such co-optation and remained content to demonstrate a high degree of control over a little corner of the world.

Local men expressed surprisingly little resistance to the position of power the FNS's director assumed within the community. Similar to the traditional ward boss or patronage politician, Breckinridge's control over jobs and other forms of financial assistance allowed her to build support and loyalty. At times, the FNS provided the area's only employment opportunities. During the depression, the FNS employed nearly one hundred men through a carefully designed jobs program. On one day alone, forty area residents solicited Breckinridge for work. She endorsed work relief programs over direct financial assistance because they would allow recipients to maintain their pride. Though the service's debts were beginning to mount, its director recommended the construction of two additional nursing centers in 1930, citing the job opportunities that these projects would provide. The FNS also hired local men to whitewash barns and haul logs. While useful, these tasks were certainly not essential in such lean economic times. However, much in the same way as the federal government, Breckinridge recognized that deficit spending could play a valuable role in boosting the economy.[115]

Not everyone, however, benefited from the FNS's largesse. Though Leslie County had a National Reemployment Office that worked to match both skilled and unskilled workers with jobs in the area and that promised employers the security of knowing that their workers had been deemed both "qualified and competent" by "a standardized government agency," Breckinridge preferred to impose her own standards when making hiring decisions.[116] Men who had not paid their annual dues did not make the service's "Grade A" list and therefore were unable to obtain positions on FNS building projects. However, Breckinridge offered those who owed money an opportunity to redeem themselves. In 1932, she sternly advised men whose accounts were delinquent to report immediately to the superintendent of Hyden Hospital to be assigned a task and thereby work off their indebtedness.[117] She had little sympathy for individuals who were not willing to help themselves.

Breckinridge often used her position of power within the community to offer moral judgments regarding those who failed to live up to her standards. Unlike the federal government, she personally knew the people she was serving and kept close tabs on their "circumstances."[118] This familiarity with patients, she claimed, allowed her to provide assistance particularly targeted to their needs and to avoid enabling individuals who were not behaving responsibly. The FNS kept a close watch on its patients, rewarding those it deemed deserving while withholding assistance from those it considered profligate.

While most FNS patients were grateful for the economic boost the organization provided Leslie County during the depression, not everyone was satisfied with the favoritism Breckinridge displayed in hiring decisions. In March 1936, she received an anonymous letter demanding that she fire the local residents who had received long-term employment from the service and replace them with others from the area who needed work. If she did not take steps to spread the wealth by April 1, the letter threatened, she could expect "an awfull explosion." The writer also threatened to set fire to the service's barns and to shoot at Breckinridge from the bushes. The unknown author added, "You better look out. . . . [R]emember the first of April is not long."[119]

After receiving this letter, Breckinridge hired a deputy sheriff to serve as a night watchman at Wendover, but she did not expect anything further to come from the threats. But after three fires were set on FNS property, with one of the blazes resulting in the destruction of the service's pump house and the evacuation of Wendover, Breckinridge sought assistance.[120] Local sheriffs concluded that the fires had been set intentionally and brought in bloodhounds from Lexington.[121] Although Breckinridge was eager to find the culprit, she was careful to prevent news of the investigation from leaking out. She particularly wanted to keep the story out of the press. She did so, she claimed, because she feared that publicity might undermine the police's efforts. She certainly had other motives for maintaining silence. The first to gain patrons' sympathy by playing up any natural disaster or accident that threatened the FNS, Breckinridge avoided news coverage of this story because she feared that it would undermine supporters' favorable impressions of the Appalachian people. She understood that donors would question her claims of patient loyalty if news of the threats spread.

Breckinridge, however, wrote to select supporters to describe the incident and to request donations to offset the costs of the investigation. In every letter, she reminded the recipient that the information enclosed was "strictly confidential."[122] She hypothesized that outsiders, not service patients, were responsible for the threats and argued that the situation was "a by-product of what we call civilization," claiming that the opening of mines and the roads coming into the area had disrupted the region's peace. "The Twentieth Century is creeping in on us in its least desirable forms," she announced.[123]

In another letter, Breckinridge blamed the threats on Leslie County natives who had left the area but were now returning. She alleged that she attempted to distribute job assignments to those who most needed work. The director asserted, however, that she had a responsibility to take into account "character, ability, and fidelity" as well as financial hardship when making hiring decisions. She contended that those moving back into the mountains were "not in the main as reliable a group as the old mountaineers, who never left the land"; hence, the returnees did not deserve FNS jobs. "You see," she confided, "the situation in here is that I control a great deal of power." She concluded that the attacks were the "price one pays for responsibility."[124]

Although Breckinridge worried that her nurses were in danger, she relished the opportunity to "liv[e] in a detective story." In letters to executive committee members, the director related all the exciting details of the case. She enthusiastically described local efforts to track down the perpetrators using bloodhounds, noting that detectives had allowed her to pet and feed the dogs. In August, she reported that "an excellent G-man" from Louisville had visited. Showing that she had absorbed the lingo, she confidently predicted that the case would soon "break."[125]

That fall, growing frustrated that the Justice Department was no closer to finding the culprits, Breckinridge contacted Eleanor Roosevelt, who encouraged the FBI to intervene. When the FBI arrived in Leslie County, agents requested handwriting samples from all of the women in the area. The service's nurses deceitfully collected these samples by instructing mothers to compile their children's Christmas wish lists. When the nurses turned over the samples, the FBI identified the handwriting and charged a woman who lived only two miles from Wendover with making the threats.

Putting aside her contempt for the perpetrator, Breckinridge asked the Department of Justice not to prosecute for several reasons. First, she believed that the members of the family were so "unbalanced" that if punished, they would express their anger by causing more damage. Second, she explained that the family was "poor and pitiful" but "not a criminal type." The case, she concluded, required "social assistance and the deepest compassion." She could take care of the situation from this point on. The FBI officially closed the case in November 1936.[126] When her theory that the person directing the threats toward the FNS was an outsider failed to hold true, Breckinridge instead portrayed the culprit as mentally unfit. Doing so allowed her to protect the glowing image she had painted of service patients as full of potential and worthy of assistance. She chose rehabilitation rather than punishment to show that the mountain peoples' innate qualities of trustworthiness and loyalty could be restored with minimal effort. Of course, her organization could best provide this needed rehabilitation.

INSTEAD OF experiencing a period of expansion, as Breckinridge had hoped, the FNS struggled to survive the 1930s. Financial hardship and her riding accident caused Breckinridge to shift from a strategy of growth to a maintenance approach.[127] Through ambitious fund-raising efforts, some successful and others not, and by cutting costs "to the very bone," the FNS weathered the depression without closing centers or significantly reducing services.[128]

Breckinridge's strong faith in the value of her plan allowed her to stay upbeat in the face of the trials these years brought. The service's record spoke to the quality of care its nurses provided and the number of lives they saved. The FNS registered its three thousandth maternity case in 1937. During its first twelve years of operation, the service lost only two women due to pregnancy-related causes at a time when the national average still hovered at 5.9 deaths per thousand.[129] Breckinridge proudly reported that her nurses maintained this low mortality rate while avoiding many of the heroic measures that doctors often employed.[130] In treating these three thousand cases, FNS nurses had performed only six Caesarean sections and had used forceps, routinely used in hospitals across the nation, only fourteen times.[131]

As the depression wore on, Breckinridge's romantic impression of the Appalachian people as poor but proud and of the mountain way of life as gritty and exciting began to fade. In its place came a more realistic understanding of the obstacles that her patients faced. Instead of offering short-term assistance, such as gifts of castor oil and shoes, Breckinridge began to investigate long-range solutions to the deep-rooted structural problems of poverty and underdevelopment. Like FDR, who promised that he would harness the power of government to provide Americans a New Deal, Breckinridge subsequently envisioned her organization in an expanded role, addressing not only health concerns but also the complex social and economic issues facing eastern Kentucky.

By the late 1930s, the FNS's financial outlook seemed less grim, with contributions increasing after 1935.[132] The executive committee voted to raise the salaries of hospital nurses by ten dollars each month starting in the summer of

1937. For the first time, Breckinridge also agreed to accept a salary. She stipulated, however, that her wages never exceed those paid to the other nurse-midwives on staff.[133] Although contributions dropped off sharply during the depression, resulting in a daily struggle to keep the service running, the organization's endowment fund increased significantly, reaching $253,000 by 1939.[134]

Subscriptions finally rebounded to their pre-1929 levels in 1940. The FNS could again think of expanding outside of Leslie County. Breckinridge, however, was nearing sixty years of age. The deprivations of the past ten years would have a lasting effect on the way she administered the organization. She became less willing to take risks and more content to demonstrate the effectiveness of her tactics in one location. Henceforth, she would encourage FNS-trained nurses to take their skills to new regions and would welcome observers from other nations who wanted to transplant her ideas, but she would never again consider creating satellite organizations, as she had in 1930.[135]

As one worldwide crisis subsided, another—ultimately even more devastating—was quickly developing. By the late 1930s, world leaders found it impossible to ignore Adolf Hitler's thirst for world domination. Following the 1938 Munich Conference, war appeared inevitable. Mary Breckinridge recognized that if fighting broke out, her staff, consisting mainly of British nurse-midwives, would be depleted. She began to consider how the Frontier Nursing Service (FNS) would cope in the event of a war. She sadly predicted that "the war could do what the depression had not been able to do, namely, close down a large area of the F.N.S."[1]

For most Americans, the announcement that war had broken out in Europe came as little surprise. On September 3, 1939, Breckinridge and FNS staff members anxiously gathered around a battery-powered radio in the living room at Wendover to hear reports that Germany had invaded Poland. War had come at last, President Franklin Delano Roosevelt announced, warning solemnly, "When peace has been broken anywhere, the peace of all countries everywhere is in danger."[2] Having witnessed the devastation that followed the first Great War, Breckinridge dreaded the suffering another conflict would bring to men, women, and children across the globe as well as the war's effects on the FNS.

Breckinridge's concern was warranted. FNS staff would have to work twice as hard to compensate for the shortage of labor that plagued the service throughout the early 1940s. Long before the war began, Breckinridge recognized that maintaining an adequate staff would prove problematic, and she began to develop an emergency plan. In 1939, eighteen of the service's twenty-two nurse-midwives were British citizens. Breckinridge warned supporters that the service would be "ripped from end to end" as these individuals returned to the "Old Country."[3] Although public health officials had endorsed the concept of nurse-midwifery for several decades, few Americans had obtained such training. Foreseeing the difficulty she would have rebuilding her staff, Breckinridge established the Frontier Graduate School of Midwifery (FGSM) in the fall of 1939. By educating its own employees, the FNS avoided closing Hyden Hospital or any of its outpost centers during the war. More important, the admission of its first class marked the beginning of the FNS's attempt indirectly to serve rural areas by training specialized practitioners.

WHEN BRECKINRIDGE hired her first staff members in 1925, no school in the United States offered training in the virtually unknown field of nurse-midwifery. Thus, she had no choice but to recruit staff from Great Britain, where the profession was well established. From the start, however, she looked forward to the day when she would create her own facility to train nurse-midwives. Such a school, she reasoned, would better allow the FNS to share its philosophy of rural health care with others throughout the nation and even the world.[4]

In the early 1930s, Breckinridge explored the possibility of setting up a professional midwifery program administered jointly by the FNS and the University of Kentucky. The university's president, FNS supporter Frank McVey, enthusiastically endorsed the plan. The curriculum Breckinridge outlined required students to be registered nurses and to take one year of university coursework before gaining one year of clinical experience at Wendover. When the depression prevented her from raising the funds for the project, Breckinridge withdrew her proposal. She remained hopeful, however, that as soon as the organization's economic position improved, she could move forward with her plan to train nurse-midwives.[5]

Unable to finance a FNS-run school, Breckinridge worked instead with the Maternity Center Association (MCA) to establish a training facility. Founded in 1918, the MCA administered a network of clinics that provided prenatal care and instruction to poor parturient New York City mothers. Encouraged by the Committee on the Costs of Medical Care's finding that the nation could provide better care to all Americans by training new nurse-midwives, several MCA leaders united in 1931 to form the Association for the Promotion and Standardization of Midwifery. Breckinridge served on the association's board of trustees. The association's work led to the creation of New York City's Lobenstine Midwifery Clinic and School in 1932. FNS nurse-midwife Rose McNaught helped to establish the training program and taught at the school for the rest of her career.[6] The creation of the MCA's nurse-midwifery school brought attention to the budding profession but did not solve the FNS's immediate labor needs. Only one of the MCA's first twenty graduates joined the staff of the FNS. As the benefits trained nurse-midwives could provide became better known, the demand for MCA graduates far outstripped the supply, leading Breckinridge to continue recruiting British staff throughout the 1930s.[7]

The announcement that war had begun in Europe in the fall of 1939 sent Breckinridge scrambling to deal with the impending exodus of British nurse-midwives. Eager to devise a solution, the director called an emergency meeting of the organization's executive committee and described for those present the challenges the service faced.[8] British nurse-midwives soon would be returning to England, and the FNS would have no means of replacing the lost staff. As physicians became scarcer, she predicted, the demand for nurse-midwives would increase. The Lobenstine Clinic alone could not possibly fill the nation's needs. Breckinridge stressed that the only way the FNS could continue to provide care to the mothers of Leslie County was for the service to establish its own training program.[9]

Aware of the severity of the situation, the executive committee authorized the director immediately to establish a training school. The committee members approved her recommendation that the new four-month program initially accept only two students at a time and that it enroll only applicants who held diplomas from approved nursing schools. The committee also endorsed her plan to provide scholarships to nurses interested in taking courses at the Lobenstine Clinic. Nurses who trained at the FNS or who accepted scholarships from the service would be required to remain with the organization for two years. Breckinridge hoped that these measures would allow her to add six new nurse-midwives to her staff by July 1940.[10]

After Breckinridge gained the executive committee's consent to create a training school, the details fell quickly into place. The FGSM opened its doors just two days later, becoming only the second program in the nation to provide such instruction. The director was able to implement her plan so quickly because she had already taken the liberty of seeking advice from the Department of Nursing and Health at Teachers College, Columbia University, and from the MCA. The FNS's two most experienced British nurse-midwives agreed to postpone their departure to oversee the first class of students.[11]

Breckinridge and her assistants patterned the school's curriculum after the British system of nurse-midwifery education. The accelerated program included classroom instruction as well as hands-on experience. The FNS's medical director and graduate nurse-midwives provided lectures. To qualify for certification, each student had to perform twenty deliveries, with at least five occurring in the hospital and five in patients' homes. Two obstetricians administered oral and written exams to the students at the end of the course. The FNS honored those who passed with a diploma, and the State of Kentucky agreed to award graduates a license to practice midwifery.[12]

In 1929, when Breckinridge first announced her plan to establish a training facility, she stressed that it would serve "daughters of leading citizens in the mountains" who wanted to become nurse-midwives.[13] The FGSM, however, would train few if any area natives. As Breckinridge later noted, several factors explain why local women did not receive this training. For one, the FGSM accepted only applicants who held nursing diplomas, and most of the region's women lacked even high school degrees. The FNS offered financial assistance to women from leading families who wanted to attend nursing schools outside the mountains, but few returned after they completed their programs of study. If they did, marriage and family obligations often prevented them from practicing their profession.[14] The FGSM recruited students from around the world but failed to educate those in its own backyard.[15]

AS SOON as the first students enrolled at the FGSM, British staff members began to submit their resignations. In January 1940, Breckinridge reported that four nurses had already returned to Britain. The departures of these individuals represented not only a loss of staffing but also a loss of friends. In the *Quarterly Bulletin*, the director expressed her sorrow at watching old friends go: "Spring would indeed be welcome if the world were at peace," she noted. Spring, however, would not come until the service's "intimate Old Country ties" were restored and "families and friends in warring nations" reunited.[16] While grieving personally for the loss of colleagues, she feared for the service's future. She predicted that the service would be "crippled" if the war spread in Europe, an assumption that proved correct. By the fall of 1940, only eight British staff members remained.[17]

Adding to Breckinridge's concern that she would not have adequate staff to keep the hospital and all the outposts open, an influenza epidemic swept through Leslie County in January 1941, further reducing the FNS's rapidly dwindling ranks. Despite the service's best precautions, twenty-two of forty-one staff members fell ill. The symptoms, Breckinridge reported, came on so quickly that "it was almost as if people were being hit with stones." The director reluctantly closed the FGSM when the instructor and two of the three students became ill.[18]

Breckinridge took immediate steps to find temporary nurses in Lexington and surrounding areas to help the service handle the hundreds of cases reported on its districts. Nurses tried to return to their duties as soon as possible, but those who attempted to resume work too soon experienced relapses. Although few nurses remained healthy, the service continued its work. According to staff member Agnes Lewis, many nurses went on calls "when they had no business going, but the patients were worse than they were, and they went."[19] Breckinridge emphasized that the FNS's "blue-gray line never wore so thin, but it held at every point." She stressed to donors that even during the crisis, "no woman was unattended during childbirth."[20]

As an emergency measure designed to keep the hospital open, Breckinridge allowed former couriers who had completed Red Cross Emergency Nurses' Training to begin serving as nurses' aides. Breckinridge had long been an advocate for stricter nurse training requirements and in the past had opposed the movement to license practical nurses.[21] She recognized, however, that in times of crisis, nurses with partial training were better than no nurses. Still, she stipulated that aides never work without the supervision of graduate nurses.[22]

BRECKINRIDGE RECOGNIZED that if the United States joined the fight overseas, her labor woes would only increase, but she nevertheless encouraged American leaders to declare war. Unlike many reformers who were pacifists, Breckinridge stood out as a vocal jingoist. Always hesitant to express her political beliefs for fear of alienating supporters, she put aside these concerns and used the service's *Quarterly Bulletin* as a vehicle through which to endorse the idea of an alliance between democratic states as outlined in Clarence Streit's book, *Union Now* (1939).[23] She further delineated her belief that America needed to enter the war in an August 1940 editorial published in the *Lexington Herald-Leader* that she had reprinted and widely distributed. Taking advantage of her freedom of speech, which she now feared was in jeopardy, she criticized American leaders for being slow to recognize and to meet the challenge of totalitarianism. She called for an international union between the remaining free democracies—the United States, Canada, the United Kingdom, Ireland, Australia, New Zealand, and South Africa.[24] She urged these free states to fight not out of hatred but out of love and of a desire to spread the benefits of democracy to "an ever widening circle of men."[25]

Just as many female pacifists cited their gender as justification for their position, claiming that women, with their special nurturing gifts, had a particular obligation to push for peace, Breckinridge justified her interest in going to war by stressing women's unique position—notably, their vulnerability. She reminded men that they had a duty to their wives and daughters, who bore and raised the nation's children, to make sure that war did not come to America's shores.[26] Breckinridge urged American leaders to abandon their isolationist stance and join the Allied fight. An ardent Anglophile, she believed that an attack against Great Britain was in essence an attack on the United States, since the two countries had a long friendship and shared similar cultures.[27] Though she did not like the thought of war, she saw it as a necessary evil. Her family had a legacy of fighting in defense of its principles; she resigned herself to the fact that the current crisis would not be resolved without bloodshed. Breckinridge expressed relief when in December 1941 the United States responded to the attack on Pearl Harbor by declaring war on Germany and Japan. The decision, she believed, was long overdue.[28]

BY 1941, war mobilization had restored the nation's financial health. The Appalachian economy, like that of the country in general, experienced marked improvement during the war. Between 1940 and 1950, per capita income in Leslie County rose from $114 to $418.[29] Laborers who had struggled to find work for more than a decade suddenly found themselves in high demand. According to Ronald D Eller, "Saw mills that had not operated in years now hummed. . . . [N]ew coalmines were opened. . . . [C]ompany towns and county seat villages bustled with life, and a throng of mineral agents, timber buyers, and land developers invaded the region anew." Thousands of young Appalachian residents joined the armed forces, and some of the highest enlistment rates in the nation were found in the mountains. Other mountain residents were drawn to northern cities such as Chicago, Cincinnati, and Dayton, whose booming war industries offered high-paying jobs, steady employment, and better living conditions. A study of outmigration during World War II found that between 1940 and 1942 alone, almost 19 percent of eastern Kentucky's population—40 percent of the men between the ages of fifteen and thirty-four—left.[30]

Men, however, were not the only ones leaving the mountains in search of better opportunities. Local women who had formerly worked for the FNS in domestic labor left in large numbers as well, in some cases to follow their husbands and sometimes in search of more exciting work for themselves. Already unable to provide the level of care to which they were accustomed, FNS nurses faced even greater burdens as hospital and clinic maids resigned their posts. The FNS had no trouble finding help when jobs were scarce, but now that the nation was experiencing a shortage of labor, service salaries could not compete with the wages offered by other employers. Nurses increasingly were forced to add tasks such as cooking and cleaning to their workloads. Breckinridge found it unacceptable that nurses should have to "come back after hours in the saddle to a cold house, a cow to milk, feed and water, a horse to groom and feed, and fires to build before she can even cook something to eat," but still she hesitated to raise wages.[31]

Although Breckinridge had worked throughout the 1930s to build Leslie County's economy, she had little sympathy for local residents who chose to improve their situations by moving elsewhere. She had developed a strong personal allegiance to the region, and she expected her neighbors to remain faithful to the area even as higher wages beckoned elsewhere. In her mind, those who chose to move were "unreliable," and she assumed that when the economy again turned sour, as it surely would, the mass exodus would reverse and people would come streaming back.[32] While Breckinridge supported road construction and limited industrial development, she tended to view the outsiders who came into the mountains as professionals deserving of high wages while relegating local men and women to low-paying domestic and manual labor positions. In 1944, Breckinridge reluctantly raised weekly salaries for maids from five to six dollars per week.[33] This modest increase did little to solve her labor woes, leading Breckinridge to demand that local FNS committees recruit women in their communities to replace the women who left. Aware that she would have to close outpost centers if the labor problems did not improve, Breckinridge threatened to close centers first in districts where maids could not be found.[34]

Professional staff earned much higher salaries than their nonprofessional counterparts; still, the wages the FNS paid nurse-midwives did not compare favorably to the sums they could earn elsewhere. Service wages never fully rebounded from the drastic cuts instituted in the early 1930s. In 1943, senior staff members earned just under fifteen hundred dollars per year. By comparison, most public health organizations paid nurse-midwives between two thousand and twenty-six hundred dollars per year. FNS nurse-midwives knew that they could earn considerably more money elsewhere, but few chose to leave, revealing their degree of commitment to eastern Kentucky and their level of satisfaction with working for the service. When staff left, however, low wages caused great difficulty in attracting new employees.[35]

If FNS nurse-midwives had wanted to leave, they certainly would have had ample opportunity to find positions elsewhere. As doctors left their communities to join the war effort, Americans became concerned that there would be no one available to provide care on the home front. Early in the war, Hazel Corbin, director of the MCA, warned that "doctors and nurses [were] being plucked from [the nation's] civilian ranks like petals off a daisy."[36] The media heightened women's fears that no doctor would be there to care for them during childbirth. In 1943, *Women's Home Companion* suggested that nurse-midwives could provide a welcome alternative for those women who lacked access to physicians, noting that ten years earlier, the midwife was "shut-out from medicine's back door"; now, however, she was "an honored occupant of its parlor."[37]

As interest in the field grew, the FNS began receiving several inquiries each month from private and public agencies that sought to add nurse-midwives to their staffs. The U.S. Children's Bureau was one such agency that became an enthusiastic advocate of nurse-midwives during the war. The Children's Bureau not only began hiring nurse-midwives to serve in rural areas that lacked physicians but also began allocating funds to encourage the training of additional nurse-midwives. Funding from the Children's Bureau aided the FGSM as well as programs established around the same time in Tuskegee, Alabama; New Orleans; and Harlem.[38]

Despite Breckinridge's claims that reform could best occur through private enterprise, during the war the FNS began to participate in several federal programs. In addition to accepting money from the Children's Bureau to pay for FGSM scholarships, the FNS also received aid through the Emergency Maternity and Infant Care program. Created in 1943 to bolster troops' morale, this program provided funds to ensure that servicemen's wives received adequate maternity care, foreshadowing the large-scale government subsidization of health care that began during the 1960s with the creation of Medicare and Medicaid.[39] While the idea of universal health care remained controversial, few Americans questioned the government's decision to provide assistance to the wives and children of men who were so faithfully serving their country.[40]

During the war, Breckinridge received her first taste of the benefits of federal funding, but she also discovered the burdens government aid would place on her organization, a discovery that did not surprise her. The FNS operated in a different environment than did most public health organizations, which were concentrated in urban areas. Federal bureaucratic restrictions often failed to account for the challenges facing organizations that served in remote geographical locations, viewing all agencies through the same lens. Breckinridge lamented the lack of flexibility government programs demonstrated, but even more, she resented the level of oversight that came with federal support and feared that such assistance would limit her autonomy.

The service's wartime participation in the Cadet Nurse Corps foreshadowed the constraints federal bureaucracy would place on the service in future decades. Congress established the corps in 1943 as an emergency measure designed to increase the nation's supply of nurses. The program, funded through the Bolton Act, encouraged young women to pursue careers in nursing. The Cadet Nurse Corps provided federal grants directly to training institutions that agreed to increase their enrollments and to condense their courses from thirty-six months to a maximum of thirty months. Many students found the benefits of the program attractive. Cadet nurses paid no tuition and received a monthly stipend. Recruitment brochures assured students that "nurses make fine wives and good mothers" and that the "marriage rate among nurses is high." Between July 1943 and October 1945, nearly 170,000 young women joined the Cadet Nurse Corps.[41]

Unlike traditional nursing students, cadet nurses were required to complete a six-month period of on-site training, choosing from among a range of participating agencies and hospitals. This arrangement ensured that despite the shortened courses of nursing study, students continued to receive three years of training, which nursing leaders argued was essential; at the same time, cadets provided labor during the latter stages of their education, helping to lessen the shortage of nurses on the home front.[42]

In 1944, the FNS eagerly accepted its first group of cadet nurses. Breckinridge hoped that the students would ease the heavy burden her nurses had been carrying for several years. She also believed that the cadet program would provide her with a new means of building support for the rural nursing methods she advocated. However, Breckinridge quickly became disillusioned with the program. She insisted that cadets focus on learning rather than on providing service and consequently refused to allow them to work without direct supervision. Instead of helping to alleviate the organization's shortage of nurses, the cadets exacerbated the problem. Overseeing students burdened FNS staff, and the student nurses ultimately provided little in the way of patient care.[43]

Although the cadet program did not ease the FNS's nursing shortage, as

Breckinridge had hoped, she continued to accept cadets for two years. In 1946, however, Breckinridge decided to discontinue the FNS's affiliation with the Cadet Nurse Corps after receiving orders from the state board of nursing to submit detailed outlines of the training being provided to students. The director explained that because her nurses were scattered throughout the countryside rather than congregated in a hospital, it was extremely difficult to coordinate their activities. Breckinridge reported that her nurses remained overburdened and that she felt it would be of little use for them to make an in-depth record of what they were teaching students. Breckinridge pointed out that cadets who chose to come to the FNS did so because they wanted to learn how rural nurses functioned, and she believed that they could best do so by shadowing more experienced nurses, not by receiving formal instruction in a classroom. The state director for nursing education acknowledged the additional burdens of compiling an outline of the FNS's instructional program but refused to adjust the policy, reiterating sternly, "An outline is one of our requirements."[44]

When the government refused to consider the FNS's special circumstances, Breckinridge terminated her organization's affiliation with the Cadet Nurse Corps.[45] Her experience with accepting government aid during the war lent credence to her long-held assumption that doing so would limit her ability to devise creative, flexible solutions to the problems she witnessed in society. In the future, she would remain wary of government programs. Her desire to protect her autonomy and the position of authority she had carved out for herself made her hesitant to accept federal funds as they increasingly became available after the war.

FOR MOST Americans, the depression ended as the war began. The FNS, however, continued to experience financial hardship throughout the early 1940s. In November 1944, Breckinridge lamented, "Every time we meet a budget with some degree of ease, the budget goes up and we have to struggle all over again."[46] The cost of necessities such as hay, hospital supplies, and food rose throughout the war without a concurrent rise in subscriptions, placing heavy fund-raising burdens on the service's director.[47]

In an effort to increase contributions, Breckinridge tailored her message to focus on the crisis facing the nation. She continued to stress her patients' worthiness, but she no longer drew attention to their pure bloodlines. Throughout the 1930s, the use of eugenic rhetoric declined as Americans increasingly connected racial purity, so enthusiastically celebrated by the German Nazi Party, with totalitarianism. Moreover, the depression forced many people to rethink Darwinian notions of economic justice. In response to this shift, Breckinridge revised the FNS's annual appeal in 1938, removing references to the Appalachian people as "pure Anglo-Saxons."[48]

Instead of continuing to rely on outdated claims that Appalachian residents' pure blood made them worthy, Breckinridge redirected her focus toward mothers and children and their right to skilled medical care. She used the war as a backdrop for the argument that women performed vital, patriotic services. Their contribution went beyond holding down farms and factories and suffering vicariously as their husbands and brothers fought to protect freedom.[49] Women, like men fighting oversees, gave their lives unselfishly in service to their nation every day. "Maternity," Breckinridge emphasized, "is the young woman's battlefield." Because women placed their lives on the line, they, like the nation's soldiers, deserved the best care available, and the FNS was offering that care.[50]

In the American mind, soldiers represented the ultimate heroes, and few wartime Americans questioned the idea that fighting men deserved both admiration and compensation. Long before the creation of a fledgling welfare state during the 1930s, the U.S. government had created a massive system of military pensions for Civil War veterans. Other groups that wanted to justify support for their constituents and to demonstrate their deserving status compared them to soldiers. For example, the American Federation of Labor promoted noncontributory old-age pensions for retired workers by arguing that they constituted an "army of labor."[51]

In the early twentieth century, both suffrage supporters and opponents invoked military rhetoric to bolster their positions. Opponents argued that politics were a man's province and pointed to women's lack of military service to justify their exclusion. Elihu Root, secretary of war under President William McKinley, for example, countered suffragists' demands, stating that women did not belong in politics because they lacked the necessary fighting spirit. Writing in 1894, Root explained, "Politics is modified war. In politics there is struggle, strife, contention . . . everything which is adverse to the true character of woman."[52]

Undiscouraged, women co-opted militaristic images such as those used by Root to justify their involvement in politics. Suffragists argued that mothers, like soldiers, provided a service to the nation by raising future generations. Like military service, motherhood demanded that those involved be willing to sacrifice their lives, as many women did while giving birth. Hence, suffragists contended, society should reward women, like men, with the right to participate in the political process.[53]

Reformers began to draw more frequent comparisons between childbirth and military service during World War I. Child welfare advocates, including a young Mary Breckinridge, advanced their cause with arguments that resembled those of the suffragists. Child welfare reformers did not push for women's rights per se but used military metaphors to encourage increased attention to the high maternal and infant mortality rates that plagued the nation.[54]

Having witnessed the interest this comparison generated during World War I, Breckinridge invoked it again when war broke out in 1939. She created a new publicity brochure and titled it the *American Appeal*.[55] In it, she urged donors not to "give one penny to the Service that [they] had intended to send to the Allies," but she stressed that contributors must also continue to support the home front.[56] "War is hard on women and children as well as men," she reminded patrons.[57] The FNS would continue to ensure that the families of servicemen had the best care possible, she promised. Although they were not fighting or producing war materials, FNS nurses' work constituted "patriotism of a high order put to practical use."[58]

Breckinridge's goal of making maternity safer for the women of Appalachia fit nicely into the agenda of Progressive Era reformers, but by the 1940s, her pledge to "save helpless mothers and babies" had begun to appear passé and overly sentimental. Breckinridge felt that using military metaphors would allow her to update the service's image. She still emphasized self-sacrifice and devotion, but she did so in a way that highlighted her patients' bravery and boldness rather than their helplessness. War came periodically and appeared more spectacular, but childbirth called women to sacrifice their lives just as bravely and without fanfare.

To prove her assertion that childbirth had been more dangerous than war, Breckinridge conducted extensive research. She painstakingly calculated casualty figures from the Mexican War, the Civil War, the Spanish–American War, and World War I. Then she estimated the average yearly number of maternal deaths, using figures from birth registration and census records. She conferred with Dr. Louis Dublin, president of the American Public Health Association, and with representatives from the U.S. Children's Bureau, the *New York Times*, the U.S. Bureau of the Census, the *Louisville Courier-Journal*, and the National Geographic Society to obtain information and to seek advice on her methodology. Based on her findings, she concluded that childbirth historically had indeed been more dangerous than military service. "Death and mutilation —mutilation and death, that is the lot of thousands of women every year throughout the generations."[59]

Breckinridge's new fund-raising pitches brought only limited success. Donations rose slightly but never approached predepression levels. Contributions to the service's endowment grew, but annual subscriptions continued to decline. Between 1940 and 1945, Breckinridge added $184,000 to the organization's endowment. The interest this fund earned allowed her to compensate for the smaller return from subscriptions. In the summer of 1945, Breckinridge reported that the endowment fund had topped the $400,000 mark. Her goal of raising $500,000 was in sight. She optimistically looked to the future, noting that $1,000,000 now seemed possible.[60]

The decline in subscriptions and the simultaneous rise in endowment contributions illustrate a shift in the FNS's support base in the early 1940s. As the service aged, so too did its donors. As many of the organization's initial benefactors who had been drawn to the FNS's racialized mission began to die, they left legacies to the FNS. Their gifts provided for the service's long-term stability, but the loss of their yearly subscriptions translated into a decline in funds for operating expenses. Recognizing that the restrictions donors placed on gifts would prohibit her from using funds in the way she felt would most benefit the service, Breckinridge requested that contributors designate their legacies as "unrestricted." She explained with great confidence that this way, three or four hundred years hence, the FNS's trustees could use the income to meet the unique needs of future generations.[61]

AS SHE did every year, Adeline Cashmore wrote to Mary Breckinridge on January 23, 1944, commemorating the anniversary of her son's passing. Twenty-six years after the young boy's unexpected death, Cashmore remembered the child she had never met and reassured his still-grieving mother that he was better off in his new home. He had escaped the cruelty and hatred of this second war and instead was "free." Cashmore rejoiced, "As the years go by and war makes us feel very old . . . I think of that young unsullied life, clothed in the very light of God and feel so thankful."[62]

Knowing that her organization had improved the lives of other women's babies helped Breckinridge cope with the grief that had once threatened to consume her. Children at whose births FNS nurses had assisted during the service's first year of operation were now old enough to fight overseas, and many had enlisted. Breckinridge reported that recruits from FNS territory proved to be "extremely healthy young men," impressing officials in their "superior fitness."[63] Although Breckie did not live to serve in World War II or to become a "leader of men," as his mother had dreamed, she could revel in the contributions of an entire generation of FNS "sons" who had answered the call of their country.[64]

Breckinridge honored the sacrifices made by local boys and FNS employees participating in the war effort by setting up a Victory Shrine Chapel at Wendover. By 1945, she had recorded the names of 934 Leslie County residents who had joined the armed services. A flag hanging in the chapel memorialized twenty-nine area men who had given their lives to defend freedom.[65] A separate list recognized the contributions of FNS staff members who had left to serve their countries. Breckinridge eagerly awaited the reunions that would take place when the war ended. More than simply colleagues and neighbors, FNS employees and patients had become her family, and her family would not be complete until everyone returned home.

The war forced the FNS to make serious readjustments in how it did business, from tailoring its fund-raising message to reflect the current crisis to dealing with shortages in supplies such as diapers and horseshoes.[66] The most serious threat, however, came as service employees departed. As the organization responded to this staffing crisis, however, the FNS' expanded its mission, increasing its long-term impact. By 1945, the FGSM had graduated thirty-six nurse-midwives. These new medical professionals went on to serve in fourteen American states as well as in such far-flung countries as Liberia, China, and India. They carried with them Breckinridge's concept of rural health care.[67] Although the FNS never established the satellite services its director envisioned, it indeed had the larger impact for which she hoped.

T he war forced members of the Frontier Nursing Service (FNS) to part with old friends, but instead of weakening the bonds staff shared, the crisis helped to strengthen the female culture that characterized the organization. The women who remained with the service from 1939 to 1945 began to see the FNS as more than a source of employment. They came to view the organization as their family and to consider Leslie County their home. Furthermore, Mary Breckinridge started to see her staff as more than just employees. During the war, she began to depend for emotional sustenance less on fellow reformers such as Lucille "Pansy" Turner and Adeline Cashmore and instead turned to her FNS colleagues for support, love, and encouragement.

WORLD WAR II required American women to become more autonomous than they had been at any previous time. Once criticized for working outside the home, women now found the media and the government suddenly encouraging them to demonstrate their patriotism by taking positions in war industries and in newly created female armed services divisions. To convince women that they could perform the skills these jobs required, advertisements drew comparisons between traditional female domestic tasks and war work. Any woman, propagandists asserted, could be the next Rosie the Riveter. One advertisement promised that cutting out airplane parts differed little from cutting out dress patterns. Women responded enthusiastically to assurances that they could perform tasks that most Americans considered men's work. The number of American women working outside the home increased by 55 percent between 1940 and 1945. By the end of the war, women comprised 40 percent of aircraft industry workers and 34 percent of all ammunition industry employees.[1]

Unlike their peers who needed the call of patriotism to convince them that it was appropriate for women to work outside the home, FNS nurses, secretaries, and couriers had been challenging societal views of acceptable female behavior since the service's inception.[2] Observers have compared joining the service to joining the Peace Corps today since it offered "excitement, adventure, and independence to the dedicated" at a time when women had few similar opportunities.[3] When Breckinridge established the FNS, she purposely created a female organization. She designed a service directed by a woman, staffed by women, and devoted to improving conditions mothers faced.

Breckinridge did not consciously seek to challenge traditional gender norms when she created the FNS. Her decision to work with mothers and children fit nicely with society's conception of the issues with which women should concern themselves. Locating the FNS in a rural area that, in the words of one observer, could "hardly be considered a woman's land," however, necessitated that Breckinridge and her nurses become independent from men. The director quickly learned that her demonstration could not succeed unless she and the women she employed stopped designating duties as specifically men's or women's work and willingly performed any task that confronted them.[4]

The rural environment in which they operated required FNS nurse-midwives to display a high level of autonomy. In theory, they were supposed to conduct only normal deliveries and to call physicians when complications arose. Breckinridge granted, however, that the "frontier nurse-midwife" often had to "hold the fort" until the medical director arrived. Doctors frequently could not reach struggling patients in time. In such cases, nurses had to be prepared to intervene to save patients' lives.[5] One FNS nurse-midwife, Grace Reeder, recalled that she and her colleagues developed close relationships with God, often relying on prayer to help them through risky cases.[6] The FNS's *Medical Routine* acknowledged that a nurse-midwife on occasion had to overstep the boundaries of her position and authorized her to "act according to her own judgment" on the condition that she immediately report her actions to a supervisor.[7] Many nurse-midwives at first were intimidated by the idea of making critical decisions on their own without physicians' help, but most of these women grew to enjoy the independence the FNS offered. One former employee admitted that after working for Breckinridge, she was sure she would be unable to return to caring for patients "on the outside," where she would be unable to "give an aspirin . . . without a doctor's order."[8]

Through her work with the FNS, Breckinridge realized that despite the strict limitations society placed on females, women could perform any task if they approached it with an open mind. Her confidence in her abilities grew as she raised increasingly large sums of money and as she built a national reputation for her work. As Breckinridge became more comfortable taking on non-traditional roles, she became more insistent that her staff too accept new assignments.

Employees frequently balked at the expectations Breckinridge placed on them, arguing that they were not equipped to handle the tasks she assigned. Staff members repeatedly observed that they found the director's demands intimidating. One of her secretaries claimed that when she first arrived at Wendover, she was so scared of her new boss that she periodically would go to her room and scream in frustration.[9] Another assistant similarly recalled that she was terrified of making a mistake. If "Mrs. Breckinridge" gave an order, she explained, "you [did] it whether you [could] or not."[10]

Employees learned quickly that their new positions required more than nursing and midwifery skills. Only two months after Gladys Peacock and Mary B. Willeford joined the service in 1926, Breckinridge sent them to construct a new nursing center at Beech Fork. When they protested that they lacked building knowledge, Breckinridge simply replied that she had known nothing when she built Wendover, and "if [she] could learn by doing, so could they."[11] The nurses' assignment took them to the middle of a forest, thirty-two miles from the nearest town. When they arrived at the site of the future clinic, twenty-five local men were there to greet them, waiting for orders. Neither the nurses nor the workmen, Peacock recalled, knew anything about construction. "We knew that they knew nothing, but fortunately they did not know that we knew nothing, and our chief job was to keep them from knowing," she explained.[12] Eager to please Breckinridge, Peacock and Willeford boldly instructed the assembled men to prepare the foundation. By the time the center was completed, the nurses had become carpentry experts. Peacock proudly recalled, "Soon we knew just as much about the requirements for a perfect joist or rafter as we did about the requirements for a blue ribbon baby."[13] Equipped with their new skills, Peacock and Willeford went on to supervise the construction of four more nursing centers.[14]

Like Peacock and Willeford, Agnes Lewis quickly discovered that it was impossible to refuse an order from Breckinridge. Lewis served as the director's administrative assistant, but her primary responsibility was maintenance and construction of FNS facilities. Many people commented that Lewis did not look like the type of person who would oversee septic tanks, retaining walls, and wells. Colleagues described her as a southern gentlewoman, small in stature and quiet in demeanor.[15] And Lewis was quick to point out that these skills, considered so unusual in a woman, did not come naturally to her. Only at Breckinridge's insistence did she find the courage to take responsibility for overseeing FNS facilities. Claiming to lack a mechanical or mathematical mind, Lewis recalled, saved her "not a bit." Breckinridge thought "that if you had a B.A. degree after your name, you ought to be able to do everything."[16] Unable to convince her boss that she did not have the skills necessary to supervise work sites and to oversee maintenance workers, Lewis resigned herself to her plight. She recognized that if she wanted to continue working for the FNS, she would have "to live with two-by-fours, number sixteen common nails, sleepers, joists, sills, and the like."[17]

Couriers especially had to step out of their comfort zone to meet Breckinridge's expectations. Working with the FNS, one former volunteer explained, forced them to leave their "sheltered existence" and "look . . . at life" in a new way. These young women arrived in "lovely riding boots and the most elegant jodhpurs" but soon found themselves rising at dawn, sleeping on cots, and standing in line to brush their teeth. Tasks they would never have imagined performing, such as leading livestock over the mountains between nursing centers, became routine.[18] The first couriers Breckinridge recruited were all young men, but by the early 1930s she had switched to using college-aged women in these roles.[19] The reasons for this change are unclear, but young women may simply have fit better in the female world she had created.

Breckinridge challenged the women she employed to abandon their ingrained ideas concerning acceptable female behavior. Society dictated that women did not perform heavy labor or supervise male workers, but the demanding nature of the FNS's work required staff to ignore traditional prescriptions regarding what women could be and do. As one of the organization's nurse-midwives proudly pointed out, an individual could not effectively serve in a rugged environment such as Leslie County without learning "to be a horsewoman, stable boy, mechanic, carpenter, plumber, acrobat, teacher and bluffer."[20] When nurses, couriers, and secretaries left the FNS, they did so with new skills and a heightened confidence in their abilities. One nurse learned that she had the "gift of the divining rod" while working for the FNS.[21] Soon after joining the service, another nurse-midwife reported, "I am learning about oil lamps when the electricity fails, about spark plugs, thermostats, distributors, radiators and stubborn jacks. . . . Think of the vast store of knowledge I'll have acquired by the time I leave here!!"[22]

ON THE eve of World War II, FNS employees were accustomed to performing tasks many women would have considered impossible. The war, however, required Breckinridge and her staff to shoulder an even greater burden. Many nonessential jobs such as painting and upkeep on buildings were abandoned during the course of the war, but Breckinridge's staff had no choice but to take on other duties. As local men enlisted or left to find employment in war industries, FNS nurses had to assume responsibility for tasks for which they had formerly paid their neighbors. Likewise, as a series of medical directors joined the war effort, FNS nurse-midwives had to accept greater responsibility for clinical care.

Couriers shouldered many of the added responsibilities. They loaded hay and sawdust, drove delivery trucks, and even learned to shoe horses. In the *Quarterly Bulletin*, Breckinridge reflected on how her staff had met the challenges the war brought, noting, "It is satisfying to know how many things women can do in wartime."[23] Breckinridge was especially proud of former couriers who joined the military. After hearing that Helen "Pebble" Stone had signed on as a pilot with the Women's Auxiliary Service Pilots (WASPs), Breckinridge praised her decision to accept such a dangerous position.[24] Years later, when looking back over her life, Stone explained that her experience with the FNS was the catalyst that inspired her to join the WASPs: "Simply living at Wendover broadened my horizons. I had never dreamed of becoming an airplane pilot but at FNS anything was possible."[25]

On one hand, Breckinridge applauded women such as Stone who accepted exciting roles; on the other, she still clung to her belief that motherhood was a woman's ultimate calling. She relived her own personal struggle of forty years earlier as she watched former courier Marion Shouse decide whether to join the Women's Auxiliary Army Corps (WAACs) or to marry a longtime suitor. Early in the war, the young woman sought the FNS director's advice on how best to contribute to the war effort. She explained that she wanted to work in some capacity that involved danger because she could not stand to sit by as others suffered. Breckinridge heartily endorsed Shouse's decision to serve overseas with the WAACs and penned a response to this effect. Before Shouse received her mentor's reply, however, she wrote again to inform Breckinridge that she had accepted her suitor's proposal. Breckinridge hastily telegraphed Shouse, applauding her final decision as enthusiastically as she had her earlier resolution. Although she affirmed new roles for women, she could not shake the lesson her parents had so carefully taught her: marriage and family were a woman's most important responsibility.[26]

BEYOND MAKING female employees more confident of their abilities, the challenges of war helped to build a sense of camaraderie among service employees. A fire destroyed the Garden House, the FNS's main office building and staff housing unit, in January 1942 but reinforced this growing unity. The financial costs of replacing the structure and its occupants' belongings seemed minimal when compared to the value of the FNS records lost in the fire, which reflected the service members' collective hard work and shared purpose. After local men and staff gained control of the blaze, Dorothy Buck, Breckinridge's assistant director, cabled their leader, who was in New York for a speaking engagement. In her telegram, Buck broke the news that despite secretaries' attempts to save the statistical files, the records from the service's fifth thousand maternity cases, which had not yet been tabulated, had been "reduced to black powder."[27] The staff spent the day following the fire dipping surviving papers into water and covering them with sawdust to stop them from smoldering. According to Buck, the process was "nearly as back-breaking as it was heart-breaking."[28] Dr. Louis Dublin, the FNS's volunteer statistician, urged Breckinridge to remember the lives the FNS had helped to save, not the records that had been lost.[29]

The FNS by the 1940s functioned as a tight-knit community, or what sociologists call a "total institution." In such environments, daily activities—work, sleep, and play—take place in one location, within the confines of the institution. Members of total institutions are surrounded by the same people day in and day out, and daily activities become carefully planned and ritualized. Perhaps most importantly, total institutions develop well-defined goals or a well-defined mission, which all participants understand and work to advance. Prisons, army barracks, boarding schools, monasteries, and even mental institutions can be examples of total institutions.[30]

Not all women felt at home in such an insular environment. Ruth Boswell, a former FNS staff member, recalled that "people at Wendover [were] a tight little group and you [had] to be a certain kind of person to fit in."[31] Many nurses, couriers, and secretaries, however, felt completely at ease within this female world and made lifelong commitments to the service, even choosing to be buried in the organization's private cemetery. For these individuals, the service became a surrogate family and Leslie County became a permanent home.[32] Breckinridge and her staff socialized informally with area residents, but FNS employees spent most of their free time with each other.[33] Nurses, couriers, and secretaries developed deep friendships that often lasted long after they moved on to new projects.

Similar goals, values, and hobbies united women who made lifetime commitments to the FNS. Employees shared Breckinridge's belief that mothers and babies were a precious resource that must be protected at any cost. They identified with the imagery so often employed by the director in fund-raising material that portrayed FNS nurses as an invading "army" set to do battle against the forces that threatened mountain women and children. Service employees were prepared to commit themselves fully to their new work, just as a soldier would sacrifice everything to defend his or her country. The service often held up the deceased Nancy O'Driscoll to illustrate the seriousness of nurses' commitment. O'Driscoll's funeral, patterned after official military ceremonies and led by a riderless horse and "a corps of nurses in uniform," reminded both nurses and observers of the importance of the organization's work and the bravery of its staff.[34]

Long-term service employees shared Breckinridge's philosophy of total dedication. Nurses such as Betty Lester internalized the FNS's mission of service. Lester explained that during her forty-three-year career with the organization, she strove to live up to the high standards that Breckinridge demanded. FNS employees, she recalled, did not smoke in other people's houses and did not drink. "We had to remember we were the Frontier Nursing Service [and] not let the service down. . . . We were very careful about that," she remembered.[35]

Those who settled permanently in Leslie County tended to regard fulfilling work as more important than monetary reward and appreciated the slower pace a rural environment offered. In an article published in the *Journal of American Nursing*, Buck advised, "Those looking for high salaries; those who find their pleasure only in concerts, plays, picture galleries—those should not seek happiness in the Frontier Nursing Service." The individuals who were most content working for the organization, according to Buck, were those who enjoyed the company of dogs and horses and those who preferred quiet wooded paths to crowded city sidewalks.[36]

Still, even women who valued the simpler lifestyle the FNS offered found the transition to their new work difficult. For many, the trip to Hyden was an unforgettable initiation. British nurses in particular had little idea of what to expect. The director sent each new employee detailed travel instructions, but they had to find their way on their own. The trip was exhausting. After docking in New York, nurses traveled to Lexington, where they were fitted for uniforms. Then they boarded a night train for Hazard or Krypton, the closest rail stations. Most, tired from their travels thus far, were surprised to learn that they still had to ride another twenty-five miles on horseback before reaching Wendover.[37]

Fifty years after she arrived in Leslie County in 1928, Lester, a Briton, clearly recalled her panic after disembarking from the train that had carried her to Krypton. Watching the train chug off around the bend, she stood quietly, "a mountain on one side and a mountain on the other . . . not a soul in sight." According to Lester, she never felt lonelier in her life.[38] Couriers met new employees at the train station and led them the remaining distance to Wendover. Helen Browne recalled that when she arrived in 1938, she was greeted by a courier holding a pair of riding pants. Challenging Browne's sense of decency, the courier instructed her to change into them "right . . . in the middle of the road." They then mounted horses and made the final leg of the journey over rough terrain, the likes of which Browne and many of her fellow newcomers had never seen.[39] One nurse recalled that after her trip ended, "nothing seemed impossible."[40]

New employees were not always prepared for what they found when they arrived at Wendover. For example, the new Hyden Hospital secretary, eager to make a good impression on her first day, came attired in her best business dress and heels. A hat with a white gardenia completed her ensemble. She did not expect that she would have to travel by jeep for five miles through the rain and wind. Nor did she foresee having to share the vehicle with several pigs. The experience did not discourage her, however. She reported that she arrived "windblown, drenched, muddy and smelly—but happy."[41]

Similarly, Lewis expressed surprise after arriving at her new workplace in 1930. When she accepted a position with the FNS, she assumed that she would be working in Lexington. After receiving travel instructions to Wendover and failing to find the obscure location on the map, she became "absolutely sick." Her dread only worsened when she arrived in Hyden. She immediately received orders to carry her suitcase and lead a small child nearly one mile up a steep mountain to the hospital. At that point, Lewis considered going home, but she decided to try out her new position temporarily. She ultimately stayed until 1967, when she retired.[42]

To ease employees' adjustments to their new roles, Breckinridge assigned senior nurses to mentor new recruits. Experienced staff helped their green counterparts plan their days, learn to ride, and find their way around the area. After this introduction, inexperienced nurses acted as "floaters," filling in wherever needed until they could prove themselves. Only when they were completely acclimated to their new surroundings were they assigned their own districts.[43]

Over time, FNS employees created a unique work culture that allowed them to adjust to responsibilities and challenges that came with serving in an unfamiliar, rural environment and allowed them to reconcile their feminine nurturing sides with the independent, strenuous work they were expected to perform. In *The Physicians' Hand: Work Culture and Conflict in American Nursing* (1982), Barbara Melosh defines "work culture" as measures employed by workers to resist or adapt to the pressures that managers, employers, or the work itself imposes.[44] In the case of FNS employees, distinctive uniforms, masculine nicknames, and daily and seasonal rituals became key aspects of the work culture that developed and facilitated the process of identity reformulation that signified their adjustment to their new environment.[45]

The ideas and habits Breckinridge and her nurses brought to the FNS from their days as students in hospital training programs heavily shaped the organization's work culture. Designed to mold young ladies into disciplined caregivers, nursing schools were highly regimented institutions. Teachers and supervisors scrutinized students' behavior in classrooms, on wards, and even in dormitories. According to Melosh, "The insularity of the schools and the intensity of hospital life comprised a powerful rite of passage." Students were required to put others' needs above their own, often for the first time in their lives. Moreover, their new role forced them to embrace sickness and death and to overcome their natural squeamishness.[46] To cope, nursing students established traditions and rituals that eased the contradictions they felt between their old ways of thinking and the new attitudes that supervisors expected them to adopt.

One way nursing students adjusted to their duties was by coining masculine-sounding nicknames for each other. Doing so allowed them to leave old identities behind and helped them to resolve the perceived conflict between their gender and their work.[47] Masculine-sounding nicknames created a sense of camaraderie among FNS nurses resembling that which developed among nursing students. FNS employees rarely called one another by their given names. Instead, they referred to each other by masculine-sounding sobriquets such as Jerry, Jim, Freddy, Sammy, and Harry, most of which the women had acquired as nursing students. Breckinridge encouraged employees to continue using these names.[48]

For couriers in particular, the nicknames ensured that their time with the service would remain vivid in their memories. The FNS provided young debutantes an opportunity to abandon temporarily their middle-class notions of how a young lady should act and to take on a completely new identity. For couriers, nicknames symbolized their brief but life-changing transformation. After couriers returned to their homes and started families of their own, their experience with the FNS remained etched in their minds. Breckinridge ensured this emotional bond would remain strong by addressing letters to couriers using their service nicknames.[49]

Like nicknames, the distinctive uniforms Breckinridge selected provided nurses a further reminder of their days as students and reinforced their new identity as FNS employees. Although they were strangers in an intensely close-knit community, by the 1940s, the FNS uniform ensured them a friendly welcome anywhere they went. In her study of the service's uniform, Donna Parker argues that standardized garments fostered an esprit de corps, "unified staff working towards a common goal[, and made] them feel like a family and team."[50] Each nurse received strict instructions that she must not "dispose of her uniform to anyone outside of the service," further emphasizing the special position held by those wearing the FNS uniform.[51]

Beyond nicknames and uniforms, rituals helped build bonds among staff members and added to the FNS's role as a total institution. Afternoon tea was a sacred event for Wendover residents. All work stopped precisely at four o'clock, when a courier rang the cowbell to summon everyone to the living room. Clad in their blue jeans and smelling "rather odorous," couriers prepared and served tea and snacks to the assembled staff. New to the ritual, each arriving group of volunteers received detailed instructions from their predecessors on how to prepare Breckinridge's tea just the way she liked it. The director sat in a special chair and dispensed cheese tidbits to the Wendover dogs, while nurses, couriers, and any guests discussed current events or books their host had recently read. The director prohibited discussion of work because she felt that relaxation was necessary if nurses were to maintain their emotional and physical strength.[52]

The distance separating the outpost centers from Wendover prohibited most nurse-midwives from participating in afternoon tea. The district nurses' experiences were very different from those of women who worked at the hospital or lived at the organization's headquarters. The outpost centers were located in the county's most isolated areas. Several centers were not even equipped with telephone connections in the 1940s. Recognizing the crippling loneliness that such isolation could bring, Breckinridge assigned two nurses to each center except when funding problems prevented her from doing so.[53]

The entire FNS staff gathered once each year, at Thanksgiving. Outpost nurses (except those who had to remain at the centers to answer emergency calls) traveled to Wendover for dinner. Before they ate, they always held a moment of silence to honor absent loved ones and then sang a song to celebrate the year's blessings. Those nurses whose schedules allowed them to leave their centers gathered on Christmas and Easter as well. The Fourth of July also provided an excuse to meet and celebrate the service's cultural diversity. American and British nurses tried to outdo each other with skits and their best renditions of their respective national anthems. Daily and holiday rituals brought FNS nurses together and reminded them of the important role they played in a larger enterprise.[54]

THE FNS functioned as a total institution by the 1940s, with a clearly defined purpose, a centralized structure, and a definite culture—a distinctly female culture. Visitors' descriptions of the service illustrate well the noticeable way gender shaped its identity. Anne Mulhauser, a courier who served during the summer of 1935, described the FNS as a "woman's world."[55] Similarly, another volunteer recalled that coming to Wendover was an eye-opening experience, allowing her for the first time to live within "a community of self-sufficient women."[56]

A young man who visited the FNS during the summer of 1939 vividly described the all-female world he found. "My time at Wendover," he reported, "was one of the few times in my life I've regretted I wasn't a woman." As a man, he was "utterly worthless, only good to be led around and ordered about" by the organization's staff. He humbly thanked Breckinridge for allowing him "on the premises" to view her work. He insisted that most women, "once they'd won success without much or any assistance from mankind," would treat male visitors as "intruders, as snakes in the manger, wrenches in the machinery, or more appropriately, weasels in the hen roost."[57]

The FNS's distinctly female nature was most evident at Wendover. The ten to twenty women who resided at the organization's headquarters at any given time most clearly experienced the FNS as a total institution. The number of residents at Wendover changed frequently as a result of courier turnover, but mainstays included Breckinridge; Buck; Lewis; Lucile Hodges, the service's bookkeeper; and Jean Hollins, resident courier. Until the early 1970s, there were no staff quarters for men or married couples.[58] On any given evening, one could find "an astonishing number of women and dogs" seated around the fireplace.[59] The sense of solidarity apparent at Wendover led one visitor to compare it to "a reunion in a college dormitory."[60]

The FNS provided a homosocial world not only for its director and its staff but also for its many female donors across the country. Breckinridge had a talent for drawing contributors in and making them feel a personal stake in the organization's work. The *Quarterly Bulletin* and fund-raising literature stressed that every donor was part of the FNS's army engaged in the fight on "the battlefield of motherhood." By reading service publications and often through visits to witness firsthand the service's work, supporters became intimately familiar with the FNS's mission and its personnel. They felt a kinship with Mac, Stevie, and the other nurses, having experienced vicariously their struggles against nature and disease. Supporters were on a first-name basis with the service's horses and responded to equine obituaries posted in the *Bulletin* with kind letters of condolence. By emphasizing the collective danger that all women faced, no matter their geographical location or class status, Breckinridge developed strong allegiances and helped reinforce her organization's female-centered culture.

MARY BRECKINRIDGE grew up in an era that celebrated same-sex friendships and encouraged close bonds between women.[61] Breckinridge married twice, but throughout her life, she looked to other women to provide emotional support, companionship, and reassurance. Whether with boarding-school classmates, fellow workers with the Comité Américain pour les Régions Dévastées de la France, or FNS donors and employees, Breckinridge spent the majority of her life within a female world. She was an intensely private person, but when she did share intimate thoughts such as her religious struggles, the debilitating depression that followed the deaths of her children, or her fears that her project would not succeed, she did so with other women. Her mother, Katherine, sought similar companionship from female friends and provided a model that Mary emulated.

Adeline Cashmore remained Breckinridge's closest confidant during the early years of the service's history, but as time went on, they began to write to each other less frequently. After Cashmore moved to India in 1936, the pair had increasing difficulty keeping in touch. In a letter to Adeline's sister, Maud Cashmore, Breckinridge lamented, "Between Kentucky and India, the communications are the slowest, I am sure, between any two points on this planet."[62] Despite lengthy silences, Adeline Cashmore continued to keep Breckinridge in her thoughts and prayers after war broke out. She looked forward to the day when they would reunite. "When this horror is over there will be so many aeroplanes on hand perhaps you will come over that way and we shall look once more upon each other," Cashmore suggested hopefully.[63] To overcome adversity during the FNS's earliest years, Breckinridge had depended on the encouragement and advice she received from the Cashmores and Pansy Turner. Knowing that her friends were praying for the service provided her with needed confidence. As the years passed, however, Breckinridge began to require less reassurance. By 1940, as she approached the age of sixty, her organization was well established and God's plan for her life appeared evident. Consequently, she relied less and less on Adeline Cashmore's words of praise and comfort.

As Breckinridge drifted away from her friends overseas, she formed stronger friendships with members of the FNS staff. From the start, she had been looking to re-create the intense bonds that she had experienced in France, but her need to establish her authority as director had prevented her from growing too close to her FNS colleagues. Breckinridge served as the matriarch of her organization —"Lord of the Place" and "Commander-in-Chief."[64] Breckinridge's relationship with most service employees was authoritative, and many of them found her demanding and intimidating.

By the 1940s, however, as she aged and as her position of authority grew more secure, she began to let high-ranking service employees into her inner circle. She particularly developed close relationships with her two assistant directors, Dorothy Buck and Anne "Mac" MacKinnon. MacKinnon had joined the service in 1928, and as superintendent of Hyden Hospital, she had become Breckinridge's confidant. As Breckinridge explained, Mac "was woven into the very fabric of the FNS," and when she left to return to Britain in 1940, her departure "maimed" the organization.[65] Buck, an American, remained with the FNS during the war, providing Breckinridge with much-needed assistance and support. Like Mac, Buck had joined the service in 1928, and her long tenure made her an important resource. However, Breckinridge valued "the Bucket's" companionship even more than her experience and history with the organization. "Never have my friendships seemed as precious to me as now," Breckinridge remarked during the war.[66]

In April 1945, Breckinridge received word that Adeline Cashmore had died in India. Breckinridge grieved the loss but continued to feel that Cashmore was with her in spirit. She explained, "I am one of those people who needed a great saint. . . . I am sure that the Frontier Nursing Service has Adeline's protection forever."[67] With her dear friend gone, Breckinridge grew to value FNS employees' companionship even more during the remaining years of her life.

SOON AFTER Adeline's death, Breckinridge found reason to celebrate. On May 7, 1945, after hearing that the war in Europe had ended, Breckinridge and her staff shared a bottle of sherry that she had been saving to honor the occasion.[68] They looked forward to the announcement of victory in Asia, when the war would finally draw to a close. Breckinridge longed for the day when old friends would come home. Only then could life return to normal.

ten *Wide Neighborhoods*

The years following World War II represented a period of significant transition for both Mary Breckinridge and the Frontier Nursing Service (FNS). One by one, FNS staff members who had left at the start of the conflict began filtering back, and each received a joyful welcome. The nurse-midwives returned eager to resume work on their districts, but changes were afoot. Leslie County was no longer the same place Breckinridge and the FNS had first come to serve. The war had given the county's economy, particularly the coal industry, a needed shot in the arm. The arrival of electricity and paved roads had eroded its isolation. Breckinridge's advancing age influenced how she viewed these changes. She was nearly sixty-five years old when the Allies signed the armistice, and with the advent of Social Security, that age had become a common milestone of retirement. Breckinridge did not retire, but her priorities gradually shifted. After 1945, she concerned herself less with expanding her organization and instituting new ideas and more with crafting a legacy for herself and holding onto power.

By 1945, the FNS not only was well known among medical practitioners, many of who had come to Wendover to study firsthand its director's methods, but also had become a household name.[1] In the 1920s, the service attracted a sizable following among middle- and upper-class women. Over the course of the next two decades, news of the brave "nurses on horseback" spread. Newspaper and magazine reports, full-length monographs, and radio broadcasts featured tales of the frontier nurses' attempts to fight poverty and disease in the mountains.[2] This publicity came at a cost, however. Too often, outsiders focused on the "unusual and picturesque" and wrote sensational and inaccurate accounts, forcing FNS staff to commit precious energy to repairing the damage.[3] Breckinridge's experiences working with authors and filmmakers in the 1940s convinced her that the price of media coverage was too high. Only she could provide a truthful, unbiased record. Her autobiography, *Wide Neighborhoods*, completed in 1952, represented her attempt to provide a definitive account of the FNS. Through this book, she attempted to solidify her spot in history.

IN THE FNS's early years, Breckinridge recognized that publicity was necessary, but from the start she worried that reporters might twist her words. The director carefully controlled everything printed about the FNS, even demanding that the service's publicity offices submit press releases for her to edit.[4] She gave the publicists she hired in the 1930s careful guidelines, cautioning them to avoid writing or saying anything that would upset physicians or the Appalachian people. In particular, she instructed her publicists to avoid romanticizing Leslie County. "After all," she astutely observed, "we are a scientific organization and however much romance may appeal to the average newspaper reader, it is not going to help us at all in real contributors who want to put their money into an organization which they feel is thoroughly conservative and efficient."[5] Breckinridge felt that as a well-bred southern woman, she had a duty never to embarrass anyone in written or verbal publicity; hence, she carefully scrutinized all accounts of her organization's work.[6]

During the 1930s, when she was still striving to establish a reputation for the service, she allowed two authors to write full-length monographs about the FNS.[7] She edited the books but became frustrated when she could not control the content of the reviews the books received. Following a November 1943 radio broadcast, Breckinridge assured readers of the *Quarterly Bulletin* that she was not responsible for the segment's content. She noted that this was the second time that the service had been "exploited over the air under the guise of giving a book review of *Nurses on Horseback*." She could not understand "how any individual or public agency [could] be so lacking in ethics as to exploit a charity for personal gain."[8] Breckinridge believed that too many authors were motivated not by a sincere desire to help the FNS but by economic and professional self-interest.

By the 1940s, when the FNS had gained a wide following, Breckinridge increasingly viewed publicity, even that written by "ladies and gentlemen" of integrity, as a liability to her organization. Every time a magazine article was published, service employees spent weeks answering the resulting "mass of useless letters," which rarely included checks. Breckinridge lamented that most came from young girls who had no nursing training but who expressed a desire to come to Appalachia and uplift its poor, downtrodden residents. More often than not, published accounts of the FNS's work contained untruths that Breckinridge and her staff had to spend time refuting for fear that these inaccurate portrayals would offend patients, donors, or staff.[9] The director eventually demanded that every author allow her to review personally every magazine article written about the service before it went into print. She made reporters sign an agreement to this effect before she would even allow them to visit Wendover. In one case, after she finished with revisions, *American Magazine* refused to publish the piece because her cuts had been so extensive.[10] Breckinridge became so wary of publicity by 1950 that she required students who wrote term papers about the FNS to submit copies for her approval before they turned in their reports.[11] Breckinridge no longer trusted anyone outside the service accurately to depict its work.

DURING THE war years, patriotic Americans seeking uplifting tales of bravery and dedication took a special interest in the FNS's work. Media outlets hoping to capitalize on the nation's fascination with such stories barraged Breckinridge with requests for interviews. Several motion picture companies expressed interest in capturing the service's story on film. Breckinridge at first welcomed the idea and actively pursued a deal with Metro-Goldwyn-Mayer (MGM), one of the nation's leading film production companies. She recognized that appearing on the big screen would significantly increase her organization's exposure, and she undoubtedly was flattered by the attention. She stipulated, however, that she would approve the project only if she were allowed to control the film's content.[12]

As the FNS and MGM grew closer to reaching an agreement, Breckinridge began to have second thoughts, remembering how often outside publicity had backfired. She used the war as an excuse to stall, explaining that her organization could not possibly embark on any new projects due to its shortage of nurses.[13] MGM representatives recognized that her excuses were in reality "adroit diplomacy."[14] Concerned that the deal would fall through, MGM's representative reassured her that he understood her "phobias" and that such worries, though "without reality," were inevitable when one undertook a completely new venture.[15] Despite MGM's reassurance that she would have editorial control over the film, Breckinridge continued to hold the filmmakers at arm's length.

In the interim, several other agents contacted her, eager to produce a movie about her work. She politely but firmly rejected these companies' offers. Raising her ire, one of these agencies, Republic Productions, informed Breckinridge that it intended to move forward with its project with or without her permission. Republic's representative initially tried to change her mind with flattery. If she refused to work with Republic, William Saal warned, she would be preventing a world that needed "good doses of humanitarianism and brotherly love" from learning about the altruistic deeds that she and her fellow workers performed. In case she remained unconvinced, Saal reminded her that she was not the originator of the broad concept of "frontier nursing." Rather, unselfish individuals had been providing this service since the birth of the United States. He would move ahead with his plan to create a film that would be "authentic, interesting and inspiring to the great world-wide audiences who cry for enlightenment," even if she chose not to cooperate.[16]

Breckinridge remained unmoved by Saal's mixture of adulation and threats and immediately took steps to respond to the "repugnant" letter.[17] Having already stated her position to no avail, she decided it would be best for the service's national chair, E. S. Jouett, to reiterate the organization's objections. She took the liberty of drafting a letter in Jouett's name, which she asked him to sign. She humbly added that she was not sure that her letter would represent his position and that he was free to make changes. She would defer to his "top legal brain."[18]

In this case, as at other times when she sought advice from the executive committee, Breckinridge framed her letter to highlight her helplessness. She could not "carry the burden alone." She found herself in "terrible" need of Jouett's help. In his response, which was just as predictable in its tone as Breckinridge's request, Jouett assured her that the draft of the letter she planned to send to Republic perfectly stated the FNS's position; he had nothing to add.[19] Cognizant of society's expectation that women should defer to men at all times, Breckinridge adopted a meek tone when corresponding with male members of the executive committee. Yet she always remembered that as the FNS's founder and director, she held a position of power.

Breckinridge became skilled at balancing the contradictory responsibilities of being both a traditional southern woman and the director of a nationally known public health organization. When necessary, she could play the role of a submissive woman, seeking men's protection. However, on other occasions, as when she dealt with reporters, she made it clear that she was the "matriarch" of her organization and maintained absolute control. Breckinridge's secretary described her as a "chameleon," equipped with an amazing ability to adjust to any circumstance in which she found herself. This ability allowed her to communicate equally effectively with the poorest residents of Leslie County and with wealthy northern donors.[20]

MGM representatives continued to court Breckinridge throughout the war. In the late 1940s, she finally agreed to go ahead with the film, convinced that she would have the control over its content that she demanded. Everything was set to begin production in the spring of 1949, but when the agent with whom she had been working left MGM, the deal fell through. Always half-hearted in her support for the project, Breckinridge was not disappointed, and she quietly let the project drop.[21]

BRECKINRIDGE'S EXPERIENCE with a young author named John Day early in the war reinforced her fear that movie producers would sensationalize the work of the FNS and do more damage than good. When Day first contacted Breckinridge about including a chapter on the FNS in the book he planned to write about life in the Kentucky mountains, she was amenable. She judged Day a good candidate to write a monograph that explored the region's culture. He had taught elementary school for several years in eastern Kentucky before deciding to embark on his literary project.[22] She was particularly swayed by the "genuine interest in forest conservation" he expressed.[23] His background and familiarity with the area led Breckinridge to believe that he would write a truthful, sympathetic account.

Breckinridge agreed to cooperate with Day as long as he signed a contract promising to submit any article or book that directly or indirectly mentioned her organization for her approval. She reserved the right to "take out of the manuscript any sections objected to by the Frontier Nursing Service or make any changes . . . in the interest of accuracy and of fairness to the Service and to the people among whom the Service works."[24] Eager to witness FNS nurse-midwives in action, Day signed the contract. He visited the service in September 1940, spending three days attending calls with the nurses and interviewing the director.[25]

Breckinridge did not hear from Day again until the following May, when she received a chapter in the mail along with a request that she check it and return it to him within two weeks so that he could meet his publication deadline. She was incensed that he would expect her to review the manuscript so quickly. In her reply to the author, Breckinridge pointed out that the service's annual meeting was fast approaching, making this the organization's busiest time of the year. In her cursory review of the manuscript, she had discovered numerous inaccuracies. It would be impossible for her to "do so extensive a piece of revision" in such a short time, she concluded. She advised Day either to leave the chapter out or to uphold his agreement to revise the chapter to her specifications.[26]

Breckinridge found several small factual errors in Day's chapter on the FNS—for example, an inaccurate estimate of the distance separating Hazard and Wendover and out-of-date budget figures—but her main complaints centered on his representation of her. She felt unfairly attacked and jumped to defend herself. She specifically pointed out that although she smoked, she never did so while in uniform or while on duty. "This obviously means that at times I go many hours without smoking." She likewise rejected Day's claim that she was strong willed and forced her employees to see things her way. In her rebuttal, she stressed that she mentioned this point not in her own defense but because it called the intelligence and courage of her staff into question. She alleged that Day had falsely obtained this impression from a young typist who had just begun work with the service and therefore had not had time to gauge accurately the relationship between Breckinridge and her employees. She insisted that she had a positive relationship with her staff. She reminded Day that she was old enough to be the mother of most of the FNS's nurses and to be the grandmother of many of the other women. The director argued that her nurses did not fear her but viewed her as most young people viewed older people—with respect.[27]

Day, however, stood his ground. Breckinridge's hostile response took him by surprise. He did not think she would allow herself "to become so vexed" by three or four statements that she would "write such a bitter and cutting tirade." He returned the chapter, revised to her specifications, but could not resist defending himself. He removed the statement that "members of the Service think as Mrs. Breckinridge thinks or else keep their thoughts to themselves." He assured her, however, that many of her coworkers were afraid of her—"or perhaps you would say in awe of you," he sarcastically added. Day stressed that he had the highest regard for the work Breckinridge was doing, and his account was by no means designed as a criticism. However, he reminded her that his goal in writing the chapter had been to "write an objective piece and not a paean."[28] Day viewed her complaints as a bid to protect the glorified reputation she had carefully built for herself and her organization rather than a defense of the truth, as she claimed. Day believed he was providing an "impersonal" account of the FNS's work, neither "mushy [n]or hypercritical."[29] Breckinridge, however, saw his attempt to be objective as challenging the persona she had so diligently cultivated.

Day was surprised that Breckinridge failed to recognize that he was paying her a compliment with such statements as, "She runs her service as a colonel runs his regiment."[30] He saw her as a strong leader and felt that she would find his description flattering. If Breckinridge were to have written her own account of her position within the FNS, it likely would have borne a strong resemblance to Day's portrayal. On many occasions, she had referred to herself and her nurses in military terms, but she always tempered this masculine imagery by highlighting her caring, self-sacrificing feminine side. The disagreement between Breckinridge and Day stemmed in large part from the young author's failure to show her the respect she felt she deserved as an older, successful woman.

THE ANTIPATHY Breckinridge felt for Day, though keen, did not approach her disgust for another young author who published an article about Leslie County in *Life Magazine* in December 1949. T. S. Hyland's essay, "The Fruitful Mountaineers," outraged Breckinridge as well as many residents of Appalachia. As in the case of Day, Breckinridge had cooperated with Hyland, trusting him to write an account that mirrored her own views. Following the publication of the article, she felt that he had betrayed her.

Hyland's report, subtitled "A Biological Joy Ride to Hell," sought to expose Appalachia's outrageously high birthrate, which, he argued, threatened American progress and prosperity. Hyland sarcastically reported that "mountaineers are probably . . . the busiest people on earth." Their birthrate, he claimed, was 48.5 per thousand, nearly double that of the United States as a whole and "equal to that of the swarming hordes of China and India." Lack of birth control was not to blame; instead, he cited area residents' inability to make appropriate decisions and their failure to take advantage of outside assistance. According to Hyland, the Kentucky mountaineers had no excuse for their behavior. They attracted more than their fair share of government aid and had access to some of the best medical care in the country thanks to Mary Breckinridge.[31]

After reading the version of the article that appeared in print, Breckinridge was shocked. Although she remained skeptical of journalists, especially after her disagreement with Day, Hyland had gained her confidence. The issues in which he claimed an interest, such as the drawbacks of government aid and the need for controlled reproduction, seemed to mirror her concerns. She had provided the young reporter a great deal of information because she believed that he was "giving serious consideration to real questions."[32] When Hyland informed Breckinridge that he was "appalled" by Day's "sensationalism" and "disgusted by . . . his stupidity," she felt as though she had found a true ally. Hyland promised to avoid Day's errors and to refute as many of his inaccurate claims as possible.[33]

In November 1949, following the terms of his agreement, Hyland sent Breckinridge a draft of his article for her approval, leading her to believe that she was reading the piece he planned to submit to *Life*. In reality, had had left out most of the controversial sections that would so enrage the people of Leslie County. For example, he explained that he would be adding a section that addressed the question of whether the people of the region were "degenerate morons," as many assumed, or a superior breed of people. Breckinridge was so confident that Hyland's conclusions would match her own that she suggested only minor changes to the article. Hyland assured her that he would make all the corrections that she requested and that he would treat this article "as carefully as if it were a Ph.D. thesis."[34]

Breckinridge first became suspicious of Hyland when her secretaries began to field phone calls from *Life* editors, asking strange questions such as, "Are there any tractors in Leslie County?"[35] Her worst fears were realized when she opened her newly arrived copy of *Life* just days before Christmas to find Hyland's article. The reporter emphasized every degrading stereotype traditionally used to describe the region. The people he portrayed were lazy and simpleminded and found their greatest enjoyment in feuding and in participating in bizarre religious practices.[36]

Not only did Hyland's article mock the Appalachian region, but he also attacked the FNS for enabling area residents' irresponsibility. Hyland indicted Breckinridge for "pampering" the people of Leslie County and for making it easy for them to have so many children. Furthermore, he scoffed at Breckinridge's fund-raising pitch that Appalachia was home to America's best stock and criticized her efforts to convince wealthy urban socialites, "amid a genteel tinkle of teacups," to foot the bill for the area's medical care. His description of Breckinridge as a "small, graciously domineering lady" who displayed "almost ruthless determination" only intensified her anger.[37]

As soon as the December issue of *Life* arrived in American homes, responses to Hyland's article began to fill the FNS's mailbox. As was usually the case, dozens of individuals wrote to inquire if the organization had any jobs available. Several women from surrounding counties wrote to ask for birth control information.[38] The article also inspired a few outraged responses, such as that from a disgruntled man in Iowa who stressed that his state already had a high birthrate and that Iowa did not need any of Kentucky's surplus population spilling over into his area of the country. The best solution, he claimed, would be to build a fence around areas such as Leslie County "so they would have to stew in their own juice."[39]

Leslie County residents expressed outrage at *Life*'s unfair portrayal of their community. Local resident Lee Daniel voiced his complaints with Hyland's account in the local weekly, *Thousandsticks*. Calling Hyland a "lazy glib tongue 2×4, one-gallus, Jack leg scum of the earth," he contended that the people of Leslie, Perry, and surrounding counties had grown weary of the slander and untruths constantly being written about them. They were tired of hearing, "Wher's your jug . . . when was your last feudin' and how many killed?" Hyland's account, Daniel recognized, would "cause many a laugh around a cocktail bar in New York," but in his estimation, it was "the most blackest and damnible lie that ever came from the bottomless pit of Hell."[40] Another editorial suggested that Hyland's piece was a "racket . . . designed to fill someone's pocket."[41]

Residents of nearby Perry County and its county seat, Hazard, also attacked Hyland's article, although for different reasons. The *Hazard Herald* ran a two-page column refuting Hyland's assertions. The *Herald*'s major concern was not that the author had maligned the people of Leslie County but that his report would lead readers similarly to characterize all Appalachian residents.[42] In his compelling study, *Two Worlds in the Tennessee Mountains: Exploring the Origins of Appalachian Stereotypes* (1997), David Hsiung argues for the inaccuracy of the assumption that Americans came to see Appalachia as isolated and backward because "outsiders" pinned these labels on the people residing in mountain areas. Instead, he blames the emergence of these derogatory descriptions on the ideological differences separating residents of more urban regions of Appalachia (nearer rail access) from those who settled in more remote locations on smaller streams. Hsiung claims that the more progressive mountain residents first assigned these labels to their less modern neighbors, unable to foresee that these derisive images would ultimately come to characterize the entire region.[43]

Hazard residents' reactions to the *Life* article well illustrate Hsiung's argument that there were "two worlds . . . in the mountains." Members of the FNS's Hazard Committee pitied their poorer neighbors, much as did members of the Detroit or Boston Committees. Hazard residents resented that they were mistaken for their unsophisticated neighbors. Mary Biggerstaff, a member of the mountain elite, castigated journalists such as Hyland for failing to distinguish between the "layers of society in the mountains." Instead, she recalled with much disdain, "They [made] hillbillies of us all."[44]

No rebuttals of Hyland's article were more vehement than the one offered by Breckinridge. In a letter to a supporter, she described the *Life* report as "the rankest piece of exploitation ever to appear in a modern magazine."[45] In her official response, which she quickly sent off to the *Hazard Herald*, she condemned Hyland's claims that the birthrate in Leslie County was nearly double that found in the rest of the nation. According to Breckinridge, Hyland intentionally inflated the numbers by comparing the 1940 census with the 1948 birthrate, which reflected the rise in population inspired by the coal boom.[46] She compiled her own figures, later printed in the *Quarterly Bulletin*, showing that families in FNS territory were only slightly larger than those found in other areas of the country.[47] She contended that Hyland set out to produce a sensational story, and "if he had told the truth he wouldn't have gotten it."[48]

If Breckinridge wrote directly to *Life* to express her displeasure, the letter has not survived. Breckinridge typically thought it best to ignore such matters rather than to draw further attention to misrepresentations. She explained, "My own feeling is that it is better to let all such things drop like a stone in a well, because they will soon be forgotten."[49] Breckinridge refused to entertain journalists again until 1953 and promised never again to deal with *Life*. Hyland's article engendered such hostility among service members that twenty-one years later, when the magazine asked to print a piece on the FNS, Breckinridge's successor, Helen Browne, refused, citing the publication's reputation for "lurid journalism."[50]

For the rest of her life, Breckinridge remained skeptical of journalists and their motives. She believed that only individuals directly linked to the FNS could accurately represent its work, and even then, she edited their pieces to ensure that no misstatements appeared in print. Breckinridge claimed that she censored media representations simply to protect her patients, but individuals such as Day sensed that her concern went deeper. The director carefully guarded her image as well as that of her organization. She very consciously presented herself in a way that allowed her to balance her feminine self-sacrificing nature with her rational business side. By the late 1940s, Breckinridge's interactions with filmmakers and authors had convinced her that she could not trust anyone but herself to represent her work and to protect her legacy.

BRECKINRIDGE RECOGNIZED that the FNS would outlive her, and she was well aware that the organization's success had won her a place in history. It had become a model for the effective provision of rural health care, with observers coming from around the globe to observe its methods. Descended from a long line of successful politicians and reformers, Breckinridge stood ready to take her place in the pantheon of her esteemed ancestors. She had read historical accounts of her famous relatives that brought to light—whether accurately or inaccurately—their faults and foibles, and now she anxiously sought to determine how future generations would remember her. She had read too many inaccurate accounts of the FNS over the preceding twenty years to trust that anyone other than herself could write a truthful history of the service. Consequently, in 1948, when Harper Brothers Publishing Company suggested that she write an autobiography, she happily consented. Her book, *Wide Neighborhoods: A Story of the Frontier Nursing Service*, appeared on bookshelves four years later.

Beyond simply telling her version of the story, Breckinridge's motivations for writing her autobiography included a desire to provide for the service after her death. Royalties from the book, donated in perpetuity to the FNS, would help to defray the organization's rising yearly operating costs. Moreover, she believed that publishing her autobiography would allow her to sustain donors' interest in the FNS's work. After her death, the book would permit her to continue to speak in person to audiences, as she had each year since the service's founding. She hoped that the book's readers, both faithful donors and those unfamiliar with the FNS, would be captivated by her story and would contribute to the worthwhile cause in the coming years.

Breckinridge claimed to want to accurately portray the events of her life in *Wide Neighborhoods*. Like anyone trying to write an account of his or her life, however, she found it difficult to reveal her most personal thoughts and feelings without destroying the public image that she had created for herself. Unfortunately, scholars who have studied Breckinridge's work have taken her autobiography at face value, failing to recognize how its author carefully crafted the story.[51] *Wide Neighborhoods* provides a useful tool for understanding how Breckinridge viewed her life and her work, but only if the book is carefully deconstructed and analyzed.

BRECKINRIDGE HAD some experience as an author, having edited the Service's *Quarterly Bulletin* for more than twenty years, and she had published her short story, *Organdie and Mull*, in 1948.[52] Much like eighteenth- and nineteenth-century female authors who denigrated their skills and defended their motives for writing, she emphasized that she agreed to publish this piece only because doing so would provide her another way to serve the FNS. When she sent copies of her "novelette" to friends, she humbly suggested that it had "the merit of shortness."[53] The novice author stressed that she wrote not to fulfill a personal need but to raise money for the FNS. She observed that if all one thousand numbered copies sold, the FNS would earn eight hundred dollars, enough to purchase a load of hay. That, she stressed, was "the pith of the matter."[54]

When informing friends that she had made plans to write her autobiography, Breckinridge adopted a similarly humble tone. FNS supporter Margaret Gage and her close friend Gerald Heard, a well-known theologian, first contacted Harper Brothers about publishing the story of the FNS. Breckinridge expressed surprise that anyone would want to read about her life and made it clear to supporters that Harper Brothers had solicited her, adopting the self-denigrating attitude she had been taught to view as appropriate for women. She stressed that she had agreed to the project not so that she could discuss her own accomplishments but so that she could demonstrate that the FNS's success had truly resulted from other, more powerful forces. "It took a child archangel, my son, and a saint, my anchoress, to get enough power into me to accomplish anything," she emphasized.[55] She pragmatically acknowledged that as the FNS's creator and director, she was the organization's best historian, so it made sense for her to record its story.[56]

In spite of her claims, however, Breckinridge was quite flattered and excited about the opportunity to write the book. She was an avid reader and looked forward to trying her hand at authorship. In addition, the idea that others would be interested in her life story stroked her ego. Still, Breckinridge worried that writing an autobiography would require her to share details that she preferred to have remain private. In spite of her very public role, she hesitated to let many people, even her own family, get too close to her. In correspondence with her closest friends, she confided her fears about discussing the painful events of her life. "One does not want to touch one's deepest experiences too fully to let the public read them," she remarked. She hoped that she could convey to readers what they needed to know "without laying bare too much." She predicted that in the process of writing, she would engage in "a lot of shrinking back."[57]

Before she started writing, she carefully considered how to deal with the unpleasant events of her life—most notably, her two marriages and her children's deaths. She assured her sister-in-law, "I am certainly not going to mention my divorce!"[58] Breckinridge candidly discussed her dilemma with her editor: "I am [an] outmoded thing, a seventy year-old gentlewoman." This status, she explained, carried with it certain inhibitions. She advised that she had no plans to discuss her marriages because she was "raised in a period, a part of the world, and a social class" where marriages were not discussed regardless of whether they constituted successful relationships or ended unhappily.[59] The question of how much information to reveal would plague Breckinridge throughout the early stages of writing.

DESPITE HER fears, Breckinridge looked forward to starting the book because it would give her an excuse to escape temporarily her exhausting fund-raising duties. "Now that I have this contract," she informed her editor, "I have a valid reason for shunting off everybody for a long time to come."[60] The burden of keeping the organization solvent, however, would prevent such a luxury unless she found alternative funding. The members of the FNS's board of trustees, eager to relieve their leader's burden, announced in 1949 that they planned to raise fifty thousand dollars among themselves to fund the organization for the next year. This announcement freed the director to devote her energies full time to her new project.[61]

Breckinridge had originally assumed that she would need approximately six months to research and write the book. With her consent, Harper Brothers set March 1951 as the intended publication date.[62] As she launched into writing, however, she quickly realized that the project would be significantly more time-consuming than she had first anticipated. Immediately following the organization's May 1950 annual meeting, Breckinridge began writing. She adopted a strict schedule, rising each morning at four o'clock. While drinking her coffee, she said her daily devotional. From five o'clock to seven o'clock, she revised the previous day's dictation. She took a break between seven and eight. From eight o'clock until lunch, she dictated new material to her secretary. At two o'clock, she returned to the book, researching the next chapter until four o'clock, when the staff gathered for tea. She went to bed at eight in the evening to ensure that she would be well rested to begin the next day's work. This demanding schedule allowed her to reach her goal of composing five thousand words each week.[63]

Breckinridge approached the story of her life much as she did any other medical problem she attempted to solve—that is, with research. She carefully searched through old letters and records to be sure that the "facts" she included were accurate.[64] She recognized that although she could usually remember events, it was often hard to recall "the accompanying feelings and thoughts of the time." However, she believed that if she based her autobiography on her detailed journals and abundant correspondence, she could write a completely factual account of the past. She felt that these documents would allow her to "return to [her] youth" and find it "unaltered, [and] unchanged by the long variations of years."[65]

She felt compelled to record painstakingly every detail because she expected this book to become the definitive account of her life. To ensure that such was the case, she planned to destroy all her correspondence and journals after completing the book. She wrote to old friends, requesting that they send back her letters so she could refer to them while she was writing. She would not return the letters, she warned. Fearful that they would one day be "combed through by others," she was adamant that her acquaintances allow her to burn them.[66]

The book consumed Breckinridge's waking and often sleeping hours. She frequently rose in the middle of the night to jot ideas on pieces of scrap paper. In the morning, when her staff came in for the daily conference, she would hand them her notes and ask, "What have I written here?" Her handwriting at its best was barely legible. Her scrawls, recorded in the dark when she was semiconscious, were cryptic. Helen Browne recalled that senior staff members would turn the notes upside down and sideways, trying to read them. If they could decipher a single word, Breckinridge could usually remember what she had been thinking.[67]

The director worked throughout the summer of 1950, eager to finish the biographical section of the book so that she could move on to what she viewed as the most important part, the founding of the FNS. By fall, she had finished discussing her childhood and young adult years. In a letter to her niece, Marvin Breckinridge Patterson, Mary Breckinridge wrote that the younger woman would be "enchanted" at how her aunt had "glide[d] over things like divorces and deaths."[68] She felt as though she had revealed just enough personal information, and all in all, she had "slid by pretty well."[69]

Although Breckinridge had hoped that writing would become easier after she finished discussing the details of her personal life, she found that the process grew more difficult. The thought of the fast-approaching deadline disturbed her, particularly after several bouts of illness slowed her progress.[70] The six months she originally anticipated needing to complete the book quickly stretched into a year. By August 1951, five months after her original deadline, she had taken to referring to the project as "that accursed book." She had grown "so desperately tired of writing" that she now joked that with luck, the project could be finished in her lifetime.[71] This would be her first and last book, she promised. "Not even for the Frontier Nursing Service will I go through this sort of thing again!"[72]

MORE THAN anything, Breckinridge feared that she would not have a well-written book to show for her efforts. In August 1951, she described what she had written thus far as "an appalling hodge-podge, with good bits, much diffuseness, and poor continuity."[73] Gage and Heard, the friends who had convinced her to take on the project, assured her that she was being too harsh on herself and that the finished manuscript would "be a real joy and inspiration and revelation to thousands and thousands of readers."[74] Another long-time friend urged Breckinridge to avoid being overly critical of her work because it was nearly impossible for someone, no matter how skilled, to write the story of his or her own life. Surely, her friend argued, the autobiography would not be the final word on Breckinridge's life. She predicted, "Some day someone else totally unrelated to you, will hit upon the theme, first falling in love with you, sight unseen. Then we shall have a properly evaluated story of your life and work."[75]

Despite friends' attempts to reassure her, Breckinridge remained discouraged. In a moment of exasperation, she composed a poem, dedicated to Harper Brothers, urging others who contemplated writing autobiographies to reconsider. She playfully quipped,

> If you should meet a publisher
> Who asks you for a book
> Be warned by one who went that way
> And take another look.[76]

Breckinridge had fallen victim to the assumption that writing the story of her own life and of her organization would be easy. She had lived through the events and therefore would certainly know better than anyone else how to tell the story, she had presumed. In reality, autobiography is one of the most difficult genres to master. Capturing one's life in print is similar to writing fiction but is more difficult. Autobiographers are required to create a character and to select events from their own lives "that will make the plot both plausible and dramatic." Furthermore, autobiographers feel compelled to write their story in a way that gains both readers' admiration and their compassion.[77] A difficult task indeed, as Breckinridge discovered.

SINCE HER youth, others' expectations had profoundly influenced her. Despite her claims to the contrary, Breckinridge remained strongly affected by societal norms in 1950, when she began to tell her life story. Consequently, the account she related was in many ways not her own but what others expected to read. This preoccupation with satisfying her audience led her to contradict herself at many points in her autobiography. She portrays herself in some instances as a soft-hearted benefactress, forsaking her own fortune and comfortable life-style to help others. At other times, however, she is a hard-nosed business-woman capable of overseeing thousands of dollars in donations.[78]

Throughout her life, Breckinridge struggled to reconcile two competing views of appropriate gender roles. The first, communicated by her parents, stipulated that women should remain in the home and serve others. The second, common among a younger generation of college-educated men and women, shunned sentimentality and encouraged women to express their opin-ions. Breckinridge constantly vacillated in her thinking about how women should behave. The knowledge that she would be writing for older, more conservative readers as well as younger, more liberal supporters exacerbated her tendency to waver between these two ways of thinking.

Autobiography by definition contradicts the traditional notion that women are inherently self-denigrating individuals. Consequently, most successful women who have attempted to tell their life stories have humbly downplayed their accomplishments, claiming that the path they took was destined, not chosen.[79] Carolyn Heilbrun asserts that women have typically found it impos-sible "to admit into their autobiographical narratives the claim of achievement, the admission of ambition, [or] the recognition that accomplishment was nei-ther luck nor the result of the efforts or generosity of others."[80]

Breckinridge adopted this unassuming tone in her autobiography. She clearly states in *Wide Neighborhoods* that she did not seek out success—it found her. She never intended to pursue a career. When she married for the first time, she completely renounced her ambitions in favor of those of her hus-band.[81] She began to work outside the home only when her plans to devote herself to her family were destroyed. She claims that she did not choose to establish the FNS but simply followed fate. Her deep sense of duty to help others, she contends, was "thrust upon me, by something inside of me that came from beyond me."[82]

Yet even as Breckinridge made these romanticized claims, she also felt the need to defend herself from those who would see her account as overly senti-mental. She discounts the notion that a call from God guided her decision to serve others. Breckinridge was a deeply religious woman, but *Wide Neighbor-hoods* offers few hints of her spirituality. This was a conscious choice. Gage and Heard had encouraged Harper Brothers to publish Breckinridge's autobiogra-phy because of her religious beliefs and were disappointed when they received the first draft and found only a brief mention of Sister Adeline Cashmore's influence on Breckinridge's life. Gage and Heard urged Breckinridge to dis-cuss her religious transformation in greater detail and to spend more time describing Cashmore. "A saint is such a rare occurrence in this poor world," Gage emphasized, "that she ought to be treated fully."[83] The author defended her cursory discussion of religion, however, claiming, "Truly, it does not seem to me to be even in good taste to talk about one's inner life except to the closest of friends."[84]

Breckinridge attributed her hesitancy to talk about her spiritual views to good manners, but more was at stake than she let on. She had always been reluctant to discuss politics and religion because she feared that doing so would alienate those who did not subscribe to her views. Religion, like politics, was a sensitive issue she preferred to avoid.[85] She certainly recognized that if she, as the director of a scientific, professional organization, discussed publicly her belief that she could communicate with the dead, she might undermine her reputation and that of the FNS. Discussion of life after death was better left to private, one-on-one conversations that allowed her directly to defend her theories.

Along with religion, economic class was another issue Breckinridge approached carefully in *Wide Neighborhoods*, providing a useful reminder that class status "is not a material thing." Rather, it is constructed, signifying "a pattern of appropriate conduct, coherent, embellished, and well articulated."[86] Breckinridge recognized that she needed to emphasize her membership in the ranks of the elite to attract financial support and to make herself and her organization appear respectable. At the same time, however, she distanced herself from her upper-class roots whenever her lineage might make her appear shallow. At times, she simultaneously left readers with both impressions. For example, she claimed that she brought none of her silver, mahogany, or china when she moved into the "Big House" because these items were not practical in her new, rugged environment.[87] While sympathetic to the dilemma, readers certainly would have recognized that by owning these items, she was a member of the privileged class, but because she denounced her comfortable lifestyle, she could avoid the charge of frivolity often leveled against the elite.

Despite her assertion that all mountain residents shared the same status, Breckinridge made subtle distinctions between herself and FNS patients throughout *Wide Neighborhoods*. She specifically highlighted her higher standard of cleanliness as a way of separating herself from the mountain "natives." During the service's early years, Breckinridge explained, she often spent the night in local residents' homes, primitive dwellings that were by her readers' standards dirty and overcrowded. She assured her audience that on these nights she always requested her own bed, which she "nearly always got." She found a bath "harder to manage" since Leslie County had only five bathtubs, two of them located at Wendover. Despite this obstacle, she took great care with her nightly routine. She "begged loan of [a] hand basin," which she filled with hot water so that she could wash herself and her underwear for the next day. "Except on rainy nights," she exclaimed, "my underwear as well as I myself was beautifully clean."[88] By providing seemingly unimportant details such as the condition of her underwear, Breckinridge articulated a class status separate from that of her mountain clients.

By discussing her family's history as slave owners and as leaders in the Confederate cause, she further delineated her class position. The information that her family had held many slaves and had been part of the Old South elite provided readers further clues that she belonged to the upper crust; doing so, however, forced her to acknowledge her family's participation in a system that many Americans had come to see as inhumane. Like her failed marriage, Breckinridge had no choice but to confront this uncomfortable issue.

Breckinridge used her discussion of her family's slaveholding experiences to reinforce her claim to an inherent compulsion to help others. She alleged that her grandfather's greatest dream was to free his slaves and that he had sent one of his bondsmen to Liberia. Recognizing that "the lot of freed Negroes in the South was a destitute and unhappy one," however, Breckinridge insisted that he did the dutiful thing and cared for those he had inherited.[89] Evidence suggests that at one time, James Carson truly intended to emancipate his slaves. He pursued a medical degree so that he could support his wife and children without slave labor. Nevertheless, extant records indicate that Carson ultimately emancipated only one slave; even more condemning, he added at least forty-two slaves to his holdings during his lifetime.[90]

While she apologized for her family's slaveholding past, she offered no excuses for her relatives' decision to secede from the Union. She clearly believed that the federal government's interference with states' rights warranted the South's drastic action. Confederates' defense of their principles, she reasoned, ultimately purified and strengthened the nation.[91] Breckinridge felt comfortable defending the Lost Cause. Enough time had passed for the nation to heal its wounds; the bloody shirt had been buried. Unafraid that she would alienate donors, Breckinridge used her family's role in the Civil War to illustrate her inherent passion and dedication to a cause.

Breckinridge claimed that by telling the "facts," she could give readers an objective, authentic account of her life. Her book contains an overabundance of details, a phenomenon many observers have considered the book's greatest weakness.[92] She failed to acknowledge, however, that the story she told between the "facts," the character she created, was in many ways an abstraction, a portrait of how she saw herself pieced together from documents that revealed her views at different points in her life.[93]

IN THE fall of 1951, after struggling for more than a year, Breckinridge finally completed a draft of her autobiography and began revisions. The main criticism lodged by her editor at Harper Brothers was that she tried to mention the names of too many supporters in the book, and the editor urged her to "tighten up" the story.[94] But Breckinridge defended her decision to acknowledge so many friends, emphasizing that she had not single-handedly created the FNS. Although she granted that mentioning as many supporters as possible would increase the book's sales, her urge to drop names was not motivated solely out of a desire to stroke donors' and volunteers' egos. She saw her relationship with local people, northeastern female supporters, and the physicians and nurses who served on the FNS's advisory boards as central not only to her success but also to the joy she had found in life, and she wanted to acknowledge their contributions.[95]

As Breckinridge fretted about how to comply with Harper Brothers' request that she cut twenty thousand words from her manuscript, the search for the book's title began. The author originally intended to name the book *As a Tale That Is Told*, a phrase that she drew from a verse in Psalms 90. She also suggested *My Candle of Experience*, which alluded to her desire to share her insight and discoveries with other potential health care reformers. However, she remained receptive to any title Harper Brothers might suggest. Her only request was that the words "mountain," "mountaineers," "highlands," "highlanders," or "mountain people" not appear in the title because they had so often graced the covers of "tawdry and trivial" books about Appalachia. When her editor suggested *Wide Neighborhoods*, drawn from a quotation Breckinridge used in the book, the author enthusiastically consented. This title appealed to her because it encompassed people all over the world—"from the Belgium Congo to Siam" and even "neighborhoods in worlds beyond 'this bank and shoal of time.' " The FNS had spread its philosophy and ideas to every corner of the globe, truly acting as a tree "yielding shade and fruit to wide neighborhoods of men."[96] Breckinridge believed that *Wide Neighborhoods* accurately described the FNS's work.

Harper Brothers finally published *Wide Neighborhoods* in April 1952, more than a year after its original publication date. If the writing process had been exhausting, the marketing phase proved even more tiring for Breckinridge. She immediately launched a speaking tour to promote sales. In the two weeks following the book's release, she spoke in seven different cities.[97] Over the course of the next two months, she autographed three thousand book jackets.[98] She signed so many copies that one of the service's trustees joked, "This is one book that will have more value without the author's signature than with it!"[99]

Wide Neighborhoods generated promising initial sales. In May 1952, Breckinridge was excited to learn that her book had made the *New York Herald-Tribune*'s list of "What America Is Reading" two weeks in a row. The first edition of five thousand copies sold out within a month of publication. By July 1952, the book was in its third printing. As pleased as she was with the income the book was generating, she noted, "The by-products of the book in new friends and substantial gifts . . . would amount to more than the royalties." About a year after the release of *Wide Neighborhoods*, sales began to taper off. During that first year, however, the book brought in just over three thousand dollars for the service. Royalties continued to average about four hundred dollars yearly until Breckinridge's death.[100]

Breckinridge's book received a mixed response from reviewers. A *New York Herald-Tribune* critic acknowledged the book's flaws, including Breckinridge's tendency to overquote and to employ too much emotion, but then proceeded to dismiss these faults, admitting that her style suited "the old-fashioned concept of dedicated service [she] describe[d]."[101] The *Little Rock Gazette* acknowledged that Breckinridge was "a much greater humanitarian than writer" but wrote off the book's problems, claiming that the story was compelling enough to survive its literary weaknesses.[102] A *Providence Journal* review noted that Breckinridge's writing was often "artless" and that the book needed further cutting. However, the reviewer conceded, "every time one begins to get impatient with its mass of detail or its interspersed sermonizing or poetizing, there will come an anecdote or an episode that is totally disarming." Breckinridge's charm outweighed her inability to write, the reviewer concluded.[103]

Breckinridge shrugged off the criticism her book received, going so far as to compile the negative comments in a column she printed in the *Quarterly Bulletin*. She defended her writing's lack of polish, emphasizing, "It's in my nature to do things, not to write things."[104] She took heart in the voluminous fan mail she received from supporters who extolled the virtues of her autobiography. Many of her correspondents proclaimed the book a classic. One contributor described *Wide Neighborhoods* as the next *Gone with the Wind*.[105] Another admirer gleefully wrote that she had been "torn between wanting to read and read until it was finished" and her desire to make the enjoyment of it last; like a child who could not help but to "chew up a lollipop because it tastes so good," she could not resist devouring *Wide Neighborhoods*.[106] Breckinridge's cousin, Dr. Josephine Hunt, claimed that she could not put the book down. It should have been titled "Wide Awake," she contended, because that is what it kept her every night.[107]

THE PRAISE Breckinridge received from supporters made the effort she had put into the book worthwhile. She now felt content, knowing that a detailed, accurate account of her life would be available for future researchers who sought information on her work. This compensation, however, was not enough to alleviate the exhaustion she felt after completing her project. According to her secretary, Lucille Knechtly, writing *Wide Neighborhoods* forced its author to live "a life time all over again."[108] Breckinridge was reminded that she was no longer a young woman and that the passing years were taking a toll. While writing her autobiography, Breckinridge admitted for the first time "that it [was] possible to be old."[109] Recording her life story—often considered a task for the end of one's life—forced Breckinridge to recognize her advancing age.

The death of Anne "Mac" MacKinnon, Breckinridge's assistant and closest friend within the service, also forced her to confront her mortality. Breckinridge had already watched one of her assistant directors, Dorothy Buck, die in 1949 after a two-year battle with ovarian cancer. The whole organization had rallied around "the Bucket," providing round-the-clock care in the last stages of her life. Breckinridge refused to take any speaking engagements so she could be with Buck during her final days.[110] Mac had returned from Britain just a month before Buck died, providing comfort to Breckinridge and sharing in the service's collective loss. When Mac died suddenly of a heart attack four years later, Breckinridge was again deeply shaken. She described her relationship with MacKinnon as one of the "deepest" life had ever given her, noting that their friendship was "closer than most of the friendships of men and women."[111] Both MacKinnon and Buck, buried side by side at Wendover, had been significantly younger than Breckinridge. Following the publication of *Wide Neighborhoods*, the author continued to deny publicly that she had any less energy or that she felt any older, but she began to concede privately that she was entering her declining years.

I n February 1951, Mary Breckinridge celebrated her seventieth birthday. Surrounded by Frontier Nursing Service (FNS) employees, friends from the local community, and relatives who made the trip to Wendover, the guest of honor thoroughly enjoyed her party, her first since childhood. She was thrilled when the staff presented her with a four-volume set of books detailing the life of her hero, Robert E. Lee. Unable to attend the party, her close friend Lucille "Pansy" Turner wrote to wish her well. "God seems to be playing a joke on me," she exclaimed. "You are much younger, I remember."[1]

Breckinridge viewed turning seventy as a great milestone in her life. She relished her new status as a septuagenarian. "I have learned to pronounce it and to spell it. You must do those things when you are one," she insisted. The FNS's feisty director emphasized the positive aspects of aging. She scolded photographers for retouching her portrait to eliminate the wrinkles on her face. Every year, they removed more and more lines. Soon, she joked, she expected "to wind up just a pair of staring eyes." Rather than seeing the wrinkles as detracting from her appearance, she viewed them as evidence of accumulated wisdom and years of hard work.[2]

Breckinridge considered her newfound freedom to speak her mind the best part of growing older. "Since I have become a septuagenarian," she explained,

"I come right out and say [that] I hate wearing corsages. . . . After all why wait to be an octogenarian to feel your oats. No, I say, assert yourself at 70."[3] Instead of reluctantly accepting the flowers presented to her at speaking engagements, she now gave them to any busboy, elevator girl, or telephone operator who happened to pass by.[4] She viewed her advancing age as liberating, allowing her to flout convention instead of constantly bowing to its demands.

This new freedom, however, came at a cost. Traveling became increasingly difficult, and Breckinridge's vision steadily worsened over the next decade, eventually making it impossible for her to read letters from friends without help. She found it harder with each passing year to maintain the fast pace to which she was accustomed.[5] Her mind remained sharp, allowing her to continue working on behalf of the FNS until the day before she died, but her body gradually began to fail.

When Breckinridge began writing her autobiography in 1950, she relinquished authority for the FNS's day-to-day affairs to her associates, Helen Browne and Agnes Lewis. After finishing the book, Breckinridge never regained complete control of the service. With the executive committee's endorsement, Breckinridge named Browne assistant director in 1952. Although grateful to be free from the exhausting job of overseeing every detail of the organization's administration, Breckinridge feared that she would lose her authority as the FNS's leader. She insisted that Browne continue to provide updates on organization matters every morning and afternoon. When her health became so poor that she could not leave her bedroom, the staff provided her daily reports at her bedside.

Feeling her power slip through her fingers, Breckinridge fought to maintain control of her organization. Directing the FNS was not just her job; it had become her life mission, her second family as well as her path to notoriety. But postwar changes necessitated that the FNS play its game in a new arena. The federal government assumed increasing responsibility for many of the services private charities had traditionally offered. As better roads and methods of communication emerged, rural areas became less isolated from mainstream culture. Breckinridge had always been an innovator, but as she aged, she grew less willing to embrace new ideas. She feared that the changes she witnessed would undermine the need for her organization. Although she wanted what was best for the people of Appalachia, she saw that new topics of concern were replacing the issues on which she had assumed a position of authority. Consequently, she spent the remaining years of her life upholding the status quo in an effort to preserve the role she had created for herself.[6]

IN 1945, following the detonation of the atomic bomb at Nagasaki, Japan, U.S. Secretary of War Henry Stimson said simply but profoundly, "The world is changed."[7] Indeed, World War II brought a significant transformation, both nationally and internationally. The United States emerged from the war as the leader of the free world. Isolationism, predominant during the 1930s, gave way to a belief that America had a responsibility to intervene in foreign affairs to maintain peace. Economically, the war brought renewed prosperity. By 1947, the United States was producing approximately half of the world's manufactured goods. However, this prosperity could not prevent the social unrest that smoldered beneath the surface from bubbling up. A second Red Scare led by Senator Joseph McCarthy developed in the 1950s, and minority groups' fight for equal rights rocked the 1960s.[8]

Perhaps the greatest change the war brought, however, was the expansion of the federal government's powers. Americans traditionally had resisted "big government," attacking especially the fledgling welfare state that developed during the 1930s. By 1945, however, a government-managed economy was firmly entrenched, and the imperial presidency had taken root. No longer would the federal government reserve heavy spending for periods of war. Government funding for health care and education increased significantly throughout the postwar period. Between 1948 and 1965, annual federal expenditures increased from $36.5 billion to $118 billion.[9]

Appalachia became a prime target for government spending after 1945. Americans had long been distressed to know that such a poor, underdeveloped region existed within the nation's borders. This disparity became even more striking in light of the nation's postwar economic boom. Even before Lyndon Johnson launched the War on Poverty in 1964, state and federal governments had made economic development in the mountains a priority. During the 1930s, New Deal programs had focused on creating infrastructure in Appalachia. Experts emphasized that new transportation networks were essential to Appalachian economic development, and the government made road construction a priority both under the New Deal and in the years following.[10]

Although highway construction did not provide the magic bullet that some observers had predicted, improved roads greatly benefited Appalachia, particularly Leslie County, which throughout the twentieth century had remained one of the region's most isolated pockets. In 1940, the county's closest rail access lay twenty-four miles away. It had only one paved road, connecting Hyden to Hazard. Streambeds served as roads, and residents continued to travel by horseback long after automobiles had transformed other areas of the country. Finally, during the 1940s, the state took steps to link Leslie County to surrounding areas, building two additional paved roads that connected Hyden to neighboring county seats, Manchester and Harlan.[11]

One way new roads benefited rural areas was by expanding access to education. Students could now travel out of their communities to attend better-funded consolidated regional high schools. In 1950, fewer than 9 percent of Leslie County males over the age of twenty-five held high school degrees, but graduation rates rose steadily after World War II. Whereas 47 percent of sixteen- and seventeen-year-olds enrolled in school in 1950, that number jumped to 69 percent in 1960.[12]

Planners' larger intent, however, was that new highways would facilitate economic development in Leslie County. New roads did indeed bring immediate change, if not the long-term prosperity many observers had anticipated. By connecting the area to national markets, new roads allowed for the large-scale extraction of minerals. This area was rich in high-quality coal, but little had been mined during the initial boom of the 1920s because the black gold could not be transported to market. Henry Ford, the owner of the bulk of the county's coal lands, chose to wait for the day when improved transportation or technology would allow for the efficient removal of the coal. As a sarcastic journalist explained, "Both the coal and the county were kept in reserve—a private colony, a little feudal fiefdom—until the great day when the call would come from Detroit."[13]

The call never came. Instead, the Ford Motor Company began to lease its lands to small, local operators. As the supply coming from other fields was exhausted, Leslie County's untapped high-quality coal appeared more attractive. Leslie County went from producing only 1.1 percent of the coal extracted from the eastern Kentucky fields in 1947 to producing 6.5 percent ten years later.[14] By 1960, mining employed nearly 50 percent of Leslie County's workers.[15] Small farms had once been the mainstay of the area's economy, but by 1960, only twenty full-time farms remained, employing less than 1 percent of the population.[16]

In the early twentieth century, coal largely had been extracted through deep-shaft mining. The years immediately following World War II, however, saw the birth of the ubiquitous truck mine. The demand for coal and the potential profits inspired entrepreneurial individuals to begin digging coal out of small seams. As Ronald Eller explains, "With as little as a one thousand dollar investment a man could open a seam of coal at the outcrop, construct a wooden bin down the hillside with which to load the coal into trucks, and transport it to regional markets or railside tipples."[17] Truck mining allowed some individuals to make fortunes overnight, but almost as soon as the boom began, it ended, as the Appalachian economy again suffered from overexpansion and devastating competition that ultimately would encourage mechanization and would result in widespread unemployment.[18]

The short-lived coal boom allowed the annual per capita income of Leslie County residents to increase nearly fourfold from 1940 to 1950. During the ensuing decade, per capita income in the county rose an additional 197 percent. Still, these gains did not match those realized in other parts of the state and the nation. In 1959, per capita income in Leslie County reached $711 but topped $2,200 in Louisville. After 1960, Leslie County workers' incomes would begin to decline again as the demand for high-quality coal diminished and as small mining operations failed to compete with huge conglomerates.[19]

As unemployment once again began to rise, many Leslie County residents looked beyond the mountains to cities such as Akron, Dayton, and Cincinnati, where steady work and higher wages, along with better housing, education, and health care, were available. Between 1950 and 1960, eastern Kentucky experienced its heaviest period of outmigration. By the end of the 1960s, one out of every three industrial workers in Ohio came from Appalachia. An estimated nine thousand people left Leslie County during the 1950s.[20]

Those who stayed turned to the government for help. The portion of the county's income that came from wage work declined from nearly 70 percent in 1959 to slightly less than 50 percent in 1967.[21] Residents increasingly relied for their livelihood on transfer payments in the form of unemployment, welfare, and disability checks instead of wages. The once self-sufficient region became increasingly dependent on outside assistance. The influx of government funds significantly improved the area's standard of living after the war, but its long-term economic future remained bleak.

DURING THE 1930s, Mary Breckinridge had emphasized that building a healthy economy for Leslie County was just as important as building healthy bodies, and she had made economic development a priority for her organization. However, her efforts in this regard, while well intentioned, did little to challenge the status quo. She had expressed optimism that investors would cheerfully acknowledge their "public spirited duty" and donate to her cause, but she became discouraged by the actual response. Still, she did not publicly critique those who had profited at the expense of the region and its people.

Especially as she grew older, Breckinridge became less willing to challenge the exploitative economic order that kept her patients impoverished. In fact, she found ways to cooperate with industrialists. In the late 1940s, when the coal boom was at its peak, she negotiated to mine a section of FNS property in exchange for twenty-five cents per ton in royalties. Around the same time, she approached several mine operators with a plan to provide routine care to their workers for a monthly fee that would be deducted from the miners' paychecks. Breckinridge contended that such an arrangement would result in very little added expense or work for the FNS since most of the miners who would participate already resided in the service's territory. The FNS established an alliance with one company in 1953, but mine operators expressed only mild interest in her plan.[22]

Coal operators had little incentive to address their workers' health needs, even when doing so would have cost little. In the early 1950s, Leslie County remained one of the country's few nonunion coal-producing areas. These miners earned significantly lower wages than those in other areas and lacked access to the benefits provided by the United Mine Workers (UMW) welfare fund. The UMW launched a campaign to bring Leslie County mines under contract, resulting in the eruption of violence. By 1953, eight organizers had been shot. Union opponents blew up cars, bombed union meetings, and destroyed union sympathizers' homes and businesses, leading one UMW representative to declare, "No union organizer's life is safe when he travels the highway in Leslie County." Union workers faced legal obstacles, finding themselves indicted, sued, and even jailed. The UMW declared it too dangerous to set up an office in Leslie County and instead conducted one-day "sorties" from surrounding towns.[23]

Breckinridge could have spoken out in defense of the workers, but she instead remained silent. Echoing union opponents, she assumed that the impetus to unionize came from outside agitators who "badgered" local residents.[24] She had long opposed unions, claiming that mountain workers "like to be free in their choice of their work, and in the handling of its remuneration."[25] While she claimed to be concerned about the economic plight of her patients, she could not fully shake the narrow, stereotypical mind-set she had brought to her work in 1925. She continued to view Leslie County residents through a simplistic lens that cast them as proud, independent, and content.

Her resistance to the UMW, while in part a reflection of her cultural assumptions, may also have resulted from a fear of competition. In 1954, the UMW opened ten Appalachian hospitals with funding from its welfare and retirement fund.[26] Breckinridge continued to defend staunchly the value of private charity, and although these UMW facilities were not run at government expense, she nevertheless viewed them as threatening individual initiative. Leslie

County residents had access to affordable health care, so the UMW's promises of inexpensive medical treatment were less attractive there than in areas that had not benefited from Breckinridge's organization.

IN HER 1952 master's thesis, former FNS employee Mary Ann Stillman Quarles argues that modernization left Leslie County in a state of "disorganization" as old values conflicted with new ways and ideas.[27] "Progress" was steadily encroaching on the sheltered world that Breckinridge and her nurses had grown to love. By 1960, 86 percent of the county's households owned radios, 56 percent had automobiles, and 26 percent owned televisions.[28] These innovations, combined with the movie theater that opened in Hyden in the early 1950s, provided Leslie County residents with a cultural link to other Americans that had never before existed. Individuals from across the nation watched the same shows and commercials, leading them to adopt similar dialects, styles of dress, and standards of morality. Changes in naming practices provided FNS nurses with undeniable proof that mainstream culture had invaded Appalachia. Most parents traditionally had chosen biblical names for their children, but beginning in the 1960s, nurses reported delivering infants named Shirley Temple, Jimmy Dean, Tammy, Elvis, and Maverick in honor of their parents' favorite television and movie stars and characters.[29]

As one who claimed to feel more comfortable living in the nineteenth century than the twentieth, Mary Breckinridge ambivalently viewed the changes occurring around her.[30] She wanted her patients to have the same opportunities as their city-dwelling counterparts, but she feared that the transformation occurring in Appalachia would undermine the distinctive values found in rural America. She respected the mountain people, seeing them as independent, unconcerned with wealth, and sincerely interested in their neighbors' well-being. She feared that as contact with outside regions increased and as newcomers moved to the area, these unique characteristics would disappear. Appalachia, she recognized, could not provide an antidote to the nation's ills if it became similarly corrupted. If Appalachia no longer appeared different from the rest of the nation, how would she continue to convince contributors, employees, and even patients that hers was a cause worth supporting?

Just as she feared, supporters of the FNS indeed expressed dismay when their mental pictures of Appalachia did not match the conditions they witnessed firsthand. In her detailed journal from 1948, a courier noted how "incongruous" it seemed to drive past homes lit by electricity. Furthermore, she expressed surprise that no one in Leslie County lived in log cabins. Most people she met did not resemble the stock characters she expected to see. When she did find a "Tom Sawyerish looking boy . . . walk[ing] up the road often with a .22 over his arm, bare feet, and a puppy that has loppy ears," she admitted, he was "more my idea of what they [mountain boys] should be than what they are." Though on one level she knew that reality often differed greatly from the image perpetuated by the media and that times were changing, she found it difficult to let go of her preconceived notions. As she left the mountains to return home, she lamented that she would be returning to a fast-paced, modern world: "Back to places where cars honk, electric lights blink and no horses."[31]

Whereas local development threatened to alienate service supporters, the expansion of the government's powers threatened to eliminate altogether the need for the organization. Other mountain reformers had found themselves "municipalized" as government began to attack the problems they had first identified, and Breckinridge feared a similar fate.[32] The FNS's director had long warned against the dangers of "big government," preferring instead for power to remain in individual hands. She particularly denounced the state's attempts to regulate and fund medical care, even though early in her career she had argued that good health care was a universal human right.

In 1945, President Harry Truman proposed the creation of a comprehensive national health care program, touching off a heated debate. Supporters cheered the president, arguing that the government had a responsibility to ensure that all citizens had access to medical care. Opponents, conversely, warned that the bill was "communistic," "un-American," and a threat to free enterprise. Led by the American Medical Association, the opposition included private insurance companies, several national drug chains, the American Hospital Association, the American Bar Association, and Mary Breckinridge.[33]

Breckinridge did not go on record publicly as opposing the national health insurance bill, but those who knew her clearly understood her feelings on the matter. Throughout the 1930s, she had resisted government intervention in medicine. In a 1949 letter to her friend, U.S. Representative Frances Payne Bolton, Breckinridge reiterated her opinion on the issue, insisting that rather than government aid, "the trail the FNS blazed" still provided the best way to meet the health needs of rural areas."[34]

The fight for national health insurance continued to rage throughout the late 1940s, but Truman's plan never passed. Nevertheless, the federal government began to earmark more and more funds to underwrite the costs of medical care for the elderly and the indigent and to pay for new hospitals and medical research. Between 1950 and 1970, government health care expenditures increased from $12.7 billion to $71.6 billion.[35]

Breckinridge understood that if government assumed responsibility for providing health care to every citizen, the need for the FNS would evaporate. At the very least, government's expansion into areas formerly controlled by private charity threatened her organization's financial health. Americans increasingly endorsed the notion that the government had a responsibility to provide "safety nets" and to address its citizens' basic needs. Individuals who had donated generously to charities began to curtail their giving, convinced that their rising tax dollars covered necessary services.[36] Breckinridge had already seen a drop in subscriptions. She feared that yearly revenues would decline further as governmental power increased.

BRECKINRIDGE COULD not prevent the metamorphosis she was witnessing, but she could control the way the FNS responded to the changes. She had always been an innovator, arguing that it was dangerous for an organization to stand still. Increasingly, however, she began to retrench.[37] She hoped that if the FNS appeared familiar and maintained its traditions, donors would continue to send their annual contributions and life would go on as normal. Her nurses had won fame for traveling miles on horseback any time of the day or night over dangerous terrain to deliver babies in dark, cold cabins. Although the image was increasingly unrealistic, the director hoped to preserve it.

The desire to protect the service's romantic reputation led her to question and in some cases to veto improvements that would have eased the lives of both her employees and her patients. In perhaps the most extreme case, Breckinridge opposed the construction of a highway bridge over the Kentucky River near one of the FNS outpost centers because, according to Helen Browne, "She didn't want Confluence area made too sophisticated." Breckinridge recognized that the value of her demonstration hinged on maintaining outpost centers in remote areas. The new bridge would destroy the Confluence center's isolated location. Despite experts' claims that constructing the bridge in this location would allow high school students more easily to reach Hyden, Breckinridge persuaded local officials to build the bridge downstream near Dry Hill instead. In later years, Leslie County residents referred to the bridge as "Mary Breckinridge's folly."[38] This incident reveals the amount of power Breckinridge wielded in the local area but also shows the ends to which she went to maintain her authority.

As new paved roads began to appear in the area during the war, Breckinridge faced a decision—should she continue using horses as the service's main form of transportation or begin using motorized vehicles? Outpost nursing centers formerly accessible only by horse now were in quick driving distance by car. While Breckinridge recognized that jeeps would "streamlin[e] the stork," simplifying travel for both her clients and her staff, she feared that the transition would undermine the service's financial stability.[39] Wealthy patrons often donated horses and paid the cost of the animals' upkeep. Breckinridge believed that contributors would express less excitement about paying for spark plugs and new tires than for hay and saddles.[40]

With coal trucks rumbling over the county's roads, however, it became dangerous for FNS nurses to rely on horses for transportation. In spite of her misgivings, Breckinridge gradually began to replace the FNS's stables with garages and its horses with jeeps. The first jeep, a gift from Clara Ford, arrived at Wendover in 1945. Like their equine predecessors, each jeep received a name; Ford's initial gift affectionately became known as Henrietta. The FNS's fleet of motorized vehicles grew significantly over the next several years, reaching fifteen jeeps by 1954. The service continued to keep a sizable number of horses for use in inclement weather, but staff members increasingly rode the animals only for recreation.[41]

Jeeps made the nurses' work easier but were also more expensive. In fact, after the war, everything seemed to cost more. A jeep cost nearly fifteen hundred dollars and lasted only four years in the harsh eastern Kentucky terrain, whereas horses provided an average of ten to fourteen years of service. As the person responsible for funding the FNS's budget, Breckinridge paid close attention to the price tags of modern conveniences. She stressed that charities must carefully abide by two important rules. First, they must always show gratitude for patrons' support; second, they must always remain solvent. Living through the Great Depression had taught her to conserve every dollar donors contributed. Even after the economic crisis passed, she remained fearful that her organization would not have enough money to sustain its work. As she aged, she became even more cautious with the FNS's funds.[42]

Salaries were one area where Breckinridge attempted to cut costs. In the service's earliest years, she offered wages that were competitive with those paid by similar public health organizations. Starting during the depression, when the crisis forced her temporarily to suspend salaries, FNS wages steadily slipped behind those offered elsewhere. In 1950, some nurses were earning the same monthly wage that the organization's original two nurse-midwives had received.[43]

Breckinridge recognized that the FNS's salaries lagged significantly behind those offered by government and by private industry. "Our present salaries [are] from one-half to one-third lower than most of the staff could get else-where," she admitted in 1955. She stressed, however that "none the less we are not short of nurses."[44] She praised her employees' willingness to work for salaries well below what they deserved: "There is no one on the staff of the Frontier Nursing Service, whether nurse or secretary, but is a part-time volunteer making a gift of from a half to two-thirds of her time."[45] In 1959, the highest-paid nursing staff member earned $200 per month. The same year, the American Nurses' Association reported that the average national salary for staff nurses in similar public health nursing services was $336 per month.[46]

The FNS executive committee urged the director to raise salaries and authorized increases on several occasions. Breckinridge, however, hesitated to increase the organization's expenses. She feared that if she paid staff more, she would become unable to balance the service's budget. She admitted that as "an old-fashioned woman," she had "a deep dread of debt."[47] Industry could raise its wages and salaries and pass the increased costs on to the consumer. Government could pass costs on to the taxpayer. Private philanthropies lacked that luxury.[48]

Breckinridge's fear of debt also led her to defer needed expansion projects. By the late 1950s, Hyden Hospital was nearly thirty years old. Despite several additions, the small, stone structure could not accommodate the patient load. Breckinridge recognized that the hospital was not large enough and that a new wing was desperately needed, but she resisted taking action. Having served as "the financial watchdog of the Service for nearly thirty-six years," she advised that the organization could not undertake such an expensive project until its endowment doubled. Acting prematurely, she feared, would put the service "on the rocks."[49]

Her reluctance to build a new hospital may have reflected more than financial concern, however. By 1950, hospital births accounted for 88 percent of all deliveries nationwide, with the number quickly rising.[50] The FNS saw a similar trend develop, although much more slowly. While in 1939, 85 percent of the service's patients delivered at home, by 1958, less than half did so. More than two-thirds of first-time mothers chose to give birth at the hospital.[51] Breckinridge was astute enough to realize that hospital births were not nearly as romantic to report as births in cold, lonely cabins. Her reluctance to expand the hospital further reflects her desire to maintain her organization's distinctiveness.

Breckinridge's coworkers urged her to modernize the organization, but their pleas were ignored. Assistant director Browne often grew frustrated by her supervisor's refusal to change with the times. The service's medical director, Dr. W. B. Rogers Beasley, while deeply respectful of Breckinridge's many accomplishments, likewise grew aggravated with her unwillingness to accept new ideas. When he left the service to pursue additional training in 1958, he warned Browne that the FNS would "fall flat on its face" unless she did something to revive it.[52]

THE STRUGGLE to create a national professional organization for nurse-midwives in the mid-1950s further illustrates how Breckinridge's views, once on the cutting edge, had fallen out of the mainstream. In 1929, Breckinridge and several of the FNS's early employees established the Kentucky State Association of Midwives to provide a support base for the few individuals working in the field. In 1941, the group changed its name to the American Association of Nurse-Midwives (AANM) to appear more inclusive, but its membership remained overwhelmingly made up of individuals affiliated with the FNS. Other nurse-midwives with no connection to Breckinridge's organization tended to affiliate with the National Organization for Public Health Nursing. When that group dissolved in 1952, many nurse-midwives found themselves without a home and began discussing the creation of a new organization to represent practitioners in the field.[53]

At the FNS's urging, leaders initially set out to reorganize the existing AANM. Divisions within the ranks of the profession, however, hampered this effort. Breckinridge and her associates' views about the functions a national organization should serve deviated sharply from those of their colleagues in other parts of the country. In particular, Breckinridge found herself locked in a struggle with Hattie Hemschemeyer, assistant director of New York's Maternity Center Association (MCA), and Sister M. Theophane Shoemaker of New Mexico's Catholic Maternity Institute.[54] The main issue on which organizers diverged was how to deal with physicians. One group believed that nurse-midwives should boldly attempt to make physicians and the American public aware of their role by undertaking a comprehensive education campaign, while the other faction, led by Breckinridge and her supporters, advocated "slow growth" by allowing doctors to discover on their own the valuable work nurse-midwives performed. The location in which members of the two factions practiced influenced the position they took on this and other issues. Those affiliated with the MCA tended to emphasize the concerns of practitioners working in urban hospital settings, while FNS representatives stressed the challenges facing those working in rural, isolated areas. Breckinridge's insistence that the organization keep dues low and allow non-nurse-midwives who supported the field to join further alienated her from other organizers.[55]

At its root, however, the struggle centered on control of the profession. Having watched her power in the FNS begin to weaken, Breckinridge was eager to secure control of the national organization representing nurse-midwives. She wanted to preserve the AANM because, as she explained, it had an established tradition, an invaluable asset for a young, experimental field. But she opposed rewriting the organization's articles of incorporation to reflect the ideas of other leaders. Breckinridge's "cool reception" frustrated Hemschemeyer and Sister Theophane, leading them to conclude that her main problem was that she was not interested in forming an organization that was "alive, progressive, dynamic, and growing."[56] Members of the Committee on Organization ultimately found it impossible to revamp the AANM and instead voted to create a separate American College of Nurse-Midwifery in 1955. The two organizations eventually combined in 1968, after Breckinridge's death, becoming the American College of Nurse-Midwives.[57]

IN ADDITION to issues related to professionalization, race was another key issue that separated Breckinridge from other nurse-midwives who attempted to create a national professional organization. Within the AANM, race had been a divisive question for more than a decade. Although its policy toward African Americans changed from time to time, the organization's basic position was that minority nurse-midwives should form a separate organization. Leaders of the MCA and Catholic Maternity Institute, however, saw this prohibition as undermining their goal of uniting all nurse-midwives under one organizational umbrella. Still, Breckinridge refused to change her policy of barring African American practitioners.[58]

Breckinridge was eager to have her theories on rural health care delivery carried throughout the world; thus, she invited health care practitioners from many nations to visit the FNS. For most of the service's history, however, she refused to entertain black observers at Wendover. Although she recognized the value of having foreign doctors and nurses witness her work firsthand, she would not accept persons of African descent, no matter their qualifications, into her home.

Breckinridge's racial prejudices had deep roots. Her parents raised her to view skin color as an indicator of innate characteristics and abilities. Blacks, she assumed, were intellectually inferior, designed by God to serve whites.

Clifton Rodes Breckinridge saw whites as the most "positive [and] masterful" race the world had ever seen, while blacks constituted the most "negative and tractable" race. He believed society could function effectively only if every individual knew his or her appropriate role and submitted to this natural order.[59]

From birth, Mary learned the complicated rules of racial etiquette that developed under slavery and subsequently strengthened as whites attempted to reinforce white supremacy and to keep blacks "in their place." As Jennifer Ritterhouse shows, white southerners expected African Americans to follow a hidden but agreed-upon transcript through which they demonstrated their subservience. Some of the rules were clear—blacks respectfully addressed whites with titles such as "Mr.," "Mrs.," or "Miss," black men removed their hats when approaching whites and always yielded the sidewalk. Other situations were murkier and required African Americans to deduce how best to avoid appearing "uppity" while ideally still maintaining some dignity. Whites directed violence against those who failed to show proper respect.[60] In the 1890s, a black man was lynched almost every other day in the South. As time passed, a complicated set of rules codified the social distance whites informally strove to impose. Raised in this Jim Crow system, Breckinridge believed that it was not just appropriate but beneficial for blacks and whites to attend separate churches and schools and sit in separate sections of movie theaters. Segregation, she argued, benefited members of both races.[61]

Invested in this Jim Crow system, Breckinridge attentively followed news of the developing civil rights movement in the late 1940s. In 1948, Breckinridge added an editorial written by the publisher of a "Negro" newspaper to her collection of clippings that endorsed continued segregation. Author Davis Lee compared the condition of blacks in the South to that in his home of Newark, New Jersey. Lee explained that although many northern states had civil rights legislation on the books, African Americans met with more discrimination there than in southern states, which had found "a workable solution" to the race question. Segregation, the author suggested, benefited the black community in several ways, primarily economically. According to Lee, the fact that "whites in the South stay[ed] with their own and the Negroes [did] likewise" was the "economic salvation of the Negro in the South," allowing blacks to control millions of business dollars. In an argument similar to that offered by Booker T. Washington several decades earlier, Lee concluded that the fight for equality "should be carried on within the race." Only when all blacks could demonstrate through their living standards, conduct, ability, and intelligence that they deserved to have whites consider them as equals would segregation end. Threats and agitation, Lee concluded, would only continue to make "enemies out of . . . friends."[62]

As humans tend to do, Breckinridge looked for ways to buttress her assumptions, and she found Lee's argument concerning the value of segregation compelling. Breckinridge, like Lee, believed that both races benefited from social and physical distance. She encouraged "brotherhood" rather than equality between the races. According to Breckinridge, God opposed uniformity and therefore purposely created inequality. She maintained, "No two people in the world are equal—nor any two nations, or races." She contended that people of every race should be encouraged to improve themselves, so that eventually they could reach a point where they could rule themselves, but remained opposed to contact between the races.[63]

Breckinridge did not subscribe to a simple black/white dichotomy but further distinguished between different nationalities of whites. When recruiting nurses, Breckinridge looked for applicants from specific groups that she deemed naturally superior. She rejoiced when Aase Johanesen, a Norwegian nurse, joined the service's ranks in 1940. "We are enchanted to have a Norwegian in our group," she reported in the *Quarterly Bulletin*. She expressed hope that the FNS would one day hire a Finn and a Greek.[64] The FNS received applications from nurses from all parts of the world, but its staff remained lily-white until after Breckinridge's death. In the 1930s, the FNS accepted several nonwhite nurses sent by the Rockefeller Foundation to gain experience, including a Spanish nurse and three Chinese nurses. The organization also accepted two "superior" Native American nurses sponsored by the Colonial Dames. Breckinridge agreed to train these nurses with the stipulation that they stay for a specified period and then return to serve their own people.[65]

Breckinridge justified her policy of hiring only nurses from certain racial and ethnic groups by noting that patients would not accept nurses of different skin colors. One of the first tasks Breckinridge assigned to Browne after naming her assistant director in 1952 was to send a rejection letter to an American-born Japanese nurse who had applied for a position with the FNS. The candidate had excellent references, but she had the wrong complexion. Claiming that she feared upsetting local residents, Breckinridge brought the issue before the organization's executive committee and the Hyden Committee. Both bodies expressed fear that the community would reject the Japanese nurse. The Hyden Committee advised against hiring her because they assumed that if anything happened to a patient under her care, it "would be blamed on the nurse's yellow skin."[66]

Breckinridge did not feel that the time was right for the FNS to begin hiring minority nurses, and she only reluctantly agreed to allow visitors of color to observe the service's work in the 1950s. An obstetrical physician from Ghana sent by the State Department became the first black guest to visit. Recognizing that her supervisor remained quite uncomfortable with the idea of sitting at a dinner table with a black man, Browne arranged his visit so that Breckinridge did not have to dine with him. The director, however, agreed to meet briefly with him. According to Browne, Breckinridge was "a little stiff at first," but she soon warmed up when the guest mentioned his four-year-old son.[67]

It is tempting to accept Breckinridge's defense that she was raised in a place and time when racial prejudices were almost universally shared. Given her background as a member of a prominent slave-owning family taught to celebrate the glories of the Old South, it may be unrealistic to expect Breckinridge to have challenged white supremacy, but she certainly had that option. She styled herself a nonconformist, particularly with regard to questioning medical authority. In some instances, she challenged the values her parents taught her—for example, when she shunned traditional theology in favor of more unorthodox spiritual views. Her willingness to think outside the box, however, did not extend to confronting racial hierarchies. Throughout her life, Breckinridge remained uncomfortable interacting with nonwhites. On several occasions, Browne confronted the director about her prejudices but received a polite reminder: "Brownie, you'll never understand. You weren't born and raised in the South."[68]

ONE AREA in which Breckinridge showed a little more flexibility in adapting to the times was her position on birth control. In the service's early years, Breckinridge opposed birth control for her patients except in extraordinary circumstances on the grounds that Appalachia was home to a superior race whose high birthrate benefited the nation.[69] Like many supporters, famous entertainer Will Rogers shared the director's interest in this "incubator country." "You can't beat Old Kentucky for a breeding ground. It's the limestone in the soil, and the corn in the jug that does it," he enthusiastically argued.[70] Breckinridge had failed in her duty to improve the nation's offspring with her own superior genes, having buried her two children, but working in Appalachia provided her with another chance to prevent race suicide.[71]

Breckinridge did not in theory oppose birth control. She saw contraception as a free speech issue and argued that the government should not deny its citizens' rights in any matter, including birth control. Although she acknowledged that eastern Kentucky's birthrate remained far too high, she challenged those who suggested that birth control would provide a "panacea" for the region's problems.[72] She claimed that providing contraceptive information to every Appalachian mother would be too expensive and that it made more sense to attack the underlying causes of poverty. Even if doctors distributed such information to every remote home, she claimed that the area's fundamentalist religious views would keep most women from using contraception. In addition, the value rural residents placed on children as a labor source would prevent a birth control program from producing significant results.[73] FNS policy required the organization to provide contraceptive information to any woman who requested it, but Breckinridge noted that few inquired.[74]

Breckinridge argued instead that birthrates would decline only when economic conditions in the region improved. In a position that seems peculiar today, Breckinridge argued that fertility corresponded in an inverse ratio to a population's access to education. Educated women's tendency to have fewer children, she claimed, did not stem from an intentional decision. Having married later, after directing their mental powers toward their careers, women had little energy left to apply to reproduction. To support her theory, Breckinridge suggested that a foundation sponsor a study in which one thousand couples, all college graduates, would agree not to limit their family size for ten years. To ensure that financial concerns did not motivate the participants to have fewer children, the foundation would offer every family a college scholarship for each child born during this period. Breckinridge predicted that such a study would conclusively support her theory that educated parents could not bear as many children as the uneducated.[75]

On one hand, Breckinridge commended eastern Kentucky for producing so many old-stock citizens; on the other hand, she recognized that birthrates must sometimes be limited. To "build up the young of a race by draining away the vitality of their mothers," she argued, would be counterproductive.[76] Service regulations permitted the FNS medical director to distribute contraceptives, but strict guidelines applied. Only patients who had delivered at least five living children were eligible to receive diaphragms, sponges, condoms, and jellies. To qualify for a tubal ligation, a woman needed to have delivered at least eight living infants.[77] The weak and feebleminded within the community, however, were not subject to the same restrictions. Breckinridge condescendingly suggested that practitioners should apply what she called "the red hat approach" in these cases. Simply offering a woman with a low-grade mentality a red hat would encourage her to submit to sterilization. If that was not incentive enough, Breckinridge suggested throwing in a red dress to persuade the woman.[78] A proponent of positive eugenics, Breckinridge felt that society should encourage the "fit" to help build the race while assisting the "unfit" in keeping their fertility in check.

By the 1950s, interest in eugenics had faded and Americans who had previously supported mountain residents' high birthrates came to associate exceptional fertility with struggling Third World nations. As T. S. Hyland's controversial 1949 *Life* article illustrates, Breckinridge's "fruitful mountaineers" now represented a threat rather than America's salvation.[79] With the introduction of new birth control technologies, family planning grew in popularity. A new organization, Planned Parenthood, promoted conscious child spacing within families as well as government population planning.[80]

Following World War II, contraception became more than a tool to limit family size; experts proclaimed it a path to economic development and political stability. Critics suddenly claimed that an easy-to-use, effective form of birth control was as important to national defense as nuclear weapons. Reflecting the period's hysteria over the Third World's population explosion, Dr. John Rock, who became known as "the father of the pill," noted that "the greatest menace to world peace and decent standards of life" was not the atom bomb but "sexual energy."[81] Bolstered by the support of a nation that viewed overpopulation as a dangerous threat and by women who demanded a more practical form of contraception that they could control, scientific labs competed during the late 1950s to patent the first birth control pill.[82]

In 1952, the Worcester Foundation began conducting clinical studies of Enovid, its entrant into this race, on rats and rabbits. Animal tests revealed that progesterone could effectively regulate ovulation with no permanent impairment of fertility. An important question remained, however: How would the compound work in human females?[83] Without testing the drug on women, it was impossible to predict its side effects or the long-term outcome of using oral contraceptives. Scientists conducted the first trials on twenty-nine sterile women in Boston beginning in 1954. The results were satisfactory, but the number of participants was too small to be conclusive.[84]

Researchers had difficulty recruiting and retaining subjects for a large-scale clinical study because the demands placed on trial participants were so great. Doctors expected them to take their basal temperature every day, perform daily vaginal smears, collect urine specimens, and undergo regular endometrial biopsies.[85] Frustrated that the process of enrolling participants was advancing so slowly, Katherine McCormick, the study's primary funding source, observed in a moment of exasperation that what they needed was a "cage" of ovulating females that could be carefully watched to ensure that they were following the procedures outlined by investigators. In a letter to longtime birth control advocate Margaret Sanger, McCormick explained that the only way to overcome the "headache" of noncooperation would be to "furnish enough nurses to go around to [patients'] homes and see that the women . . . accomplish the tests regularly and correctly."[86]

Rock, the physician overseeing the clinical trials, saw Breckinridge's organization as the perfect "cage" in which to conduct his study. His wife, Nan, had served with Breckinridge in the Comité Américain pour les Régions Dévastées de la France and had remained a loyal supporter of the FNS. Rock believed that FNS patients would make perfect subjects. First, the region had an extremely high birthrate. Second, the organization had more than thirty years of detailed medical records on its patients. Third, service nurses could, as McCormick suggested, visit patients on a regular basis to ensure that they were taking the medication and collecting the necessary data.[87]

Despite her eagerness to cooperate with the husband of a longtime supporter, Breckinridge initially resisted Rock's proposal to promote birth control in the area. Beasley, the service's medical director and a firm supporter of the plan, convinced Breckinridge to take the issue before the local committee. When the Hyden Committee voted by secret ballot to participate in the trials, Breckinridge invited Dr. Rock to begin administering the pill to FNS patients.[88]

In 1958, FNS nurses recruited one hundred women to join the clinical study of Enovid. Beasley oversaw the trial, personally visiting participants for the first three months. Following this initial period, nurses made monthly visits to inquire about side effects, to encourage patients to continue taking the medication, and to deliver new supplies of pills.[89] According to FNS nurse-midwife Elsie Maier, women in the region were excited to have access to the pill because "they really didn't want to have any more children." She blamed what little opposition she witnessed on patients' conservative religious beliefs.[90]

Pleased by the study's results, the FNS formally established a family planning program in 1961. Searle Pharmaceuticals continued to provide Enovid to FNS patients free of charge until 1964.[91] When the company discontinued this policy, the FNS began to offer intrauterine devices as an inexpensive alternative and began to train students at the Frontier Graduate School of Midwifery to insert the devices.[92]

The FNS's efforts in the family planning arena proved extremely successful, leading to a sharp decline in Leslie County's birthrate. In the mid-1950s, the service averaged 500 deliveries per year.[93] In contrast, in 1970, the FNS registered only 276 maternity patients.[94] The county's birthrate dropped from forty-one births per one thousand population in 1959 to twenty-two per one thousand in 1968.[95] By 1971, 70 percent of the FNS's postpartum patients accepted some form of birth control.[96]

AS SHE approached her eightieth birthday, Mary Breckinridge could not help but recognize that the world had changed significantly over the course of her lifetime. Everywhere she looked, she saw reminders. Urbanization; industrialization; the invention of cars, radios, and televisions; and two great wars had permanently altered the face of America. Although many of these changes came to Leslie County later than other areas of the country, the area's community looked very different from 1925. By 1960, horseback travel was a thing of the past; coal trucks rumbled by at alarming speeds. Few of her neighbors earned their livelihood through subsistence farming.

Breckinridge's coworkers recognized that the FNS had little choice but to change with the times. Much to their dismay, however, the organization's director proved inflexible in her responses to the transformations she witnessed. Though concerned with her patients' best interests, her fear of destroying the image of the service's work she had so carefully built and her desire to protect her power base prevented her from accepting new ideas. The FNS eventually adapted to the postwar environment in which it functioned, but these changes did not occur until after its founder's death.

In her autobiography, journalist and social activist Mary Heaton Vorse declares that as one ages, "The size of the earth over which one may roam shrinks day by day, until it decreases to the house—to one's room—to one's bed; and finally to the narrowest space of all."[1] The final five years of Mary Breckinridge's life brought a similar shrinking of her sphere. She curtailed her travel considerably beginning in the late 1950s, when Helen Browne began attending Frontier Nursing Service (FNS) speaking events in the director's stead. Breckinridge conducted her last fund-raising tour in February 1961. By then, she found even local travel difficult. The service began to host area committee meetings at Wendover instead of at the outpost centers so that the director would not have to "make the rounds."[2] In her younger years, she had found it no trouble to ride thirty miles on horseback; now she found it "wearisome" to ride five miles to Hyden Hospital by jeep.[3]

The director's eightieth birthday, like her seventieth, inspired a grand celebration. At dawn on February 17, 1961, a member of the staff stood on the mountain above Wendover and played "Happy Birthday" on the coronet so Breckinridge could hear its strains waft into her bedroom window. Later in the day, more than sixty well-wishers gathered for a dinner that consisted of the guest of honor's favorite foods—spoon bread, turkey hash, turnip greens, and spring onions. Following the meal, her friends served a round cake with eighty red candles, a replica of the cake Breckinridge's father had had at Wendover on his eightieth birthday. Dr. W. B. Rogers Beasley offered a toast, saluting Breckinridge for the inspiration she provided not only as a teacher but also as a friend. Instead of bringing gifts, FNS employees, as instructed, brought articles they had written for the *Quarterly Bulletin*.[4]

SHORTLY AFTER her eightieth birthday, Breckinridge presented her resignation to the FNS executive committee. She would not step down immediately, she announced, but rather whenever committee members decided such a move was necessary. In case of her death or incapacitation, the aging director wanted to be sure that the service would keep functioning without missing a beat. She made it clear that Browne was to take over when the time came.[5]

Breckinridge's action was symbolic. She certainly did not intend to surrender control of the organization any time soon. She still had much that she wanted to accomplish. In a letter to a fellow nurse, she declared that old people like her "linger[ed] on this planet but for one purpose . . . that of protecting and serving the young."[6] As long as she could continue working, Breckinridge planned to oversee the FNS.

Her eyesight had been failing for several years, but she continued, with the help of her staff, to edit the organization's *Quarterly Bulletin*. In 1960, the director began to write a new column, "Before We Step into the Wings." She used this editorial section as a forum to wax nostalgic on life when she was a young girl and to discuss the changes she had witnessed throughout the years. She also used the column to provide periodic updates on her health.[7]

The pace of Breckinridge's days slowed considerably following her eightieth birthday. She still spent a great deal of time corresponding with service contributors and overseeing the organization's publicity. She continued to rise early and to receive daily briefings on FNS business. She spent her afternoons working in the gardens outside Wendover. She found her chickens a source of great joy. According to former courier Nancy Dammann, Breckinridge could identify each one of her chickens by sight. Those who proved to be good mothers won Breckinridge's affection, and to their good fortune, they avoided "the Wendover pot."[8] The service's blacksmith likewise recalled the tender care Breckinridge provided her chickens, noting that they "got took care of just like some babies."[9]

BRECKINRIDGE INCREASINGLY had to rely on others for help to get through her daily routine. By 1962, she could no longer read a newspaper by herself.

Staff members had to read her mail to her every morning. The loss of her eyesight bothered her deeply—even more than her back injury—because it placed a heavy burden on her associates.[10]

Although considerably slowed by her poor health, Breckinridge did not allow it to stop her from reaping honors. In recognition of her long tenure of service to the region, the Leslie County Development Association held the first annual Mary Breckinridge Festival in September 1962. The celebration, attended by more than two thousand local residents, featured a parade, a basket lunch, and speeches by former staff members and local leaders. The FNS director proudly presided over the parade. Nurse-midwife Vanda Summers described the sight in dramatic detail: "High on a hill [stood] a horseback figure silhouetted against the blue sky. The figure was our beloved Mary Breckinridge . . . waiting to greet the parade as it advanced in perfect order to pay its respects."[11] In a more light-hearted depiction of the scene, Breckinridge joked that her horse, Doc, was nearly as old as she was but fortunately was "blessed with better eyesight."[12] Agnes Lewis reported that the day was a great success. Her only regret was that the Leslie County officials had not decided to sponsor the event a year earlier, when the honoree would have "been more equal to a large crowd, a parade, and dinner."[13]

Soon after this celebration, Breckinridge received disturbing news. During an annual physical, her doctor discovered three malignant tumors in her bladder. Doctors removed them and ordered radiation treatments. Breckinridge did not complain about her illness but rather gleefully reported that the experience provided "an old nurse" an opportunity to better understand the new medical technology and to see illness from a patient's perspective. She spent five weeks at the new University of Kentucky Medical Center in Lexington. The time away, she noted, interfered with her ability to carry her share of the service's work but nevertheless had its small comforts. Members of the FNS Bluegrass Committee hosted a four o'clock tea in her room each afternoon, allowing her to feel completely "at home."[14]

Breckinridge attended the second annual festival held in her honor in the fall of 1963, but by this time, she was too weak to mount her horse.[15] Although doctors had controlled her bladder cancer, she developed leukemia, which proved resistant to treatment. She began receiving periodic blood transfusions, significantly increasing her energy level. Despite her troubles, she remained in good spirits. In January 1964, after receiving a transfusion from Browne, she joked that the British blood coursing through her veins made her want to sing "God Save the Queen."[16] Breckinridge attended the FNS's annual trustees' meeting in Louisville in June 1964. It was the last time she would travel outside Leslie County.[17] She recognized that her days on earth were growing short.

Although she still had a number of goals she wished to accomplish, to some extent she looked forward to death because it would finally reunite her with her children. Throughout all the years she led the FNS, she had always kept a portrait of Breckie by her bedside. When she traveled, the first thing she did was unpack his picture and set it on the nightstand.[18] To recall her short years with her son, she explained, was "to step into a sort of fairyland full of sunshine and laughter."[19] Anticipating the reunion that was to come, Breckinridge selected a painting of a young blond-haired boy for the cover of the autumn 1964 issue of the *Quarterly Bulletin*. She explained that she had treasured this picture through the years because it reminded her of her small son. In the inside cover she included a poem, "Little Boy Blue," that describes a small child's playroom that has been abandoned suddenly. The toys have collected dust while waiting for their owner to return. The poem concludes with a question: "What has become of our Little Boy Blue?" Breckinridge, like the poem's author, hoped soon to learn what had become of her children. Death, she believed, would allow them again to play together.[20]

Breckinridge grew steadily weaker throughout the fall of 1964. Writing to a faithful supporter, Lewis remarked, "Mrs. Breckinridge is editing the Bulletin . . . and finding it very fatiguing. I doubt her trying to edit too many more issues." Lewis continued, "It breaks my heart to see her trying so hard to carry on."[21] Breckinridge continued to work on service business as much as her strength allowed. She refused to turn over complete control of the organization to her coworkers. The staff kept her informed of the day-to-day details. Browne recalled that she "didn't get senile in any way," but her mind "got tired." She could think clearly in the mornings, but her periods of lucidity became shorter and shorter.[22]

In the winter 1965 issue of the *Quarterly Bulletin*, Breckinridge provided an update on the status of her health. She continued to receive treatment for her bladder tumors and her leukemia. She also had fallen. In her ever-valiant style, she refused to seek treatment in Lexington after the fall because she did not want to shirk her share of the work and overburden her associates. "I am always happiest when I am busy," she remarked. "Idleness has never agreed with me. So, add your gratitude to that of this old nurse that my days of usefulness are not yet quite ended."[23]

By this point, Breckinridge only rarely left her bedroom. She quietly celebrated her eighty-fourth birthday by having her staff carry her outside in her wheelchair to visit her pet geese and cat.[24] She recognized that "time was running out," but she hoped that she would live until her eighty-fifth birthday. By then, she planned to have "all of her loose ends tidy and in order for Brownie to take over."[25]

IN MAY 1965, a month before the FNS's fortieth annual meeting, Breckinridge expressed optimism that she would be able to attend. On May 15 she confided to a close friend that she feared her poor health might prevent her from presiding, but she hoped to be where she belonged—giving her yearly report on the service's work.[26] After writing this letter, Breckinridge complained that she was tired and skipped dinner. That evening, she fell into a deep sleep from which she never awoke. Lewis and Browne, her close friends and valuable assistants, were at her bedside when her "days of usefulness" finally ended. She "stepped into the wings" the following afternoon.[27] Lewis took comfort "in the thought that Bucket and Mack and others who had been with the Frontier Nursing Service, as well as Mrs. Breckinridge's own family[, gave] her a royal welcome into that land beyond the veil."[28]

The FNS held a memorial service at Leslie County High School so that local residents could pay their final respects to the woman who had worked so hard on their behalf. The ceremony was simple, in keeping with Breckinridge's wishes. No eulogies were said during the brief, thirty-minute service. At no time was her name or that of her organization mentioned. Her body was then taken to Lexington, where mourners gathered for a second service, equally brief. Outfitted in her winter riding uniform, Breckinridge was buried with pictures of her children and locks of their hair. That day, the executive committee named Helen Browne the new director of the Frontier Nursing Service.[29]

When Breckinridge died, she left the FNS with an endowment of more than $2 million. All told, she raised almost $10 million for the organization over the course of her lifetime. This money allowed the Service to care for nearly 58,000 patients, to provide 248,000 inoculations, and to deliver safely more than 14,500 babies.[30] Numbers, however, can never fully gauge the impact Breckinridge's work had on peoples' lives. One FNS patient summed up the contributions of the service and its director to the region: "I think they was a awful lot of children that's growed up healthy that wouldn't have been done if they hadn't been here."[31]

Conclusion

Mary Breckinridge's life was rich with complexity and at times was marked by seeming contradictions. She was highly visible and comfortable speaking to crowds, but she was intensely private, developing few close personal relationships. She was often selfless, crediting friends and supporters for her accomplishments. At other moments, she could be highly egocentric, keenly aware of her image and her distinguished heritage. She embraced yet feared change. She upheld tradition but consciously flouted convention. She had a flair for the dramatic but remained practical in the extreme. She was simultaneously a visionary who believed a single person could change the world and a grounded realist who recognized that change would not come overnight. Above all else, Mary Breckinridge was human, neither completely saint nor sinner but always a little of both.

She was born into a world divided by strict racial, class, and gender hierarchies. White, female, and the product of a prominent southern political dynasty, she understood well the responsibilities this status entailed. Eighty-four years later, she left a world where many of the traditional social structures had crumbled or were beginning to crumble. De jure segregation was dead; de facto segregation was under attack. Women had long ago won the vote and now redirected their fight toward equal pay and equal rights legislation. Protesters laid siege to wealth and privilege, demanding that America fulfill its promise as a land of opportunity for all.

For Breckinridge and the other women of her generation, negotiating these changes proved difficult. Emily Newell Blair, a contemporary of Breckinridge's, titled her autobiography *Bridging Two Eras*, recognizing the challenges she faced as she tried to reconcile the older ideas she had learned as a young girl with the new ideas that she felt compelled to adopt later in life. Although Breckinridge never described her struggle as concisely as Blair did, she felt similarly torn between protecting the ideals of the era in which she came of age and embracing the changes that she witnessed as she grew older.

Making the shift from dutiful daughter to New Woman caused many women of this time to question their identities and their purposes in life. As director of the Frontier Nursing Service (FNS), Breckinridge sought to reconcile two very different interpretations of women's proper role. She was an extremely talented, fiercely driven professional living in an era when blind ambition, though applauded in men, was viewed as highly inappropriate in women. Establishing the FNS afforded Breckinridge a position of power, yet the service's focus on women and children protected her from appearing self-serving. Professional motherhood proved to be a very flexible ideology, and Breckinridge often privileged one aspect of her role over the other, depending on her audience.

Breckinridge's initial plan for an organization staffed by nurse-midwives was quite innovative for its time. In a period when doctors fought against anything that resembled "socialized medicine," Breckinridge proposed making health care a government responsibility. She challenged the status quo and argued for an expanded welfare state well before the New Deal. However, her desire for power ultimately undermined her goal of using government as an equalizing force. She initially pursued public funding for her project but was unwilling to share control, and rather than follow the recommendations of state agents and foundation boards, she took a different path. Seeking private rather than public funding allowed her to keep a tight rein on her organization's message, but doing so significantly limited her plan's scope. While she did tremendous good in Leslie County, Kentucky, her work did not have the far-reaching impact she originally intended. Her voice, which urged the government to take responsibility for health care, fell silent just as viable opportunities to develop such a system emerged in the 1930s.

DURING THE course of Breckinridge's life, Appalachia was "discovered," "created," "uplifted," and "rediscovered." From the beginning, Breckinridge promised that she would never exploit the people of the mountains, but despite her pledges to provide only positive publicity, her efforts directed additional negative attention to the area. To show why Appalachia needed help, she had to spotlight its residents' poverty and ill health. By so doing, however, she helped to reinforce Americans' stereotypical notions about the region.

Breckinridge's hierarchical view of society, which emphasized gender, race, and class distinctions, clearly shaped the way she treated her patients. On the one hand, she stressed that the Appalachian people represented the best humanity had to offer—they were racially pure and retained pioneer values. Honest, hospitable, and loyal, they refused handouts and worked hard. They had a great deal of potential; they just needed help to fulfill their destiny. On the other hand, despite her deep admiration for the Appalachian people, Breckinridge had difficulty accepting them as her equals. Despite her claims to be working through rather than for the residents of Leslie County, few if any local men and women held positions of authority within the service. She carefully distinguished between her "worthy" and "unworthy" neighbors but hired even the community's "best" residents only to perform menial labor. Instead of training local women to serve as nurse-midwives, she brought in outsiders to provide care. Breckinridge assumed that FNS representatives had the answers to the problems that plagued eastern Kentucky, and they needed to convince their patients that their ideas were better.

In spite of her class biases, however, Breckinridge does not deserve the condemnation that critics such as David Whisnant have leveled against "fotched-on" women who served the mountains in the early part of the century. Instead of bringing real improvement, Whisnant argues, reformers selfishly directed their energies toward transforming the area's culture into a model that conformed to middle-class standards. The situation, as Breckinridge's story shows, was much more complicated. We must not write off her efforts as simply a product of self-interest but instead must recognize the ways her personal ambitions intersected with a genuine desire to serve others.

Modernization was transforming Appalachia during the early twentieth century. The process was not forced on the mountains but, as recent scholarship has demonstrated, was facilitated and often embraced by many mountain residents.[1] In his study of coal towns, Crandall Shifflett challenges the standard "mythical" impression of mountain life, stressing that "mountain families had little time and energy for telling tales or making baskets. They probably strung more beans than dulcimers. Mostly life was a cycle of endless labor." Mountain residents sought advancements they hoped would improve their lives. "Roads, railroads, towns, stores, electric lighting, indoor plumbing, weekly garbage pickup, better medical and dental care, and other forms of 'modernization,' especially jobs, would have been welcomed by farm families to relieve the isolation, laboriousness, and misery of mountain life and work," Shifflett explains. "To suggest otherwise is nonsense."[2]

Even when Breckinridge's patients spoke out against the way they were portrayed in service publications, they consistently expressed gratitude for the FNS. Over and over, patients declared the FNS one of the best things ever to happen to Leslie County, and they consistently expressed appreciation for the improved health care the nurses brought.[3] Of course, it is not enough to point to local residents' acceptance of mountain reformers and their projects to justify and excuse their actions. We must note when reformers failed to challenge the dominant culture when given the opportunity to do so, and we should scrutinize their role in reinforcing mountain stereotypes. Still, we must not overlook the good they did. Considering the forces working against them, it is unlikely that the female reformers Whisnant criticizes could have prevented the industrial, economic, and cultural transformations occurring in the mountains, but in spite of their limitations, Breckinridge and her fellow mountain workers made life better for the people they served.

In her synthesis of American female reform, *Natural Allies: Women's Associations in American History* (1991), Anne Firor Scott emphasizes, "At the most elemental level a child with shoes is better off than a child without shoes, no matter what complex motivation provided the gift."[4] Leslie County residents appreciated the assistance the FNS provided. Judge George Wooten praised Breckinridge's willingness to dedicate her life to improving conditions within his community, noting, "When you've got a weedy row to hoe you don't mind someone comin' in to help ya, do you?"[5]

BRECKINRIDGE WAS a complex woman, but her medical philosophy was simple: every individual deserves affordable health care, highly trained nurses can effectively provide routine checkups, and prevention is essential. The demonstration that she launched in 1925 led to a reduction in the number of infant and maternal deaths in Leslie County. Her organization stopped the spread of infectious diseases, waged a successful war on intestinal parasites, and made contraception widely available for the first time. Breckinridge's ideas have helped to shape health care not only in eastern Kentucky but worldwide.

In 1923, when Breckinridge first proposed to the American Child Health Association the creation of an organization of nurse-midwives dedicated to serving rural mothers and babies, she boldly predicted that although the concept seemed radical at the time, the ideas on which it was based eventually would be "commonplace."[6] And indeed, many of her theories have gained currency. Breckinridge played a key role in selling nurse-midwifery to the American public. Once an alien concept linked in the public's mind with the untrained granny, by the late 1970s nurse-midwives were lauded as offering patients a more nurturing, woman-centered birth experience.[7] Breckinridge's tiered approach helped lead to the creation during the late 1960s of a new type of caregiver, the nurse-practitioner. Her emphasis on prevention is now firmly entrenched even within cost-cutting HMOs.

As the United States searches for ways to control the rapidly rising cost of health care, the potential of the community-focused system Breckinridge endorsed becomes ever more apparent. Breckinridge's ideas concerning rural health care continue to demand consideration as our society searches for practical, cost-effective ways to ensure that all individuals have access to care.

L etters of sympathy poured into the Frontier Nursing Service (FNS) offices following Mary Breckinridge's death, and national newspapers printed glowing tributes to the director. That summer, the Smithsonian Institution created an exhibit in honor of her years of service to the women and children of eastern Kentucky. The display, located in the History and Technology section of the nation's largest museum, included numerous photographs, the director's riding uniform, and a pair of FNS saddlebags, capturing the spirit of the organization Breckinridge had established and nurtured. Yet in showcasing these artifacts, the display signaled the beginning of a new era for the FNS.

In the spring of 1966, when the new exhibit was unveiled, the service's Washington Committee hosted a reception. Helen Browne viewed the ceremony as an opportunity for supporters to celebrate the past and, more important, to catch a glimpse of the organization's future. Browne carefully planned every detail of the evening—from the seating arrangements to the refreshments to her attire. She sought to assure the audience that the FNS would continue to promote the objectives its esteemed founder had endorsed. At the same time, however, she was eager to describe her exciting new plans for the organization. After a great deal of consideration, Browne decided to break tradition and attend the event in street clothes instead of her winter riding uniform. She wanted to focus the meeting on the future. Business attire would allow her to demonstrate the service's new, modern attitude, while the riding uniform would serve only to reify the past, she concluded.[1]

BROWNE RECOGNIZED that the FNS had reached a crossroads. Leslie County had changed a great deal since Breckinridge began her work there forty years earlier. On the surface, Hyden looked little different from any other American small town. Its residents, however, remained devastatingly poor. As part of his Great Society, President Lyndon Johnson had launched the War on Poverty in 1964. The Economic Opportunity Act that he maneuvered through Congress led to the creation of numerous commissions and agencies designed to rehabilitate impoverished areas such as Appalachia. Many optimistic Americans believed it was only a matter of time before all the nation's citizens had equal access to jobs, education, and medical care.

One of the great victories of the War on Poverty came when House Resolution 6675, creating the Medicare and Medicaid programs, was signed into law in July 1965. This legislation followed decades of debate concerning the government's role in health care provision. Medicare ensured that the elderly had access to adequate medical care, while Medicaid was designed to protect the financially and medically needy.[2]

Following Breckinridge's death and the passage of this bill, many FNS supporters questioned whether the organization needed to continue operating. Some observers suggested that it would be more practical for the government, which was active in the region through volunteer groups such as VISTA and the Job Corps, to assume responsibility for the services the FNS always had provided. Browne debated whether the organization she had inherited should continue functioning independently. She addressed the question on everyone's mind—"Are we still needed?"—in an editorial published in the *Quarterly Bulletin*. After a great deal of contemplation and after discussions with coworkers and local residents, she decided that the FNS still had much to contribute to the region. If nothing else, Browne argued, the organization had a responsibility to help its patients adapt to the new government services being introduced.[3] Many of the eager volunteers who invaded the region in the late 1960s had little knowledge of the mountain culture. Browne felt that her nurses had a responsibility to provide a buffer between government agencies and the local people.[4]

The new director recognized that her organization's ability to continue functioning depended not on her pronouncement that the FNS was still relevant but on supporters' willingness to continue sending donations. In 1966,

Browne hired a professional fund-raising agency to assess contributors' impressions of the organization and attitudes concerning its future. The agency found that although many FNS supporters believed that the government could more efficiently provide medical services to the people of eastern Kentucky, most felt that the service was still needed because its staff provided the "human touch" that was lacking in health care at the time.[5]

Convinced that the service's faithful donors would continue to support the organization's work, Browne began to initiate long-needed changes. For nearly a decade, the FNS had been frozen in time. The new director recognized that to survive, the service would have to adopt new ideas and methods to keep pace with the times. Although she had lost a close friend, she expressed relief that she had at last been freed to make the adjustments that would allow the FNS to remain viable.[6]

Staff needs were Browne's first concern. She immediately raised salaries and instituted a retirement plan.[7] She also took steps to enlarge the service's medical team. The medical director had long been unable to keep up with the patient load. Breckinridge had recognized the need to recruit a second physician but had hesitated to do so because of the high cost. In 1966, Browne finally hired the service's first assistant medical director. The same year, she also hired a dentist. The FNS's medical team expanded considerably over the next ten years. By 1975, the organization employed two family practitioners, a pediatrician, and an obstetrician/gynecologist.[8]

An even more pressing issue was how to reorganize the FNS to make it eligible to receive Medicare and Medicaid reimbursements without jeopardizing the high level of care its nurses prided themselves on providing. When dealing with the federal government, Breckinridge had often noted that her service did not fit the model of most public health organizations. She found herself hamstrung by bureaucratic policies on numerous occasions. Browne faced similar obstacles. Medicare and Medicaid had strict rules concerning reimbursement. Every patient had to be seen by a physician. Nursing care and health maintenance services were not covered. At the FNS, nurses provided the bulk of day-to-day care and had always made disease prevention a high priority. Browne recognized that the organization could not survive without government aid, but to accept Medicare and Medicaid funds, she would have to compromise the service's mission.[9]

To comply with federal regulations, the FNS created a Home Health Agency in 1966 to coordinate visits to homebound patients. Nurses could no longer make routine house calls. Every treatment they provided had to be specifically sanctioned by the medical director. If the nurses were visiting one member of a family, they were prohibited from bandaging a cut or treating the cough of another. Sick individuals were advised to visit the clinic for care. Home deliveries, once the service's hallmark, became rare.[10]

With the introduction of Medicare and Medicaid funding, the FNS began to shift from a personalized community health care provider to a standardized, high-tech medical system. The influx of government funds led to a dramatic increase in the organization's operating budget. In 1964, the FNS had a budget of $325,000. By 1970, that number had more than doubled, surpassing $800,000. This rise in income allowed the organization to purchase equipment and hire staff that hospitals in more prosperous regions had long taken for granted.[11] In 1965, Browne announced that the FNS planned to build a new modern hospital as a tribute to its late director. In the two months following her death, donors—without solicitation—sent more than $40,000 in her memory. Browne felt that a new hospital would be a fitting way to memorialize Breckinridge's contributions to the region and to "perpetuat[e] her pioneer work."[12]

Although the new hospital, growing staff, and modern equipment were designed to ensure better health care for the residents of Leslie County, many people, particularly service employees, viewed negatively the organization's transformation. As the FNS grew larger in the 1970s, employees who had worked with the organization before Breckinridge's death complained that it no longer had the "family atmosphere" it had previously possessed.[13] Service members soon would be reduced to delivering "medical care like everybody else." Nurse Molly Lee explained that by demanding that the FNS modernize, the government had "ruined [its] simplicity."[14]

Like the staff, many local residents disliked the growth they witnessed. FNS patient Carolyn Gay noted that after Breckinridge's death, patients and nurses no longer developed personal relationships. Employees increasingly came to view working with the service as just a job, no longer putting "heart and soul into it like [Breckinridge] did."[15] An equal number of Leslie County residents, however, embraced the changes, eager to see the FNS offer the range of services available in urban hospitals. Criticism of the service, largely absent during Breckinridge's lifetime, became common after 1965. Former courier Nancy Dammann suggested that watching television led patients to become more critical as they sought the quick cures available on hospital soap operas.[16]

Most of the complaints directed toward the FNS concerned not the limited range of services it offered but local residents' lack of input into decision making. Breckinridge had consulted the local committees on some issues, such as whether to distribute birth control. However, on most issues, she told committee members what she planned to do and expected their stamp of approval. One local resident recalled that "what Mary Breckinridge wanted happened, thank you. The mountain people just said 'Lovely' and accepted it very happily."[17] Following the leader's death, residents became more vocal, criticizing the FNS for failing to interact with its neighbors and for ignoring community officials' input. Many area residents also condemned the service for hiring locals to perform only menial labor.[18] In 1975, a reporter for the *Louisville Courier-Journal* claimed that the FNS's "mystique" was beginning to crack. The reporter noted that the service's maternalistic attitude, which patients accepted in 1925, was not tolerated fifty years later. In 1975, in response to complaints, the FNS established an advisory committee composed of twenty-four local residents who represented a cross-section of the community.[19]

In the midst of growing local unrest, the FNS moved forward with its plan to build a new hospital. When the service built Hyden Hospital in 1928, it cost $30,000. The new Mary Breckinridge Hospital would cost nearly one hundred times that amount. Browne hoped that a large chunk of the expense would come from the federal government, with additional funds from FNS patrons and local residents.[20]

Raising money would occupy much of Browne's time between 1966 and 1975, when the new facility finally opened its doors. Although she had little experience writing grants and meeting with government officials, she had no choice but to learn. She submitted a request for funding through the Hill-Burton Hospital Construction Act in 1966, but the service's application was denied after she received only five minutes to present the organization's case. Despite the rejection, Browne had architects proceed with drawing plans for the new hospital.[21]

Although she had little luck with the government, the level of private donations exceeded Browne's expectations. Professional fund-raisers predicted that the service would be able to raise only $1,750,000. FNS administrators optimistically set a goal of $2,800,000. They then raised the first $2,000,000 in less than one year.[22] Local residents contributed nearly $50,000.[23] Private donors and foundations chipped in another $3,000,000, and the Appalachian Regional Commission provided an additional $1,200,000. The structure, including equipment and furnishings, cost just under $3,000,000. The surplus revenue would help defray the increased expenses of operating the new hospital.[24]

The Appalachian Regional Commission agreed to fund the FNS's project not because commission members recognized the need for a new hospital in Leslie County but because they were impressed by the organization's potential to train rural medical practitioners.[25] As it had for the previous thirty years, the FNS continued to offer instruction in midwifery. This field experienced a tremendous surge in popularity in the early 1970s. Empowered by the feminist movement and by a declining respect for organized medicine, women began to demand a greater say in their health care.[26] However, demand by women only partially explains the renewed interest in midwifery. The need to provide care to poor individuals who lacked access to physicians' services played an equally important role in the field's popularity. Nurse-midwives, experts hoped, could provide affordable, safe care during normal pregnancies. Overburdened with Medicaid cases that provided only meager reimbursements, physicians began to look more favorably on midwives. By 1973, nurse-midwives had gained the legal right to practice in seventeen states.[27]

In the early 1970s, the number of schools offering midwifery training expanded considerably, but the FNS's long-established program, although it offered only a certificate, not a master's degree, as did many of the new programs, remained popular. In 1973, Browne reported that the FNS received on average two hundred inquiries each month from individuals who wished to study at the school, and the school maintained a two-year waiting list.[28]

In 1970, the FNS began offering a new program to train family nurse-practitioners (FNPs). The nurse-practitioner movement that swept the country during the 1980s and 1990s was in its infancy at this point. Mary Breckinridge had long understood that properly trained nurses could effectively treat minor illnesses and provide preventative care under physicians' direction. The medical community was slow to adopt her theory, but as medical costs rose and the nation faced a shortage of doctors in the 1960s, many people began to look to highly trained nurses to assume responsibility for some of the routine duties traditionally performed by physicians.[29]

The FNP training program "formalized what FNS nurses had been doing for years."[30] The FNS accepted students who held associate's degrees, hospital diplomas, or bachelor's degrees in nursing. The FNS's one-year curriculum consisted of training in diagnosis, assessment, and management of common family health problems. The program was administered jointly by the service's medical director and Gertrude Isaacs, a nurse-midwife who held a doctorate in nursing.[31] Isaacs praised the program for allowing nurses, who had for too long been "hiding [their] light under a bushel," to demonstrate fully their skills.[32]

Nurse-practitioners gained legitimacy in the 1970s, but agencies still were unable to recoup their fees because private insurance plans as well as Medicare and Medicaid refused to reimburse for their services. The FNS played an important role in changing these policies. In 1976, the FNS urged supporters to write to their congressional representatives in support of House Bill 2504, which would make nurse-practitioners' and physician's assistants' fees reimbursable. Isaacs testified before the House Ways and Means Subcommittee regarding the need for this legislation, particularly in rural areas.[33] Finally, in December 1977, President Jimmy Carter signed the Rural Health Clinic Services Act, allowing nurse-practitioners, certified nurse-midwives, and physician's assistants to be reimbursed under Medicare and Medicaid.[34]

Responding to the decline in births in Leslie County and recognizing the needs of students across the United States, the FNS adapted its training programs in the 1990s to provide distance education. Students now remain within their own communities, working with established practitioners who serve as preceptors. In 2003, the FNS began to offer master's degrees and added a post-master's track two years later. By 2007, the FNS training programs had more than two thousand alumni, including practitioners in all fifty states and ten foreign countries. Assisting medically underserved areas remains as central to the organization's mission as ever. Breckinridge's goal of improving health care lives on as the service graduates new practitioners who carry its founder's philosophy of providing rural health care throughout the world.[35]

Notes

Abbreviations

EC   Executive Committee
FNSCBC   Frontier Nursing Service Collection, Southern Appalachian Archives,
            Hutchins Library, Berea College, Berea, Kentucky
FNSCUK   Frontier Nursing Service Collection, University of Kentucky Special
            Collections, M. I. King Library, Lexington
FNSOHC   Frontier Nursing Service Oral History Collection, University of Kentucky
            Special Collections, M. I. King Library, Lexington
FNSQB   *Frontier Nursing Service Quarterly Bulletin*
HEB   Helen E. Browne
KCB   Katherine Carson Breckinridge
MB   Mary Breckinridge
MBT   Mary Breckinridge Thompson
PC   Prewitt Collection, Mary Breckinridge Series, uncataloged, University of
            Kentucky Special Collections, M. I. King Library, Lexington
SB   Sophonisba Breckinridge
WN   Mary Breckinridge, *Wide Neighborhoods: A Story of the Frontier Nursing
            Service* (1952; Lexington: University Press of Kentucky, 1981)
WPAR   Works Progress Administration Research Project Records, Kornhauser
            Health Sciences Library, University of Louisville, Louisville, Kentucky

Introduction

1. "Mary Breckinridge, 1881–1965," *FNSQB* 41 (Summer 1965): 17.

2. "She Hath Done What She Could," *Hazard Herald*, May 20, 1965, FNSCUK, box 370.

3. Breckinridge and representatives of the organization even today prefer to call it simply Frontier Nursing Service. For its founder, doing so reinforced the universality of her project and her expectation that it would be replicated in rural areas throughout the country. Because her goal of expanding nationwide never occurred and the service instead became a unique, singular organization, I choose to call it *the* Frontier Nursing Service.

4. Forty-year total, FNSCUK, box 156, folder 11.

5. "American" appeal, May 1942, FNSCUK, box 29, folder 14.

6. "Mary Breckinridge Served Long and Well," *Louisville Courier-Journal*, May 18, 1965.

7. "Mrs. Mary Breckinridge Designated Outstanding Citizen by Newspapers," *Thousandsticks*, January 29, 1953, FNS scrapbook, fall 1951–June 1954, FNSCUK, box 45.

8. Bob Hope Woman of the Week citation, April 9, 1954, FNSCUK, box 364, folder 25. See FNSCUK, box 364, for more information on her honors and awards.

9. Articles about the service include Anne G. Campbell, "Mary Breckinridge"; Crowe-Carraco, "Mary Breckinridge"; Dye, "Mary Breckinridge"; Klotter, *Breckinridges of Kentucky*, chapter 17, 18. The FNS has attracted the attention of many graduate students, particularly those in the field of nursing, who have produced benign narrative accounts of the FNS's work. See, for example, Snihurowycz, "Frontier Nursing Service"; Tirpak, "Frontier Nursing Service"; Criss, "Culture and the Provision of Care." Three other dissertations, while more analytical, again look at the FNS from a specific angle and do not investigate the full picture of Breckinridge's work: Altizer, "Establishment"; Blackwell, "Ability 'To Do Much Larger Work' "; Harris, "Constructing Colonialism."

10. This collection consists of 292 cubic feet of materials contained in more than six hundred carefully inventoried boxes. Due to privacy issues, some of the collection dealing with patients' medical records is restricted.

11. MB to Lucille "Pansy" Turner, January 2, 1951, FNSCUK, box 346, folder 13.

12. In the 1970s, researchers collected 194 interviews that now make up the FNS Oral History Collection, housed in the University of Kentucky Special Collections, M. I. King Library, Lexington.

13. For an overview of the Progressive Era, see Wiebe, *Search for Order*. The body of scholarship on women's Progressive Era reform is substantial. See, for example, Aiken, *Harnessing the Power*; Allen F. Davis, *American Heroine*; Allen F. Davis, *Spearheads for Reform*; Fitzpatrick, *Endless Crusade*; Frankel and Dye, *Gender, Class, Race and Reform*; Hall, *Revolt*; Odem, *Delinquent Daughters*; Payne, *Reform, Labor, and Feminism*. Recent scholarship has expanded the scope of inquiry to focus on reform efforts outside northeastern cities. See Baldwin, *Cora Wilson Stewart*; Curry, *Modern Mothers*; Pascoe, *Relations of Rescue*; Sims, *Power of Femininity*.

14. Kornbluh, "New Literature," 178, 181–82.

15. See, for example, Skocpol, *Protecting Soldiers and Mothers*; Muncy, *Creating a Female Dominion*.

16. See especially Gordon, *Pitied but Not Entitled*; Ladd-Taylor, *Mother-Work*. See also Koven and Michel, *Mothers*. The articles in this groundbreaking volume investigate maternalism from a variety of perspectives and offer comparisons of how maternalism shaped public policies in various countries.

17. On this idea of an entering wedge, see Skocpol, *Protecting Soldiers and Mothers*, 379.

18. For examples of the various projects female Appalachian reformers tackled, see Barney, *Authorized to Heal*; Blackwell, "Ability 'To Do Much Larger Work' "; Forderhase, "Eve Returns to the Garden"; Searles, *College for Appalachia*; Stoddart, *Challenge and Change*; Tice, "School-Work and Mother-Work."

19. Whisnant, *All That Is Native and Fine*, 11.

20. Ibid., 263.

21. Searles, *College for Appalachia*, ix. Searles notes that his main goal in documenting Alice Lloyd's story is to challenge Whisnant.

22. Stoddart, *Challenge and Change*, 4, 231.

23. Searles, *College for Appalachia*, 14, 146, 158.

24. Stoddart, *Challenge and Change*, 230.

25. Searles, *College for Appalachia*.

26. Albert Steward quoted in Tice, "School-Work and Mother-Work," 216.

27. Ibid., 193.

28. Ibid.

29. Ibid., 216.

30. Ibid., 217.

31. See, for example, Cavender, *Folk Medicine*, which examines medical care delivery in the context of socioeconomic change.

32. Barney, *Authorized to Heal*.

33. Much of the historiography of medicine centers around doctors' calculated campaign to establish their professional and economic dominance. Starr, *Social Transformation*, offers the most detailed account of physicians' struggle to establish their "sovereignty." E. Richard Brown, *Rockefeller Medicine Men*, likewise emphasizes doctors' less altruistic motives. Nursing historians have offered an alternative perspective, emphasizing the factors that limited nurses' quest to establish themselves as professionals. See Reverby, *Ordered to Care*; Melosh, *"Physicians' Hand."*

34. The sociological literature on professionalization is extensive. Select examples include Friedson, "Are the Professions Necessary?"; Bledstein, *Culture of Professionalism*; Larson, *Rise of Professionalism*.

35. See Borst, *Catching Babies*; Leavitt, *Brought to Bed*; Litoff, *American Midwives*; Wertz and Wertz, *Lying-In*.

36. Ettinger, *Nurse-Midwifery*, 194.

37. HEB, interview by Dale Deaton, March 27, 1979, 79OH174FNS75, FNSOHC.

38. Freedman, " 'Burning of Letters Continues,' " 185.

Chapter One

1. Klotter, "Family Influences," 121.

2. Hess, *America's Political Dynasties*, 239.

3. J. W. Brock to W. C. P. Breckinridge, March 18, 1884, quoted in Klotter, *Breckinridges of Kentucky*, ix.

4. Taney, *Kentucky Pioneer Women*, 76.

5. William C. Davis, "John C. Breckinridge," 198.

6. Klotter, *Breckinridges of Kentucky*, 11, 315. Klotter's interpretation has heavily shaped my portrait of the Breckinridge family. For a discussion of the sense of responsibility that came with being a Breckinridge, see pp. 303–24.

7. William C. Davis, "John C. Breckinridge," 199.

8. According to Wyatt-Brown, the tradition of recording family lineage through the naming of children was a distinctly upper-class, southern phenomenon: "The relation of the dutiful child to ancestors and to community was thus made clear [through the selection of names]; one could not easily escape to pursue one's own hopes under such circumstances" (*Southern Honor*, 122). On the Breckinridge tradition of naming children after kin, see Terry, "Family Empires," 250–51.

9. Klotter, *Breckinridges of Kentucky*, 3–13. For a supporting view of the Breckinridge family's ascent through the frontier elite, see Terry, "Family Empires."

10. Harrison and Klotter, *New History*, 49, 70.

11. Klotter, *Breckinridges of Kentucky*, 3–13; Alexander Brown, *Cabells and Their Kin*, 232–33.

12. William C. Davis, "John C. Breckinridge," 198.

13. Klotter, *Breckinridges of Kentucky*, 95–136; William C. Davis, "John C. Breckinridge," 209.

14. Bolin, "Sins of the Fathers," 39.

15. Ibid.; *WN*, 6. On "virulent rebel institutions" and for a description of Washington and Lee's role in providing a Lost Cause education, see Charles Reagan Wilson, *Baptized in Blood*, 152.

16. Bolin, "Clifton Rodes Breckinridge," 413–16.

17. Bolin, "Sins of the Fathers," 35–52; MB to Harold M. Carlson, May 8, 1945, FNSCUK, box 340, folder 3.

18. John Q. Anderson, "Dr. James Green Carson," 251–54; *WN*, 6–7; Airlie Plantation Deed, Airlie Plantation Records, 1846, 1862, 1868, 1951, series G, part I, reel 11, Texas History Center, University of Texas, Austin. For more details on Carson's Louisiana holdings, see Menn, *Large Slaveholders*, 175–76.

19. John Q. Anderson, "Dr. James Green Carson," 251–54.

20. Minnie Murphy to Robert C. Reinders, May 7, 1951, Airlie Plantation Records, 1846, 1862, 1868, 1951, series G, part I, reel 11.

21. Ronald L. F. Davis, *Good and Faithful Labor*, 26.

22. D. Clayton James, *Antebellum Natchez*, 159.

23. Woodman, *King Cotton*, 244; Roark, *Masters without Slaves*, 77; Ronald L. F. Davis, *Good and Faithful Labor*, 139.

24. John Q. Anderson, "Dr. James Green Carson," 263.

25. "Annals of Hazelwood," in *Family Records, William Waller Carson, Knoxville, Tennessee, 1845–1930*, 289, FNSCUK, box 369, folder 4.

26. Genealogy chart compiled by MB, September 3, 1948, FNSCUK, box 369, folder 1.

27. Letter from Clifton Breckinridge quoted in Bolin, "Clifton Rodes Breckinridge," 414.

28. Ibid., 416.

29. Ibid.; David W. Hacker, "Dealing with the Russians," *Arkansas Gazette*, July 3, 1955, FNSCUK, box 369, folder 3. Though Bolin does not make this point, this nickname paid tribute to Clifton Breckinridge's distinguished predecessor, Stephen A. Douglas, often called the Little Giant.

30. Although Mary Breckinridge's parents could have afforded to purchase a house, her father preferred renting because he felt "Washington real estate wasn't safe." He had seen his father's house confiscated when he decided to join the Confederacy and consequently hesitated to purchase real estate (MB to Marion Shouse Lewis, May 21, 1943, FNSCUK, box 62, folder 6; *WN*, 7–8).

31. MB, "Description of a Rural Community Known to Me," FNSCUK, box 366, folder 12.

32. Joe Carson, "I Remember . . .," typescript, FNSCUK, box 369, folder 2.

33. Klotter, *Breckinridges of Kentucky*, 315; MB, "Description of a Rural Community"; *WN*, 3–4, 8; MB to Waller Carson, November 7, 1946, FNSCUK, box 340, folder 6. For additional details about Oasis, see drafts of *Wide Neighborhoods*, FNSCUK, box 350, folder 1.

34. My understanding of the lore passed down by the Breckinridge family is shaped by Brundage's collection of essays on collective memory in the South, *Where These Memories Grow*.

35. Hall, " 'You Must Remember This,' " 463.

36. Charles Reagan Wilson, *Baptized in Blood*, 100.

37. Clifton R. Breckinridge speech, in Southern Society for the Promotion of the Study of Race Conditions and Problems in the South, *Race Problems*, 171–73.

38. For a fascinating look at how southern children—both white and black—learned the rules of racial etiquette, see Ritterhouse, *Growing Up Jim Crow*.

39. For a similar example of a southern family that measured status by heritage rather than monetary wealth, see Fosl, *Subversive Southerner*, 18.

40. Woodward, *Origins of the New South*, 157.

41. Phipps, " 'Their Desire to Visit the Southerners,' " 222–25; Cook, "Growing Up," 40. Cook notes that although former planters and their children viewed themselves as poor, most still had more resources than their fellow southerners, black and white.

42. Cook, "Growing Up," 12–13.

43. Welter, "Cult of True Womanhood," 152. For black women's attempts to uphold prescribed gender roles, see Jones, *Labor of Love*, 59.

44. See, for example, Wolfe, *Daughters*; Scott, *Southern Lady*.

45. Foster, *Ghosts*, 137.

46. Ibid., 4; Wolfe, *Daughters*, 134–35; Friedman, *Enclosed Garden*. Despite these restrictive expectations, Wolfe and Friedman argue, southern women actually had an easier time entering the public arena than their northern counterparts. Since the southern heritage placed a strong emphasis on women's duty to care for others, the region's women were better able to expand their caring from the home to the community.

47. Bolin, "Clifton Rodes Breckinridge," 408, 425.

48. KCB to Susanna Preston Lees, September 15, 1895, quoted in Willis, "Arkansan in St. Petersburg," 18.

49. Ibid., 25; "Minister Breckinridge May Resign," *New York Times*, December 21, 1894.

50. Willis, "Arkansan in St. Petersburg," 16. For additional references to their strained finances, see KCB to MB, April 15, 1897, February 14, 1899, PC.

51. *WN*, 9–11. Mary never shared a close bond with Lees. On occasion, the sisters lost track of one another, prompting Mary to send a self-addressed envelope to Lees requesting notification the next time she moved (MB to Lees Dunn, April 13, 1942, FNSCUK, box 339, folder 7). Mary's relationships with her brothers, both career military officers, were closer, but a sense of duty as much as sincere affection seems to have underscored those connections.

52. *WN*, 1, 10–12. Mary noted that she dealt with "sadness" by writing poetry. In her autobiography, she remembers writing a great deal of poetry during her years in Russia. See MB to KCB, February 19, 1899, PC.

53. *WN*, 7.

54. Ibid., 5.

55. Ibid., 8–9.

56. Ibid., 16, 20.

57. MB to Katy Carson, October 4, 1896, PC.

58. *WN*, 21.

59. Ibid., 19.

60. Ibid., 20.

61. Ibid., 21.

62. MB, typescript of *Wide Neighborhoods*, FNSCUK, box 351, folder 1; *WN*, 22. Katherine Carson Breckinridge's correspondence expressed her preference that Mary study languages rather than mathematics (KCB to MB, September 12, 1897, PC).

63. *WN*, 22.

64. Ibid., 24.

65. MB to KCB, September 15, 1897, PC.

66. KCB to MB, September 12, 1897, PC.

67. Ibid., 29. She describes her sense of estrangement from her classmates in MB to KCB, February 9, 1898, PC.

68. MB to KCB, February 19, 1899, PC.

69. Miss Low's School Yearbook, 1898, FNSCUK, box 366, folder 5.

70. *WN*, 46.

71. Ibid., 26.

72. MB, typescript of *Wide Neighborhoods*.

73. Rosenzweig, *Anchor of My Life*, 6.

74. Kessler-Harris, *Out to Work*, 113; Woloch, *Women and the American Experience*, 275. For a concise overview of the options becoming available to the New Woman, see Evans, *Born for Liberty*, 147–52.

75. Solomon, *In the Company of Educated Women*, 45, 47, 56, 60, 63.

76. Antler, " 'After College What?,' " 10.

77. Gordon, *Pitied but Not Entitled*, 153. Statistics show that as many as 50 percent of college women from this era chose not to marry at a time when more than 90 percent of the general population committed to such unions. For some educated women, marriage would come later in life, but many would remain perpetually single or would form single-sex relationships known as Boston marriages.

78. Emotional breakdowns among talented women of this generation appear to have been quite common but remain understudied. Historians have documented crises experienced by individual women such as Jane Addams, but a more comprehensive investigation of the ways New Women coped with the distance separating their goals and options is needed.

79. *WN*, 45.

80. Mrs. Samuel Preston Davis Sr., "Arkansas Society."

81. "Katherine Carson Breckinridge," in *Family Records*, 160–61.

82. "Mrs. S. P. Lees," in ibid., 169.

83. Surprisingly, no full-scale biography of Sophonisba Breckinridge has appeared to date. For more information on her education and career, see Goan, "Establishing Their Place." Sophonisba and Mary were distant cousins. Both were descendants of John Breckinridge. For more details on their connection, see Klotter, *Breckinridges of Kentucky*, xv–xviii.

84. W. C. P. Breckinridge to SB, October 8, 1884, Breckinridge Family Papers, reel 1, box 739, University of Kentucky Special Collections, M. I. King Library, Lexington.

85. Desha Breckinridge, "Mary Curry Desha Breckinridge," *Lexington Herald*, June 25, 1918.

86. W. C. P. Breckinridge to SB, March 30, 1885, Breckinridge Family Papers, reel 1, box 739.

87. *WN*, 32–33.

88. Klotter, *Breckinridges of Kentucky*, 9, 319.

89. MB to KCB, September 8, [1897], PC.

90. KCB to MB, September 12, 1897, PC.

91. *WN*, 40.

92. Loren Nunn Brown, "Work of the Dawes Commission."

93. *WN*, 41–43.

94. Ibid., 45, 36–37. For a young woman, the loss of sexual purity was the worst fate possible. Organizations such as the Women's Christian Temperance Union warned that men had natural "animal instincts" that they constantly struggled to keep in check. Any departure on women's part from society's dictates of modesty and decorum could lead men to lose control. To prevent such travesties, chaperones became a required feature of interactions between unmarried gentlemen and ladies by the 1880s. See Odem, *Delinquent Daughters*, 24–25; Rothman, *Hands and Hearts*, 185–86, 208.

95. *WN*, 26.

96. MB, *Organdie and Mull*. Breckinridge intended this short story to be a fund-raiser for the FNS.

97. MB to Mrs. Stephen Bonsal, November 9, 1948, FNSCUK, box 69, folder 8.

98. MB, *Organdie and Mull*, 34.

99. *WN*, 47–48.

100. Ibid., 46–50. For dates of her first marriage, see Breckinridge Genealogy, FNSCUK, box 369, folder 1. Breckinridge took her husbands' names both times she married. She resumed using her maiden name, however, later in life. For clarity, I have chosen to refer to her as "Mary Breckinridge" throughout this volume ; her employees called her "Mrs. Breckinridge."

101. MB, journal excerpt, PC.

102. *WN*, 51.

103. Mary Breckinridge Morrison, "Women of Thackeray," copy in FNSCUK, box 356, folder 1.

104. The school was eventually renamed Lees-McRae College to recognize Susanna Lees's contributions ("S. P. Lees," in *Family Records*, 168–72, 304–7).

105. *WN*, 51.

106. Ibid. Breckinridge explains in her autobiography that following Morrison's death, she did not consider going to college because she had renounced all her professional aspirations when she married him. She was drawn to nursing simply because it would allow her to serve others.

107. Reverby, *Ordered to Care*, 77.

108. *WN*, 52. During this era, most schools of nursing required applicants to submit letters from their physicians and other community leaders testifying to their physical and moral fitness. St. Luke's was no exception. See *History of the St. Luke's Hospital Training School*, 30.

109. Kalisch and Kalisch, *Advance*, 135.

110. Donovan, *Different Call*, 36–37; *History of the St. Luke's Hospital Training School*, 25.

111. Starr, *Social Transformation*.

112. Ibid., 73–74, 151, 154–56.

113. Roberts, *American Nursing*, 15.

114. Ibid.; Melosh, *"Physician's Hand,"* 32.

115. Reverby, *Ordered to Care*, 60.

116. Sandelowski, *Devices and Desires*, 44.

117. *History of the St. Luke's Hospital Training School*, 32, 34, 54–56, 72.

118. Melosh, *"Physician's Hand,"* 52, 66–67.

119. *WN*, 56–57.

120. Registered nurse certificate issued to Mary Breckinridge Morrison by the State of New York, May 28, 1910, FNSCUK, box 364, folder 2.

121. *WN*, 58–59.

122. Mary Breckinridge Morrison, "Poetry of the Southern United States," copy in FNSCUK, box 356, folder 2.

123. KCB to MB, September 12, 1897, PC.

Chapter Two

1. Pinkley-Call, *Pioneer Tales*, 45–46; Rayburn, *Eureka Springs Story*, 16, 33.

2. Allard, *Who Is Who*, 226; Rayburn, *Eureka Springs Story*, 71; Schaefer, *I Didn't Know That Either!*; Susan Schaefer, telephone interview by author, June 14, 2001.

3. For example, using the pen name "Progressive Citizen," she carried on a running correspondence regarding an ordinance to ban dogs within city limits, which she emphatically opposed. See clippings in FNSCUK, box 357.

4. It is doubtful that Mary ever intended to work as a nurse, but if she had, doing so would have been impractical after her marriage as a consequence of her class status and the demanding nature of the work. Hospitals hired few graduate nurses, relying instead on students for labor. Trained nurses thus had few opportunities except in private duty service, which required that they hire themselves out to families who could afford to pay for in-home nursing care. In the early twentieth century, such work had not completely shed its association with domestic service, requiring the nurse to remain on duty around the clock and resulting in a chaotic, unpredictable schedule (Kalisch and Kalisch, *Advance*, 186–88).

5. Ibid., 259–63. For more information on the professionalization of medicine, see Starr, *Social Transformation*, 102–12.

6. Miller, "Arkansas Nurses," 165, 156–57. The liberal law that Breckinridge helped to pass in Arkansas helped the FNS in later years. Kentucky had a reciprocal agreement with Arkansas, and Arkansas had low standards for licensure, making it easier for British nurses, who were highly trained but did not always use the same methods as American nurses, to become licensed. See MB to Jessie Greathouse, March 23, 1948, FNSCUK, box 196, folder 8.

7. MBT, "Report." Correspondence concerning Breckinridge's professional affiliations during these years is located in FNSCUK, box 336.

8. Rheta Childe Dorr quoted in Baker, "Domestication," 91.

9. MBT, "Motherhood—A Career," November 1916.

10. *WN*, 62.

11. Wiebe, *Search for Order*, 169.

12. For more information on the development of the child welfare movement in the United States, see Meckel, *Save the Babies*; Ladd-Taylor, *Mother-Work*.

13. Dye and Smith, "Mother Love and Infant Death," 332.

14. Meckel, *Save the Babies*, 103; Julia Grant, *Raising Baby*.

15. Evans, *Born for Liberty*, 127.

16. Woloch, *Women and the American Experience*, 300, 606.

17. Laurel Thatcher Ulrich quoted in Julia Grant, *Raising Baby*, 15.

18. For more information on the scientific housekeeping movement, see Graham, "Domesticating Efficiency," 643–48.

19. Evans, *Born for Liberty*, 181.

20. Muncy, *Creating a Female Dominion*, 113.

21. Meckel, *Save the Babies*, 101–3; Klaus, *Every Child a Lion*, 32; Ehrenreich and English, *For Her Own Good*, 183–86.

22. For more information on the U.S. Children's Bureau, see Lindenmeyer, *"A Right to Childhood."* Ladd-Taylor, *Raising a Baby*, is a good source for viewing how mothers responded to the Children's Bureau. Muncy, *Creating a Female Dominion*, provides an excellent discussion of the political opportunities the Children's Bureau opened up for women.

23. Ladd-Taylor, "Hull House Goes to Washington," 117. The Children's Bureau initiated its campaign to improve reporting of births in 1913. Its volunteers conducted a door-to-door survey of areas that were not included in the Federal Birth Registration Area (that is, areas known to have less than 90 percent of births recorded). These efforts led to the addition

of fifteen new states to the Birth Registration Area by 1920. For more details on this campaign, see Muncy, *Creating a Female Dominion*, 58–62.

24. Meckel, *Save the Babies*, 238, 240. By comparison, in 2004, the U.S. infant mortality rate was 6.8 per 1,000 live births and the maternal mortality rate was 13.1 per 100,000 live births (National Center for Health Statistics, "Deaths: Final Data for 2004," <http://www.cdc.gov/nchs/>, accessed October 30, 2007).

25. *WN*, 45.

26. See MBT, "Motherhood—A Career," November 1916, 40.

27. Bederman, *Manliness and Civilization*, 99.

28. Ladd-Taylor, *Mother-Work*, 46–47.

29. *WN*, 60.

30. MBT, *Breckie*, 138.

31. Ibid., 151.

32. Julia Grant, *Raising Baby*, 44.

33. MBT, *Breckie*, 47, 151; *WN*, 61; Breckinridge's scrapbook of her son's life, PC.

34. Pickens, *Eugenics*, 136; *WN*, 60; MBT, *Breckie*, v, 40. She usually kept Breckie inside on extremely cold nights, but on one occasion, he did wake with frostbite.

35. *WN*, 65.

36. Ibid., 66.

37. MBT, *Breckie*, 58–59.

38. Ibid., 113. Breckie's scribbles decorate Breckinridge's correspondence in FNSCUK, box 336, folder 3.

39. *WN*, 62.

40. Copies of these articles are located in FNSCUK, box 355.

41. MBT, "Motherhood—A Career," November 1916.

42. In future chapters I will explore Breckinridge's views on eugenics and the ways she applied them to the FNS. For more information on eugenics, see Chesler, *Woman of Valor*, 122–23; Gordon, *Woman's Body, Woman's Right*, 270; Higham, *Strangers*, 150–53; Pickens, *Eugenics*, 126–27.

43. MBT to Elizabeth Harrison, August 28, 1917, MBT to John Dewey, August 28, 1917, FNSCUK, box 336, folder 3; *Crescent College Bulletin* 11 (July 1918): 2.

44. Elizabeth Harrison to MBT, September 5, 1917, William Hard to MBT, October 11, 1917, FNSCUK, box 336, folder 3. Harrison was a leader in the kindergarten movement, and Hard worked in a Chicago settlement house and was particularly interested in the legal rights of women and mothers.

45. Julia C. Lathrop to MBT, June 3, 1918, reprinted in *Crescent College Bulletin* 11 (July 1918): 1.

46. MBT to Murray Auerbach, September 16, 1917, FNSCUK, box 336, folder 3.

47. *Crescent College Bulletin* 11 (July 1918): 1.

48. MBT to SB, June 19, 1917, FNSCUK, box 336, folder 3. Sophonisba Breckinridge served as vice president of the National American Woman Suffrage Association. See Barr, "Profession for Women," 245–51. Breckinridge probably was also influenced by another

cousin, Madeline McDowell Breckinridge, who served as second vice president of the National American Woman Suffrage Association in 1914. For more information on the suffrage movement in the South, see Ida Clyde Clarke, "What Woman Suffragists Are Doing in the South," *Southern Woman's Magazine*, November 1914, 14–15. Breckinridge's membership in nursing organizations may also have influenced her to support the suffrage movement. Lewenson, *Taking Charge*, argues that many nurses supported female suffrage because they believed doing so would aid their attempts to strengthen training requirements.

49. Baker, "Domestication."

50. MBT, "Effect of Woman's Suffrage on the Home," *Eureka Springs Daily Times-Echo*, June 21, 1917, FNSCUK, box 357, folder 9.

51. Cott, *Grounding of Modern Feminism*, 4.

52. MBT, "Woman's Great Service," *Eureka Springs Daily Times-Echo*, January 16, 1918, FNSCUK, box 357, folder 9.

53. *WN*, 181.

54. MBT, "Woman's Great Service."

55. Ladd-Taylor, "Toward Defining Maternalism," provides a succinct description of the differences separating maternalists and feminists.

56. *WN*, 61.

57. Clara D. Noyes to MBT, July 3, 1917, FNSCUK, box 336, folder 3; MBT, "Red Cross Busy at Work," *Eureka Springs Daily Times-Echo*, October 16, 1917, FNSCUK, box 336, folder 3.

58. See news clippings in FNSCUK, box 357, folder 4.

59. *WN*, 69–71.

60. Carson Breckinridge to MBT, February 18, 1916, <http://www.mcu.usmc.mil/MCR Cweb/ftw/files/pap1418.txt>, accessed May 2001.

61. MBT, *Breckie*, 171–72.

62. Ibid.

63. Ibid., 176, 178, 179, 182, 185, 191; "Breckinridge Thompson," *Eureka Springs Daily Times-Echo*, January 24, 1918; "Breckinridge Thompson," *Fort Smith Times-Record*, January 26, 1918. Breckie was originally buried beside his sister in Fort Smith, Arkansas. Mary Breckinridge later had their bodies moved to Lexington, Kentucky, and they are now buried beside her at the Lexington Cemetery.

64. J. Fred Bolton, editorial, *Eureka Springs Daily Times-Echo*, February 25, 1918, in Breckinridge's scrapbook of her son's life, PC.

65. MB to "Chela" [Margaret Gage], January 10, 1952, FNSCUK, box 352, folder 1.

66. MBT, *Breckie*, 93–94.

67. Ibid., 29.

68. *Good Housekeeping*, May 1917, quoted in Rosenzweig, *Anchor of My Life*, 5.

69. *WN*, 66.

70. MBT, *Breckie*, 196.

71. Ladd-Taylor, *Mother-Work*, 49.

72. Ladd-Taylor, "'My Work Came Out of Agony and Grief,'" 324.

73. MBT to SB, May 23, 1918, FNSCUK, box 336, folder 4.

74. Jane A. Delano to MB, February 4, 1918, MBT to Jane A. Delano, March 2, 1918, FNSCUK, box 336, folder 4.

75. MBT to Ella Phillips Crandall, February 26, 1918, FNSCUK, box 336, folder 4. See also Allard, *Who Is Who*, 226.

76. MBT to SB, May 23, 1918, FNSCUK, box 336, folder 4.

77. *WN*, 75. For more information on the "brother / sister rule," see Zeiger, *In Uncle Sam's Service*, 58, 146. Zeiger argues that the government designed this ruling to "staunch the disruptive flow of feminine emotionalism across the Atlantic."

78. MBT, *Breckie*, vi, 188, 195, v.

79. Braude, *Radical Spirits*, 16, 19, 25, 27.

80. Ibid., 33–34, 51.

81. MBT, *Breckie*, 195.

82. Lathrop's friendship with Sophonisba Breckinridge led Mary Breckinridge to begin her work with the Children's Bureau. For more information, see MB, draft of *Wide Neighbor-hoods*, FNSCUK, box 350, folder 3.

83. Muncy, *Creating a Female Dominion*, 96–98.

84. Reports of Thompson's trips and meeting announcements are in FNSCUK, box 336, folder 5. See also "Frontier Nursing Service," *Woman's Almanac* (1940), reprint in FNSCUK, box 35, folder 21; MBT to KCB, August 25, 1918, FNSCUK, box 336, folder 4.

85. "Care for Children," *Wilmington Morning News*, July 1, 1918, FNSCUK, box 336, folder 5.

86. "Child Welfare Worker Heard," *Moline Daily Dispatch*, August 24, 1918, FNSCUK, box 336, folder 5.

87. "Aid Infants, Save Nation," *Chicago Daily Journal*, August 21, 1918, FNSCUK, box 336, folder 5.

88. MBT to KCB, September 7, 1918, FNSCUK, box 336, folder 4; report of South Dakota trip, FNSCUK, box 336, folder 5.

89. Ethel Swan to MBT, August 31, 1918, Alice H. Wood to MBT, August 31, 1918, FNSCUK, box 336, folder 4.

90. MBT to KCB, September 16, 1918, FNSCUK, box 336, folder 4.

91. *WN*, 75–76; Gribble, " 'We Hope to Live through It,' " 26, 16. Nurses were in high demand during the epidemic, as many people recognized that trained care could mean the difference between life and death. During a ten-month period from 1918 to 1919, more Americans died from the influenza than died in World Wars I and II, Korea, and Vietnam combined. Many nurses lost their lives.

92. Bangs, *Loss or Gain*, 5.

93. For more on CARD's origins and its contributions, see Chuppa-Cornell, "U.S. Women's Motor Corps," 467.

94. MB, "Program of Work in Organizing a Nursing System in a Rural Section of the Devastated Areas in France—Described in Terms of Geographical, Historical, Racial, Industrial and Economic Forces," FNSCUK, box 366, folder 12.

95. MBT, "Goats: Vic-sur-Aisne," FNSCUK, box 336, folder 6; *WN*, 84–85.

96. The thrill she felt is reflected in MB to KCB, July 18, 1920, FNSCUK, box 336, folder 7.

97. *WN*, 75–110; Klotter, *Breckinridges of Kentucky*, 255–56.

98. *WN*, 95–97. These plans fell through soon after she returned to the United States in 1921. See Breckinridge's correspondence with her mother during 1920 in FNSCUK, box 336, folder 7.

99. *WN*, 63. Breckinridge mentions her relationship with Thompson only briefly in her autobiography and makes no reference to her divorce or the causes that led to it.

100. *Mary B. Thompson v. R. R. Thompson*, divorce suit filed in Sebastian County, Arkansas, May 14, 1920, PC.

101. MBT to KCB, July 23, 1919, FNSCUK, box 336, folder 6; MBT to KCB, January 28, 1920, FNSCUK, box 336, folder 7.

102. The number of divorces in America increased steadily after the Civil War. According to O'Neill, "Divorce in the Progressive Era," one in twenty-one marriages dissolved in 1880, but by 1916, the rate had increased to one in nine.

103. Nowhere in the suit does Breckinridge elaborate on the "indignities" Thompson committed, but her associates have speculated on the nature of his indiscretions. John Marshall Prewitt, her nephew-in-law, hypothesized that Richard Thompson became involved with a female student, noting that Mary's father, Clifton Rodes Breckinridge, considered Thompson "a first class cad" (John Marshall Prewitt to William J. Marshall, March 28, 2002, PC). For additional speculations on Breckinridge's divorce, see HEB, interview by Dale Deaton, March 27, 1979, 79OH174FNS75, FNSOHC; HEB, interview by Carol Crowe-Carraco, March 26, 1979, 79OH173FNS74, FNSOHC; Emily Saugman, interview by Dale Deaton, March 7, 1979, 79OH166FNS67, FNSOHC.

104. MBT to KCB and Eleanor [Blaydes], FNSCUK, box 336, folder 7.

105. Genealogy chart compiled by MB, September 3, 1948, FNSCUK, box 369, folder 1. Breckinridge's niece, Katherine Breckinridge Prewitt, recalled that her aunt removed the stitching from the *T* in her monogram on a tablecloth she later gave to Prewitt (Katherine Prewitt, interview by author, November 10, 1998). Dick Thompson went on to serve as Arkansas state senator from 1925 to 1939 and ran several businesses around Eureka Springs (Allard, *Who Is Who*, 226).

106. MB, memorandum having reference to Mr. Day's chapter called "Frontier Nurses," June 4, 1941, FNSCUK, box 59, folder 12. Breckinridge challenged the idea that she "took back her name," claiming instead that it "it was given to [her] by the courts." See also MB to Clifton Breckinridge, July 14, 1920, FNSCUK, box 336, folder 7.

107. Beatrice Williams, interview by Anne Campbell, January 26, 1979, 79OH148FNS55, FNSOHC.

108. MB to KCB, March 6, 1921, FNSCUK, box 336, folder 8.

109. MB to KCB, March 28, 1921, FNSCUK, box 336, folder 8.

110. MB to KCB, July 3, 1921, FNSCUK, box 336, folder 8.

111. Breckinridge expresses her homesickness in MB to Mrs. Edgar Tufts, March 29, 1921, FNSCUK, box 336, folder 9; MB to KCB, April 1, 1921, FNSCUK, box 336, folder 8.

112. MB to KCB, March 28, 1921, FNSCUK, box 336, folder 8.

113. MB to KCB, April 1, 1921, FNSCUK, box 336, folder 8.

114. MB to KCB, October 17, 1920, FNSCUK, box 336, folder 7.

115. For description of the Brackens, see *WN*, 67–68.

116. C. E. A. Winslow to MB, March 1, 1923, FNSCUK, box 337, folder 2; MB to C. E. A. Winslow, March 6, 1925, FNSCUK, box 337, folder 6; Elizabeth Scarborough to MB, December 20, 1921, FNSCUK, box 336, folder 8.

117. In a draft of *Wide Neighborhoods*, Breckinridge notes that her mother had a very unhappy childhood and that it was only natural for a "homesick refugee" to be emotionally scarred by the experience. The difficulties of Katherine Breckenridge's childhood made her aloof and detached. See MB, typescript of *Wide Neighborhoods*, 6. For additional descriptions of Katherine Breckinridge's reserved demeanor, see "Annals of Hazelwood," in *Family Records, William Waller Carson, Knoxville, Tennessee, 1845–1930*, 290, copy in FNSCUK, box 369, folder 4.

118. For more details on Sophonisba's breakdown, see Barr, "Profession for Women," 103.

119. MB to Anne Morgan, January 10, 1922, FNSCUK, box 337, folder 1.

120. *WN*, 113.

121. Pansy [Lucille Turner] to MB, February 9, 1924, FNSCUK, box 337, folder 3.

122. MBT to Ella Phillips Crandall, February 26, 1918, FNSCUK, box 336, folder 4.

123. *WN*, 114.

Chapter Three

1. MB, "Outline for a Demonstration of a Children's Public Health Service in Owsley County, Kentucky," [1923], 1, FNSCUK, box 348, folder 3.

2. MB, "Memorandum Concerning a Suggested Demonstration for the Reduction [of] the Infant and Maternal Death Rate in a Rural Area of the South," [February 1923], 2, FNSCUK, box 348, folder 3.

3. The rise resulted in part from the movement of birth from home to hospital, where intervention was more likely. The rise also could have resulted from better reporting and record keeping. See Leavitt, *Brought to Bed*, 27, 182.

4. Only two of the twenty-two reporting countries (Belgium and Chile) had higher maternal death rates than the United States. See Van Blarcom, "Provisions," 697.

5. Meckel, *Save the Babies*, 156.

6. Ibid., 142.

7. For a discussion of the Sheppard-Towner Act, see Ladd-Taylor, *Mother-Work*, 167–69; Ladd-Taylor, " 'Grannies' and 'Spinsters' "; Ladd-Taylor, " 'My Work Came Out of Agony and Grief' "; Muncy, *Creating a Female Dominion*, 108; Skocpol, *Protecting Soldiers and Mothers*, 508–10.

8. MacKaye, "Untamed America," 327.

9. Gavit, "Rural Social Settlements," 5–6.

10. Quoted in Poole, *Nurses on Horseback*, 166.

11. Van Blarcom, "Provisions," 698.

12. For a discussion of this problem, see Pearl, "Distribution of Physicians," 1024.

13. Muncy, *Creating a Female Dominion*, 98.

14. MB to SB, May 23, 1918, FNSCUK, box 336, folder 4.

15. MB, "Outline." Established in 1909, the American Child Health Association served as an umbrella organization, bringing together public health officials, doctors, nurses, philanthropists, and social workers. For a history of the American Child Health Association, see Van Ingen, *Story*.

16. MB, "Outline," 2.

17. MB, "Memorandum," 1. Breckinridge was not the first individual to recognize the benefits nurse-midwifery would bring to the United States. A few public health officials had suggested the value of nurse-midwives as early as 1911. See Litoff, *American Midwives*, 122–24.

18. See Litoff, *American Midwife Debate*. Breckinridge saved many articles relating to this debate, including Rude, "Midwife Problem," and Hardin, "Midwife Problem," copies in FNSCUK, box 362, folder 3.

19. Historians have found no evidence linking midwifery to high infant mortality rates. Because birth and death records were sketchy before the early twentieth century, it is difficult to determine whether midwives really endangered women's lives, as opponents claimed. See McGregor, *From Midwives to Medicine*, 37. Ulrich found that eighteenth-century midwife Martha Ballard averaged only 6.1 maternal deaths per 1,000 live births, a figure that compares favorably to U.S. rates in the 1930s (*A Midwife's Tale*, 173). Scholars tend to blame physicians for keeping infant and maternal death rates high. Doctors' interventionist methods spread disease and often slowed the natural course of labor. See Litoff, *American Midwife Debate*, 5–6.

20. Leavitt, *Brought to Bed*. Leavitt argues that women were not pawns in the medicalization of childbirth but instead actively sought out the safer and less painful births they believed male physicians could offer. For a very different feminist perspective, see Shorter, *Women's Bodies*; Donegan, *Women and Men Midwives*.

21. Kobrin, "American Midwife Controversy," 197–99.

22. Leavitt, *Brought to Bed*, 43.

23. Ibid., 267–68. The women who continued to rely on midwives were overwhelmingly from rural areas or were African American or eastern European immigrants. In some cases, they did so because they were more comfortable having a female present, but in many instances, the difference in cost influenced such decisions. See Ladd-Taylor, *Mother-Work*, 23.

24. Kobrin, "American Midwife Controversy," 198–201.

25. Litoff, *American Midwife Debate*, 7.

26. MB, "Memorandum," 1.

27. Ibid.

28. Robb, "Brief Sketch."

29. Buhler-Wilkerson, *False Dawn*, 12–19.

30. MB, "Outline," 4.

31. Ibid.

32. See John M. Dodson, "Preventive Medicine and the General Practitioner," *Kentucky Medical Journal* 21 (March 1923): 115–21, reprinted from *Journal of the American Medical Association*, January 6, 1923.

33. Meckel, *Save the Babies*, 164–66.

34. Van Blarcom, "Provisions," 700. Even as medically supervised births became more common, doctors had little contact with patients, no matter their economic status, before labor. This situation resulted in part from the high cost of such services as well as from the lack of understanding of fetal development and Victorian modesty, which deemed physical exams improper (Meckel, *Save the Babies*, 159–61). John C. Campbell, *Southern Highlander*, 213, specifically notes that in the mountains, even trained physicians seldom saw a mother until she was in labor.

35. MB to Anne Dike, March 28, 1925, FNSCUK, box 337, folder 6.

36. MB, "Outline," 2.

37. John C. Campbell, *Southern Highlander*, 218, 221.

38. *Berea Quarterly for the Southern Mountains* 26 (October 1912): 3.

39. Bradley, "Hobnobbing," 91–92. Essayist Will Wallace Harney, "Strange Land" (1873), first described Appalachia as "a strange land and a peculiar people." For the most comprehensive account of the creation of Appalachia, see Shapiro, *Appalachia*.

40. Martin, "To Keep the Spirit."

41. "A Duel Ends in Two Deaths," *New York Times*, November 16, 1895, reprinted from the *Louisville Post*, November 11, 1895.

42. J. W. Williamson, *Hillbillyland*, 207–13.

43. Tice, "School-Work and Mother-Work," 203.

44. Billings and Blee, *Road to Poverty*, 9.

45. Batteau, *Invention of Appalachia*. See also Brodhead, *Cultures of Letters*, 119–20. I thank Dwight Billings for referring me to this useful source.

46. Becker, *Selling Tradition*, 42–43.

47. Eller, *Miners, Millhands, and Mountaineers*; Darlene Wilson, "Felicitous Convergence."

48. *Berea Quarterly for the Southern Mountains* 26 (October 1912): 3.

49. For more information on Neville's and Stewart's work, see Cornett, "Angel for the Blind"; Baldwin, *Cora Wilson Stewart*.

50. Whisnant, *All That Is Native and Fine*, 19.

51. Cora Wilson Stewart promoted a similar image in her *Country Life* readers (Baldwin, *Cora Wilson Stewart*, 98).

52. Quoted in Baldwin, "Cora Wilson Stewart," 85–86.

53. "Address of President Frost," *Berea Quarterly for the Southern Mountains* 25 (April 1911): 16.

54. "A Social Survey in the Mountains," *Berea Quarterly for the Southern Mountains* 28 (April 1914): 7.

55. "Program and Summons," *Berea Quarterly for the Southern Mountains* 28 (April 1914): 29.

56. MB, "Outline," 2.

57. MB, "Memorandum," 2.

58. Organizational meeting minutes, May 28, 1925, FNSCUK, box 2, folder 2.

59. MB, "Outline," 2.

60. *WN*, 157–59.

61. For a discussion of the responsibility the Bluegrass elite felt for eastern Kentucky, see Whisnant, *All That Is Native and Fine*, 37.

62. MB to Ella Phillips Crandall, October 20, 1923, FNSCUK, box 348, folder 3.

63. *Child Welfare in Kentucky*.

64. Veech, "For Blue Grass and Hill Babies." For details on the restrictions placed on lay midwives, see Midwife Annual Permit, FNSCUK, box 348, folder 4.

65. MB to Anne Dike, March 28, 1925, FNSCUK, box 337, folder 6; *WN*, 158. In 1926, Kentucky's General Assembly amended the state's medical practice law to address the lack of trained physicians in rural areas. This legislation enabled practitioners who did not hold degrees from recognized institutions to gain certification in specific counties. Breckinridge and her nurses benefited from this change. For more information, see Ellis, *Medicine*, 67.

66. Annie Veech, "Public Health Service," *Louisville Civic Opinion*, December 9, 1922, WPAR, box 11, folder 83.

67. Annie S. Veech to Owsley County Doctors and Citizens, July 27, 1923, FNSCUK, box 348, folder 3.

68. MB, draft of "Midwifery in the Kentucky Mountains: An Investigation," FNSCUK, box 348, folder 1.

69. Ibid. Chapter 6 analyzes Breckinridge's class biases, which come through clearly in this document, and further investigates how Breckinridge's expectations shaped her findings.

70. *WN*, 116.

71. Alfred Binet first introduced the IQ test in 1905. These tests, often used to confirm racist assumptions, were based on the idea that intelligence was biologically determined. Institutions employed Binet's test to identify the "feebleminded" (Pickens, *Eugenics*, 151–52; Kline, *Building a Better Race*, 26; Goldberg, *Discontented America*, 149).

72. MB, "Frontier Nursing Service," 3.

73. MB, "Midwifery in the Kentucky Mountains: An Investigation in 1923," *FNSQB* 17 (Spring 1942): 31. Woodyard went on to test 810 more FNS children, coming to the conclusion that mountain children were even more intelligent than she first believed. See also *WN*, 120–21.

74. William Hutchins to Anna S. Veech, July 3, 1923, FNSCBC, box 1, folder 1.

75. For insight regarding the kind of area she hoped to find, see MB, draft of "Midwifery in the Kentucky Mountains."

76. MB to Anne Dike, March 28, 1925, FNSCUK, box 337, folder 6.

77. *WN*, 157–58.

78. "A Statement of Facts by the Frontier Nursing Service, Inc.," [1925], FNSCUK, box 330, folder 7.

79. See 1920 U.S. Census data taken from <http://fisher.lib.virginia.edu/collections/ stats/histcensus/>, accessed October 31, 2007.

80. Bradley, "Hobnobbing," 94.

81. For a glimpse into how most Americans were living in the 1920s, see Allen, *Only Yesterday*.

82. Willeford, *Income and Health*, 17.

83. Quarles, "Comparison," 103.

84. See 1920 U.S. Census data taken from <http://fisher.lib.virginia.edu/collections/ stats/histcensus/>, accessed October 31, 2007.

85. For firsthand descriptions of the mountain subsistence economy, see Brewer, *Rugged Trail*, 37; Stidham, *Trails*, 89–114. See also Eller, *Miners, Millhands, and Mountaineers*, 90–91; Rehder, *Appalachian Folkways*, 166, 210–15; *Thousandsticks*, industrial ed., December 24, 1908.

86. "Farmers Institute," *Thousandsticks*, November 1, 1906.

87. "Facts for the Investor to Consider: The Material is Here," *Thousandsticks*, industrial ed., December 24, 1908.

88. H. C. Chappell, "Our Streets," *Thousandsticks*, January 3, 1907.

89. Leslie County did not have a state-sponsored health worker until 1919, when Jean Tolk arrived from Chicago. Assisted by Zilpha Roberts, a local schoolteacher, Tolk traveled through the county, teaching about proper sanitation and providing basic health care. When Tolk left to do missionary work in 1923, Leona Pace and Nola Pease took over and continued to offer nursing care until 1924. See Stidham, *Trails*, 158; Brewer, *Rugged Trail*, 37.

90. Klotter, *Breckinridges of Kentucky*, 259. For statistics on the number of hospitals and health care workers in Kentucky in the early part of the century, see Chambers and Lynn, *Medical Service*, 23. Oral history interviews support Breckinridge's claim that no doctors were practicing in the area by the time the FNS began work. Doctors who had been working in the county may have moved to Hazard, drawn by the steady salaries offered by mining companies. See Mary Biggerstaff, interview by Dale Deaton, February 12, 1979, 79OH150FNS57, FNSOHC; Ott Bowling, interview by Dale Deaton, May 24, 1979, 79OH216FNS115, FNSOHC; Sherman Wooten, interview by Dale Deaton, November 7, 1979, 82OH09FNS152, FNSOHC.

91. Cavender, *Folk Medicine*, 24.

92. MB, draft of "Midwifery in the Kentucky Mountains," 11. For a discussion of the risks posed by "quack" doctors, see J. E. Ruse, "The Protean Quack," *Kentucky Medical Journal* 23 (May 1925): 255–56.

93. *Thousandsticks*, June 14, 1906.

94. "Notice," *Thousandsticks*, May 31, 1906.

95. Barney, *Authorized to Heal*, 27.

96. MB, "Outline," 3.

97. Barney, *Authorized to Heal*, 133–34.

98. Annie Veech to MB, October 31, 1923, FNSCUK, box 348, folder 3.

99. *WN*, 124–25.

100. Annie Veech to MB, October 31, 1923, FNSCUK, box 348, folder 3.

101. Ibid.

102. MB to Annie Veech, November 14, 1923, FNSCUK, box 348, folder 3.

103. A. S. Veech, "A Practical Solution of Kentucky's Midwife Problem," 1, FNSCBC.

104. Annie Veech to MB, October 31, 1923, FNSCUK, box 348, folder 3.

105. For a look at the role physicians intended interested women to play in public health efforts, see "The Interest of Women in the Maternity and Infancy Program," *Kentucky Medical Journal* 21 (October 1923): 519.

106. Annie Veech to William Hutchins, May 6, 1927, William Hutchins Papers, Southern Appalachian Archives, Hutchins Library, Berea College, Berea, Kentucky. On Veech's professional credentials, see "Veech Gets Health Post," *Louisville Times*, April 5, 1937, WPAR, box 11, folder 83. For a discussion of female physicians' struggles to gain legitimacy, see Moldow, *Women Doctors*; Morantz-Sanchez, *Sympathy and Science*.

107. MB to Annie Veech, November 14, 1923, FNSCUK, box 348, folder 3.

108. MB to Ella Phillips Crandall, November 14, 1923, FNSCUK, box 348, folder 3.

109. MB to Annie Veech, November 14, 1923, FNSCUK, box 348, folder 3.

110. MB to Ella Phillips Crandall, November 14, 1923, FNSCUK, box 348, folder 3.

111. MB, "Outline."

112. MB to Ella Phillips Crandall, October 20, 1923, FNSCUK, box 348, folder 3.

113. Ella Phillips Crandall to MB, February 12, 1924, FNSCUK, box 348, folder 3.

114. *WN*, 131–46, 149–51; Scotch notebook, FNSCUK, box 366, folder 13.

115. *WN*, 152.

116. MB to Father Cary, March 7, 1925, FNSCUK, box 343A, folder 2. I have found no evidence that doctors ever formally diagnosed Breckinridge as clinically depressed, but her symptoms suggest that she suffered from more than just normal grief. Her claim that she would not have "remained long outside of an insane asylum" had she not received help when she did illustrates the debilitating level of her pain. See MB to Francis Massie, March 5, 1964, FNSCUK, box 158, folder 9.

117. Adeline Cashmore had embarked on a career in social work until she felt called by God to become an anchorite with the Church of All Saints in York, England. In August 1905, she abandoned all her worldly possessions and went into seclusion. For more biographical information on Cashmore, see the records in FNSCUK, box 343B, folders 10, 11, 12.

118. Margaret Gage, interview by W. B. Rogers Beasley, October 16, 1978, 79OH28FNS29, FNSOHC.

119. MB to Father Cary, March 7, 1925, FNSCUK, box 343A, folder 2.

120. In her study of female voluntary associations, Scott, *Natural Allies*, 33, illustrates this particular point by noting that religious references began to disappear from the Boston Fragment Association's minutes and that the organization abandoned reading from Scripture, which had always been a standard component of its meetings, in the 1890s.

121. *WN*, 154.

122. Ibid., 155.

123. Breckinridge's notes on scrap paper concerning face-to-face meetings with Adeline Cashmore, FNSCUK, box 343B, folder 13.

124. Adeline Cashmore to MB, January 4, 1925, FNSCUK, box 343A, folder 2.

125. Adeline Cashmore to MB, January 9, 1925, FNSCUK, box 343A, folder 2.

126. *WN*, 365.

127. Ibid., 156.

128. Adeline Cashmore to MB, December 29, 1924, August 2, 1925, FNSCUK, box 343A, folder 1.

129. Adeline Cashmore to MB, May 12, 1925, FNSCUK, box 343A, folder 2.

Chapter Four

1. *WN*, 157.

2. MB to Anne [Dike], May 6, 1925, FNSCUK, box 337, folder 6.

3. *WN*, 159–60; Klotter, *Breckinridges of Kentucky*, 258–59. Members of the original committee included, among others, physicians Scott Breckinridge and Josephine Hunt; college presidents Frank McVey and William Hutchins; newspaper editor Desha Breckinridge; mountain reformers Linda Neville, Katherine Pettit, May Stone, and Lucy Furman; and judge and gubernatorial candidate Edward C. O'Rear.

4. "Edward Clay O'Rear," in Southard, *Who's Who*, 307.

5. "The First Meeting," *FNSQB* 1 (June 1925): 4; organizational meeting minutes, May 28, 1925, FNSCUK, box 2, folder 2.

6. Harris, "Constructing Colonialism," 47. Breckinridge's control over decision making will be discussed in more detail later in this chapter.

7. Woodford County physician Alexander J. A. Alexander became chair; Julia D. Henning and Judge O'Rear served as vice chairs; Lexington banker C. N. Manning accepted the position of treasurer; and one of Breckinridge's cousins, Mrs. W. H. Coffman, became secretary.

8. "May Day Is Child Health Day," *Kentucky Medical Journal* 23 (April 1925): 199.

9. *WN*, 159; "First Meeting," 4; organizational meeting minutes, May 28, 1925, FNSCUK, box 2, folder 2.

10. *WN*, 161–62; EC meeting minutes, June 9, 1925, FNSCUK, box 2, folder 5.

11. MB, draft of *Wide Neighborhoods*, FNSCUK, box 350, folder 3; "First Meeting," 6; organizational meeting minutes, May 28, 1925, FNSCUK, box 2, folder 2.

12. Edna Rockstroh, interview by Dale Deaton, December 1, 1979, 79OH38FNS45, FNSOHC.

13. *WN*, 161.

14. Organizational meeting minutes, May 28, 1925, FNSCUK, box 2, folder 2.

15. MB, "Adventure in Midwifery"; "The Survey," *FNSQB* 1 (October 1925): 5.

16. *WN*, 163. Although Breckinridge loved data and strove whenever possible to present hard evidence to prove her worth as a professional, she never published specific results of her findings. I will investigate this omission in chapter 6.

17. Breckinridge may have first recognized the importance of establishing local support when working with the Children's Bureau. Bureau agents' first task when targeting new areas was to seek the cooperation of local women's organizations as well as the support of local

leaders, including physicians, ministers, school officials, and businesspersons (Klaus, *Every Child a Lion*, 232).

18. *WN*, 172. Her decision to court the area's "leading citizens" put her in line with foundation funding guidelines that emphasized the importance of securing the support of local elites. In this way, foundations ensured that their money supported ventures that corresponded to the foundations' capitalist interests. By getting the "right" people on board, Breckinridge likewise attempted to avoid too directly challenging the status quo. See E. Richard Brown, *Rockefeller Medicine Men*, 57. Breckinridge appears to have had little trouble convincing the area's most prominent men and women to support her plan. Many Appalachian historians have shown that local elites often were willing to ally with outside industrialists, politicians, and reformers as a way of reinforcing power. For example, Barney, *Authorized to Heal*, argues that physicians relied on local elites in their attempts to reshape Appalachian culture and to convince patients that medical care was a commodity that they must purchase. See also Weise, *Grasping at Independence*, 229; Waller, *Feud*; Conti, "Cultural Role"; Gaventa, *Power and Powerlessness*; Arnett, "Eastern Kentucky," 258.

19. Members of the Leslie County Branch of the Kentucky Committee for Mothers and Babies, FNSCUK, box 2, folder 4; resolutions passed by the Leslie County Branch of the Kentucky Committee for Mothers and Babies at its opening meeting at Hyden, August 29, 1925, FNSCUK, box 335, folder 9. For information on L. D. and Rebecca Lewis, see Stidham, *Trails*, 40–41; Brewer, *Of Bolder Men*, 177–78.

20. *WN*, 166; MB, "Adventure in Midwifery," 2.

21. Julia D. Henning to Ann [Coffman], September 5, 1925, FNSCUK, box 33, folder 6.

22. MB, "Adventure in Midwifery," 2.

23. MB, "Outline for a Demonstration of a Children's Public Health Service in Owsley County, Kentucky," [1923], 4, FNSCUK, box 348, folder 3.

24. Anne G. Campbell, "Mary Breckinridge," 271, calls the FNS "CARD reborn."

25. EC meeting minutes, September 14, 1926, FNSCUK, box 2, folder 16.

26. "Frontier Nursing Service Primer," *FNSQB* 8 (Summer 1932): 13; *WN*, 167, 175; Freda Caffin and Caroline Caffin, "Experiences of the Nurse-Midwife in the Kentucky Mountains," reprinted from *Nation's Health* 8 (December 1926), FNSCBC, box 1, folder 4.

27. "Frontier Nursing Service," *Woman's Almanac* (1940), FNSCUK, box 35, folder 21.

28. "The First Centers of Nurse-Midwifery," *FNSQB* 1 (October 1925): 12; general meeting minutes, October 9, 1925, FNSCUK, box 2, folder 8. In chapter 6, I will call into question Breckinridge's claim that patients so eagerly welcomed the nurses.

29. EC meeting minutes, October 14, 1925, FNSCUK, box 2, folder 9; EC meeting minutes, December 30, 1925, FNSCUK, box 2, folder 10. Residents of Wolf Creek again petitioned the service for a center in 1927, but Breckinridge refused their request. The committee cited the area's close proximity to Wendover and past difficulties in obtaining support as reasons for not building there. Wolf Creek finally received a center in 1960.

30. MB, "The Nurse on Horseback," *Woman's Journal* (February 1928), reprinted in *FNSQB* 19 (Winter 1944): 6.

31. *WN*, 174.

32. MB, "Nurse-Midwife," quoted in Ettinger, *Nurse-Midwifery*, 63.

33. MB, memorandum for midwifery records, [October 19, 1929], FNSCUK, box 51, folder 16.

34. "Thirty Years Onward: Frontier Nursing Service, Inc., 1925–1955," 13, 15, FNSCUK, box 29, folder 27.

35. MB to members of the Frontier Nursing Service, April 13, 1928, FNSCUK, box 338, folder 2; MB to Pebble [Helen Stone], April 26, 1938, FNSCUK, box 12, folder 9; Committee on Records, *Record Routine*, June 1930, FNSCUK, box 27, folder 7; MB, memorandum for midwifery records.

36. Greeley, "Beyond Benevolence," 49. For more information, see Tice, *Tales of Wayward Girls*, 1–3.

37. Using funds from a Carnegie Foundation grant, Breckinridge created a Records Department in 1931 to oversee nurses' record keeping.

38. This was not by choice but by necessity. Several years passed before the committee won the trust of local women, who continued to enlist the help of granny midwives, much to Breckinridge's frustration.

39. *WN*, 257–60; "First Centers of Nurse-Midwifery," 12. The prevalence of these afflictions is discussed in *Child Welfare in Kentucky*, 146–47.

40. Mary B. Willeford and Marion S. Ross, "How the Frontier Nurse Spends Her Time," *FNSQB* 12 (Spring 1937): 5.

41. Caffin and Caffin, "Experiences of the Nurse-Midwife," 2.

42. "The County Fair," *FNSQB* 7 (Autumn 1931): 19; "The Cleveland Clinic on Grassy Branch," *FNSQB* 9 (Summer 1933): 13–14.

43. "Medicine for the Mountaineers," *International Altrusan* (December 1935), FNSCUK, box 35, folder 15.

44. "The Wealthiest Nation in the World: Its Mothers and Children," *FNSQB* 4 (March 1929): 3.

45. "The Summer's Work," *FNSQB* 6 (Autumn 1930): 11; *WN*, 260.

46. Caffin and Caffin, "Experiences of the Nurse-Midwife," 2.

47. Martha Prewitt Breckinridge, interview by Carol Crowe-Carraco, March 30, 1979, 79OH176FNS76, FNSOHC.

48. Elizabeth B. Stevenson, "The Relief Nurse," *FNSQB* 9 (Spring 1934): 12.

49. MB, "A Frontier Nursing Service," *American Journal of Obstetrics and Gynecology* 15 (June 1928): 6, FNSCUK, box 356, folder 6.

50. Medical Advisory Committee, *Medical Routine*, August 27, 1928, FNSCUK, box 27, folder 1; Louisa B. Chapman, "Fits," *FNSQB* 24 (Autumn 1948): 14. The organization's *Medical Routine* resembled the "standing orders" on which other public health nurses, such as those who worked with New York's famous Henry Street Settlement, relied. See Buhler-Wilkerson, *No Place Like Home*, 110.

51. Medical Advisory Committee, *Medical Routine*.

52. Freda Caffin to Hazel [Corbin], April 3, 1927, FNSCUK, box 52, folder 4.

53. MB, "Frontier Nursing Service," 6.

54. William Allen Pusey, "The Future of Medicine," *Kentucky Medical Journal* 24 (October 1926): 497. The fear of government interference in health care survives into the present. The United States, unlike many European nations, still has no national health insurance. For more information on physicians' protests, see Starr, *Social Transformation*. For a specific look at how doctors' resistance to state medicine interfered with reform efforts during a slightly later period, see Grey, *New Deal Medicine*.

55. For Breckinridge's impressions of how national physicians viewed her organization, see MB to Mrs. Codman, December 17, 1934, FNSCUK, box 328, folder 9. For information on Lobenstine, see Ettinger, *Nurse-Midwifery*. Welch's accomplishments are described in "Patriarch's Party," *Time*, April 14, 1930. See also *WN*, 206, 304, 313.

56. MB, "Adventure in Midwifery."

57. "Our First Medical Affiliation," *FNSQB* 7 (Winter 1932): 30.

58. Barney, *Authorized to Heal*, 136–37.

59. Ettinger, *Nurse-Midwifery*, 50. Like Barney, Ettinger stresses that doctors would not have welcomed Breckinridge's nurses as eagerly if she had chosen to locate her service in a city.

60. MB to Samuel McKee, January 18, 1928, FNSCUK, box 338, folder 2, quoted in semiannual meeting minutes, May 11, 1928, FNSCUK, box 2, folder 26.

61. MB to Mr. Hoskins, January 26, 1928, FNSCUK, box 338, folder 2.

62. MB to Al [Logan], January 19, 1928, January 26, 1928, FNSCUK, box 338, folder 2.

63. MB to Dr. Keith, January 18, 1928, FNSCUK, box 338, folder 2.

64. Josephine Hunt to "Whom It May Concern," January 18, 1928, FNSCUK, box 344, folder 1.

65. "County Society Reports—Perry," *Kentucky Medical Journal* 24 (June 1926): 310.

66. "The Organization of the Frontier Nursing Service, Inc., 1946," *FNSQB* 22 (Autumn 1946): 17.

67. MB to members of the nursing staff, February 1, 1929, FNSCUK, box 51, folder 16; MB, "Nurse-Midwife," 1; MB, "Where the Frontier Lingers," 12; MB, "Adventure in Midwifery." Copies of these articles are located in FNSCUK, box 356, folders 11 and 3.

68. Pansy [Lucille Turner] to MB, January 27, 1926, FNSCUK, box 337, folder 8.

69. Adeline Cashmore to MB, July 6, 1925, FNSCUK, box 343A, folder 1.

70. Rosenzweig, *Another Self*, 27.

71. Simmons, "Companionate Marriage."

72. MB to Julia D. Henning, February 24, 1928, FNSCUK, box 338, folder 2; amendment of articles of incorporation of the Kentucky Committee for Mothers and Babies, 1928, FNSCUK, box 1, folder 3.

73. MB to Anne Dike, July 20, 1926; EC meeting minutes, June 29, 1926, FNSCUK, box 2, folder 14.

74. *WN*, 109, 112, 157.

75. For information on the Kentucky River gift, see EC meeting minutes, October 5, 1925, FNSCUK, box 2, folder 6. For information on the Kentucky Union gift, see MB to C. N. Manning, August 6, 1927, FNSCUK, box 28, folder 1; EC meeting minutes, June 29, 1926,

FNSCUK, box 2, folder 14; EC meeting minutes, October 10, 1927, FNSCUK, box 2, folder 23.

76. Wendover Guest Book, FNSCUK, box 42, folder 1; MB to Kitty [Jessie Carson], November 24, 1926, FNSCUK, box 328, folder 1.

77. "Third Annual Report," *FNSQB* 4 (June 1928): 43; "The Autumn News in Leslie County," *FNSQB* 3 (November 1927): 5.

78. *WN*, 193.

79. Ibid., 210; Dammann, *Social History*, 20.

80. *WN*, 210–19.

81. The original structure had two wings, one for midwifery patients and one for all other patients ("Reflections and Renovations," *FNSQB* 51 [Summer 1975]: 27).

82. *WN*, 221.

83. Leslie County Branch meeting minutes, March 28, 1928, FNSCUK, box 2, folder 25. The FNS paid $1,500 in expenses for the trip by MacKenzie and his wife. In light of the fact that the travel expenses for Breckinridge and her secretary for 1926–27 totaled only $1,227.45, the fledgling organization clearly sacrificed heavily to have the MacKenzies attend (semiannual meeting minutes, October 24, 1927, FNSCUK, box 2, folder 24; "Annual Report," *FNSQB* 3 [May 1927]: 5).

84. *WN*, 222–24; Thruston Morton, interview by Carol Crowe-Carraco, October 24, 1978, 82OH37FNS180, FNSOHC.

85. "Prayers Answered: Vision of Those Working for Mountain Folk Being Realized," *Lexington Herald*, July 2, 1928, J. A. Stucky Papers, box 2, folder 10, Southern Appalachian Archives, Hutchins Library, Berea College, Berea, Kentucky.

86. *WN*, 222–24; MB to Anne [Coffman], July 4, 1928, FNSCUK, box 338, folder 2.

87. Leslie MacKenzie, "Dedication Address," *FNSQB* 4 (September 1928): 8.

88. MB to Anne [Wilson], July 4, 1928, FNSCUK, box 338, folder 2; "Visitors Travel Today to See Hyden Hospital," June 27, 1928, *Louisville Courier-Journal*, WPAR, box 11, folder 38; *WN*, 224–25. Breckinridge believed that the Appalachian people needed "music and fireworks as much as they need midwifery!"

89. MB, "Rounds," *FNSQB* 5 (September 1929): 4.

90. *WN*, 228.

Chapter Five

1. EC meeting minutes, February 9, 1926, FNSCUK, box 2, folder 11.

2. E. Richard Brown, *Rockefeller Medicine Men*; Rothstein, *American Medical Schools*, 162.

3. For more information on Appalachian reform projects' difficulty in securing foundation support, see Searles, *College for Appalachia*, 110–11. Searles points out that mountain projects such as Berea College, Caney Creek Junior College, and the FNS had to seek funding from individual donors, often petitioning the same contributors.

4. A reprint of this article, published in October 1926, is located in FNSCUK, box 356, folder 3.

5. "Third Annual Report," *FNSQB* 4 (June 1928): 5.

6. See Commonwealth Fund, "Foundation History," <http://www.cmwf.org/aboutus/aboutus_show.htm?doc_id=224821>, accessed November 2, 2006.

7. Director's report, November 8, 1928, FNSCUK, box 2, folder 28; director's report, May 21, 1929, FNSCUK, box 2, folder 29.

8. Special grants report to the executive committee, February 14, 1929, 21–23, Commonwealth Fund Collection, box 2, folder Volume 1929, Rockefeller Foundation Archives, Rockefeller Archive Center, Sleepy Hollow, New York. No explanation of why the Commonwealth grant fell through appears in any of the records contained in the FNS Collection.

9. MB to Kitty [Jessie Carson], November 24, 1926, FNSCUK, box 328, folder 1.

10. See Breckinridge's correspondence from this year, FNSCUK, box 337, folder 8.

11. Staff meeting minutes, July 31, 1958, FNSCUK, box 212, folder 5; MB to Anne Dike, July 20, 1926, FNSCUK, box 337, folder 8.

12. MB to Al [Alice Logan], December 7, 1927, FNSCUK, box 52, folder 5.

13. Smiley, *Rethinking the Great Depression*, 4.

14. Statement of donations and subscriptions paid, May 1, 1926–April 30, 1927, FNSCUK, box 233, folder 2.

15. Whisnant, *All That Is Native and Fine*, 110.

16. MB to Freda Caffin, February 1, 1926, FNSCUK, box 52, folder 2.

17. "Fifth Annual Report," *FNSQB* 6 (Summer 1930): 4, 69–73.

18. MB to Kit [Jessie] Carson, January 1, 1927, FNSCUK, box 328, folder 1. Carson's newspaper clippings are located in FNSCUK, box 330, folder 2.

19. MB to Kitty [Jessie Carson], November 24, 1926, FNSCUK, box 328, folder 1.

20. See, for example, Elizabeth B. Boyd, interview by Linda Green, April 10, 1979, 79OH184FNS83, FNSOHC; Roger Egeberg, interview by Dale Deaton, April 27, 1979, 79OH190FNS89, FNSOHC.

21. For a discussion of Breckinridge's fund-raising efforts, see Altizer, "Establishment," 16.

22. "Mrs. Thompson Speaks," *Fort Smith Times-Record*, October 31, 1917, FNSCUK, box 357, folder 8; Marvin Breckinridge Patterson, foreword to *WN*, xiii.

23. Thruston Morton, interview by Carol Crowe-Carraco, October 24, 1978, 83OH37FNS180, FNSOHC.

24. Patterson, foreword, xiv.

25. Sue Grandin and Patsy P. Lawrence, interview by Anne Campbell, January 26, 1979, 79OH147FNS54, FNSOHC.

26. Lucille Elfenbein, "Favors Asserting Self at 70," *Providence Evening Bulletin*, April 24, 1952, FNS scrapbook, fall 1951–June 1954, FNSCUK, box 45.

27. Janet Geister to HEB, November 6, 1954, FNSCUK, box 196, folder 2.

28. Albert B. Chandler to MB, November 20, 1959, FNSCUK, box 364, folder 28.

29. Morton, interview by Crowe-Carraco.

30. Gladys Crooker, "Mrs. Breckinridge Tells of Frontier Nurse Service in Mountains of Kentucky," *Providence Bulletin*, January 25, 1936, FNSCUK, box 334; Agnes Lewis to Marvin Patterson, June 15, 1966, FNSCUK, box 208, folder 3; Mary Martin and Phoebe

Hawkins, interview by Anne Campbell, May 23, 1979, 79OH229FNS121, FNSOHC; Patterson, foreword, xiii.

31. Lucille Knechtly, interview by Dale Deaton, July 9, 1979, 82OH18FNS161, FNSOHC.

32. *WN*, 183; MB to Dr. Adair, December 22, 1949, FNSCUK, box 65, folder 3.

33. Waugh, *Unsentimental Reformer*, 114.

34. "Kentucky Mountains in New York," *Louisville Courier-Journal*, January 19, 1931, WPAR, box 11, folder 39.

35. FNS, "Special Appeal" (1931), FNSCUK, box 29, folder 3. For lists of supporters, see *FNSQB*.

36. "Nurse on Horseback Rides the Lonely Kentucky Trails," *New York Times*, January 18, 1931. For "angels on horseback," see Poole, "Nurse on Horseback." For "heroines of the highlands," see "Kentucky Frontierswomen," *New York Times*, May 13, 1931, WPAR, box 11, folder 39. In 1968, a reporter still used this description, modifying it slightly to "angels on horseback and jeep." See Josephine Rich, "Nursing Hill Country Style," *MD's Wife* (January 1967): 5–9, FNSCUK, box 37, folder 10.

37. "'Here Shall You See No Enemy but Winter and Rough Weather,'" *FNSQB* 1 (February 1926): 4.

38. Poole, "Nurse on Horseback."

39. "An Irish Heroine," *Lexington Herald*, July 24, 1931, reprinted in *FNSQB* 7 (Autumn 1931): 5–6.

40. "A Day in the Life of a Frontier Nurse-Midwife," 1926, FNSCUK, box 29, folder 1.

41. MB to Elizabeth Bruce, September 23, 1926, FNSCUK, box 337, folder 8.

42. MB, "Midwifery in the Kentucky Mountains," FNSCUK, box 348, folder 1.

43. Katherine Trowbridge, "A Courier Looks at Life," *FNSQB* 7 (Spring 1932): 13.

44. Poole, "Nurse on Horseback."

45. Frances Fell, "A Christmas 'Least One' on Hell-fer-Sartin," *Public Health Nurse*, December 1930, 606, FNSCUK, box 35, folder 5.

46. For a discussion of the intellectual and cultural transformation taking place at the turn of the twentieth century, see Bederman, *Manliness and Civilization*; Lears, *No Place of Grace*; Hoganson, *Fighting for American Manhood*, 35. On the emergence of the "black beast," see Joel Williamson, *Crucible of Race*, 111.

47. Bederman, *Manliness and Civilization*, 12–14.

48. Kraut, *Silent Travelers*. On the danger of importing autocracy, see Klaus, *Every Child a Lion*, 20.

49. Higham, *Strangers*, 204, 282–84. For more information on the conservative backlash that developed in the 1920s, see Goldberg, *Discontented America*, 40–44.

50. Chesler, *Woman of Valor*, 122–23; Gordon, *Woman's Body, Woman's Right*, 270; Haller, *Eugenics*. These studies focus on the movement's earliest years. For a study that investigates the movement's impact through the 1960s, see Kline, *Building a Better Race*.

51. Katz, *In the Shadow*, 188–90.

52. Nies, "Eugenic Fantasies," 69.

53. Madison Grant, *Passing of the Great Race*, 48, 263.

54. Ibid., xxxiii.

55. Katz, *In the Shadow*, 190.

56. Gordon, *Woman's Body, Women's Right*, 133–34; Dyer, *Theodore Roosevelt*, 15.

57. Higham, *Strangers*, 147; Dyer, *Theodore Roosevelt*, 143–67.

58. Frost, *For the Mountains*, 5.

59. MB, "Is Birth Control the Answer?," 160, FNSCUK, box 356, folder 10.

60. DeJong, *Appalachian Fertility Decline*.

61. Semple, "Anglo-Saxons," 150–51. Semple (1863–1932) published several well-received articles on Appalachia, and her work continues to shed light on turn-of-the-century impressions of the region. For a brief biography, see Semple, "Anglo-Saxons," 145–46.

62. MB to Kitty [Jessie Carson], November 24, 1926, FNSCUK, box 328, folder 1.

63. Her hierarchical ranking of the white races resembled the perspective of Madison Grant, *Passing of the Great Race*.

64. *WN*, 169.

65. MB to Anne [Dike], May 6, 1925, FNSCUK, box 337, folder 6.

66. "Will You Fill Her Saddlebags?" (1931), FNSCUK, box 29, folder 3.

67. MB, "Adventure in Midwifery," 3.

68. Samuel Tyndale Wilson, *Southern Mountaineers*, 9.

69. "Waiting to Serve," *FNSQB* 3 (November 1927): 2.

70. Caffin and Caffin, "Experiences of the Nurse-Midwife," 1.

71. "Frontier Nursing Service Primer," *FNSQB* 8 (Summer 1932): 19.

72. W. A. Hifner Jr. to C. N. Manning, May 24, 1935, FNSCUK, box 282, folder 6.

73. "America's Own," *FNSQB* 2 (June 1926): 5.

74. Elizabeth Perkins, "Response," *Thousandsticks*, April 7, 1927, FNSCUK, box 39, folder 1.

75. Elizabeth Bishop Perkins will, June 17, 1952, FNSCUK, box 295, folder 11.

76. Anne Morgan to Irwin Kirkwood, Mrs. August R. Meyer, J. W. Perry, Mrs. Ford S. Harvey, and R. A. Long, September 15, 1926, FNSCUK, box 330, folder 9.

77. Clara Ford to MB, April 17, 1926, FNSCUK, box 330, folder 7.

78. Information from annual reports printed in the summer editions of the *FNSQB*.

79. According to Eller, *Miners, Millhands, and Mountaineers*, 149, the Fordson Coal Company, a subsidiary of the Ford Motor Company, owned 165,000 acres of land in eastern Kentucky by 1920.

80. "Second Annual Report," *FNSQB* 3 (May 1927): 11.

81. Quoted in Greenleaf, *From These Beginnings*, 140.

82. Ibid., 141. Greenleaf does not mention the Fords' interest in the FNS.

83. Becker, *Selling Tradition*, 39, 15.

84. Raine, *Land of Saddle-Bags*, xxxiii.

85. See Whisnant, *All That Is Native and Fine*, 184.

86. "A Barrier Made Frontier," *Mountain Life and Work* 1 (October 1925): 1.

87. J. A. Stucky, unpublished article, 1914, J. A. Stucky Papers, box 1, folder 11, Southern Appalachian Archives, Hutchins Library, Berea College, Berea, Kentucky.

88. MB, "Where the Frontier Lingers," 10; MB, "The Rural Family and Its Mother," reprinted from *The Mother*, April 1944, FNSCUK, box 356, folder 15.

89. The *Berea Quarterly* is filled with this kind of rhetoric. See, in particular, "Address of Governor Wilson," *Berea Quarterly for the Southern Mountains* 15 (April 1911): 27–28.

90. For a discussion of Americans' fear of becoming "soft," see Bederman, *Manliness and Civilization*; Lears, *No Place of Grace*.

91. Bederman, *Manliness and Civilization*, 207.

92. Alfred Allan Lewis, *Ladies and Not-So-Gentle Women*, 160.

93. Raine, *Land of Saddle-Bags*, 5.

94. "Field Notes," *FNSQB* 14 (Autumn 1938): 29. In fiscal year 1932–33, 111 guests visited Wendover, staying a total of 1,841 days ("Annual Report," *FNSQB* 9 [Summer 1933]: 6).

95. Julia D. Henning to Ann [Coffman], September 5, 1925, FNSCUK, box 33, folder 6. The belief that the mountains offered an opportunity to experience life in its truest form persisted well past the 1920s. In 1940, a New York reporter remarked, "Some people think this Frontier Nursing Service of Kentucky supplies the last opportunity for the younger generation of Americans to show that they have not grown soft with easy living." She confidently predicted that "given a task to do and a sturdy horse to ride, any of them can measure up to the same sort of hard living that made heroines of their great-grandmothers" (*New York Herald-Tribune*, April 1, 1940, reprinted in "Old Courier News," *FNSQB* 15 [Spring 1940]: 24).

96. Virginia McKee, interview by Carol Crowe-Carraco, April 26, 1979, 79OH192FNS91, FNSOHC.

97. Figure derived from annual reports printed in the *FNSQB* between 1925 and 1930.

98. "Fourth Annual Report," *FNSQB* 5 (June 1929): 1.

99. My analysis here is influenced by Whisnant's work and by Shelby's arguments in " 'R' Word."

Chapter Six

1. *WN*, 19.

2. Breckinridge had met Henri and Juliette Carni while living in Arkansas. Juliette had served as a nanny and a "second mother" to Mary's son, Breckie. Breckinridge's papers include little mention of Juliette. She and her family apparently came to live in Leslie County and remained there until her death in 1927 eight days after the birth of her daughter, Mary Breckinridge Carni. The FNS did not count this death in its tabulation of its first thousand maternity cases since Juliette had been diagnosed with complications early in her pregnancy and had been sent to Lexington for treatment. See *WN*, 65–66, 178; Freda Caffin to Josephine Hunt, February 15, 1927, FNSCUK, box 52, folder 4.

3. Julia D. Henning to Ann [Coffman], September 5, 1925, FNSCUK, box 33, folder 6.

4. MB to Anne Dike, March 28, 1925, FNSCUK, box 337, folder 6.

5. MB to Anne [Morgan], May 6, 1925, FNSCUK, box 337, folder 6.

6. The FNS collection contains no data keys or summary of the study she and her

assistants conducted of births and deaths in the area, although this information is present for her study of midwives, which she conducted around the same time. She supposedly sent the information she collected on to Dr. Philip E. Blackerby, chief of the Kentucky Bureau of Statistics, but I have not been able to uncover her results through this source.

7. MB, memorandum having reference to Mr. Day's chapter called "Frontier Nurses," June 4, 1941, FNSCUK, box 59, folder 12.

8. MB to Kitty [Jessie Carson], November 24, 1925, FNSCUK, box 328, folder 1. *WN*, 163, notes that in the original canvass, she found that there had been 10 percent more births and 17 percent more deaths than had been reported to the state, but she does not put these numbers into any context by providing the official figures or by comparing her findings to state and national rates.

9. John C. Campbell, *Southern Highlander*, notes, however, that the true death rate might have been underrepresented.

10. Bromley, "What Risk Motherhood?," 13.

11. A. S. Veech, "A Practical Solution of Kentucky's Midwife Problem," 1, FNSCBC. She notes that improper feeding and poor sanitation resulted in a high infant mortality rate. Ironically, Veech appears to be basing her findings on the results of Breckinridge's study.

12. See data keys from 1925 midwifery study, FNSCUK, box 348, folder 2.

13. MB, "Midwifery in the Kentucky Mountains," FNSCUK, box 348, folder 1.

14. Data keys from 1925 midwifery survey.

15. MB, "Midwifery in the Kentucky Mountains."

16. Ibid., 9.

17. MB, "Adventure in Midwifery."

18. Harris, "Constructing Colonialism," 24, contends that Breckinridge's report of her findings had the tone of "thinly veiled condescension."

19. Sklar, "*Hull-House Maps and Papers*"; Linda Alcoff quoted in Tice, *Tales of Wayward Girls*, 9; Nicholas B. Dirks, Geoff Eley, and Sherry B. Ortner, quoted in Abel, "Valuing Care," 35.

20. "A Day in the Life of a Frontier Nurse-Midwife," 1926, FNSCUK, box 29, folder 1.

21. Shawe, *Notes*, 105.

22. Buhler-Wilkerson, *False Dawn*, ix.

23. Ibid., 21.

24. FNS guidelines, October 19, 1929, FNSCUK, box 51, folder 17; MB to MacAlpen, January 11, 1929, FNSCUK, box 338, folder 3.

25. Buhler-Wilkerson, *False Dawn*, 5.

26. *WN*, 178–80; Christmas appeal, 1925, FNSCUK, box 31, folder 1. Breckinridge chalked up the lower-than-expected attendance to inclement weather.

27. "Day in the Life." For "hoot owl hollows," see MB to Anne Dike, March 28, 1925, FNSCUK, box 337, folder 6.

28. MB to Anne [Dike], May 6, 1925, FNSCUK, box 337, folder 6. To really "brace" oneself against the primitive conditions, Breckinridge recommended frequent trips to the Bluegrass.

29. Dammann, *Social History*, 18; *WN*, 187. Breckinridge joked, "The downstairs tub received so many visitors that I threatened to give it a guest book." The mounted animals were a product of Breckinridge's hunting excursions as a young girl in Mississippi. The one convenience Wendover lacked was electricity. The building was not wired until 1948, when a donor provided the funds to do so.

30. Hudson, " 'God Held the Torch,' " 101.

31. *WN*, 241; MB, "Adventure in Midwifery," 2.

32. Dammann, *Social History*, 76.

33. MB to Anne Coffman, August 1, 1925, FNSCUK, box 53, folder 6.

34. MB to Cabell Breckinridge, August 2, 1925, FNSCUK, box 337, folder 6.

35. MB, "Adventure in Midwifery," 3.

36. "For the Last Quarter," *FNSQB* 2 (October 1926): 2.

37. MB, "Outline for a Demonstration of a Children's Public Health Service in Owsley County, Kentucky," [1923], FNSCUK, box 348, folder 3.

38. "First Annual Report," *FNSQB* 2 (June 1926): pullout section.

39. Borst, *Catching Babies*.

40. Stidham, *Trails*, 148.

41. See data keys from 1925 midwifery survey. Nowhere in her midwifery report does Breckinridge refer to "granny" midwives. While her decision to avoid such terminology was certainly intentional, her motives for doing so are unclear. Because Breckinridge was concerned with how communities would receive her nurses, she chose the name nurse-midwife rather than something like "obstetrical nurses" in recognition of people's familiarity with midwives. See MB, "Nurse-Midwife."

42. Stidham, *Trails*, 148.

43. Data keys from 1925 nurse-midwifery study.

44. MB, "Midwifery in the Kentucky Mountains," 17.

45. Ibid., 20.

46. Many experts now conclude that lying on one's back during labor is the most dangerous position because it limits blood flow to the baby and can slow contractions. Although many hospitals continue to limit women's mobility through monitoring devices, a greater appreciation of gravity's role in making labor more efficient has again arisen. See Boston Women's Health Book Collective, *New Our Bodies, Ourselves*, 447.

47. Dorothy F. Buck, "The Pages Turn Back," *FNSQB* 18 (Spring 1943): 4–5.

48. Gladys Peacock to Alice Logan, October 14, 1927, FNSCUK, box 52, folder 5; Billy to MB, July 2, 1929, FNSCUK, box 338, folder 4.

49. MB to Maud Cashmore, August 14, 1929, FNSCUK, box 338, folder 4.

50. [Freda Caffin] to Josephine Hunt, March 8, 1927, FNSCUK, box 52, folder 4.

51. Freda M. Caffin to Annette B. Cowles, March 7, 1927, March 12, 1927, FNSCUK, box 52, folder 4.

52. Buck, "Pages Turn Back," 4–5. See also Bertha Howard, interview by Sadie Stidham, July 26, 1979, 82OH144FNS186, FNSOHC.

53. Mary B. Willeford to Freda Caffin, March 13, 1927, FNSCUK, box 52, folder 4.

54. Jean Tolk, interview by Dale Deaton, November 8, 1978, 79OH78FNS34, FNSOHC.

55. Freda Caffin to Annie S. Humphrey, December 30, 1926, FNSCUK, box 52, folder 3. For a discussion of "bold hives" and the methods used to treat it, see Cavender, *Folk Medicine*, 136.

56. Freda Caffin to Annie S. Humphrey, December 30, 1926, FNSCUK, box 52, folder 3.

57. Edith Reeves Solenberger, "British Maternity Nursing on an American Frontier," reprinted from *The Cripple*, April 1930, 3, FNSCUK, box 35, folder 3.

58. *WN*, 173. On p. 169, Breckinridge inaccurately notes that "Kentucky mountaineers . . . are all of British descent."

59. Solenberger, "British Maternity Nursing," 3.

60. Ott Bowling, interview by Dale Deaton, May 24, 1979, 79OH216FNS115, FNSOHC. According to Bowling, relations between patients and nurses improved only after the FNS began hiring American nurses. British nurse-midwife Helen Browne concurred, explaining that her patients "didn't understand [her] any more than [she] understood them to start with" (HEB, interview by Carol Crowe-Carraco, March 26, 1979, 79OH173FNS74, FNSOHC).

61. Bertram Ireland to Alexander Alexander, Report of Survey, September 1, 1925, FNSCUK, box 337, folder 6.

62. Ibid.

63. "A Simple Deduction," *FNSQB* 24 (Winter 1949): 51.

64. Kraut, *Silent Travelers*, 217.

65. Dammann, *Social History*, 67, contended that Breckinridge made nurses wear their uniforms any time they went out to ensure their safety in an area known for being violent.

66. Betty Lester, interview by Dale Deaton, July 27, 1978, 82OH12FNS155, FNSOHC.

67. MB to Anne [Dike], May 6, 1925. For more information on Appalachian residents' reaction to seeing women dressed in pants, see Solenberger, "British Maternity Nursing," 1–8; John D. Muncy, interview by Sadie Stidham, May 15, 1979, 79OH213FNS112, FNSOHC.

68. Quoted in Shawe, *Notes*, 35.

69. Parker, "Made to Fit a Woman," 53–64.

70. MB to Freda Caffin, January 18, 1926, FNSCUK, box 52, folder 2.

71. Altizer, "Establishment," 14, 16. Finding newspapers to cover the service's work was not difficult. Desha Breckinridge, Mary's cousin, served as publisher and editor of the *Lexington Herald* from 1897 to 1935. Moreover, the editor of Leslie County's paper, *Thousandsticks*, served on Hyden's local committee.

72. MB to Freda Caffin, January 21, 1926, FNSCUK, box 52, folder 2.

73. MB to Arthur McCormack, January 21, 1926, FNSCUK, box 52, folder 2.

74. MB to Ethel DeLong Zande, January 20, 1926, Pine Mountain Settlement School Collection (microfilm), reel 68, Southern Appalachian Archives, Hutchins Library, Berea College, Berea, Kentucky. Breckinridge was likely reacting to tension that had developed between Pine Mountain organizers and Alice Lloyd. Lloyd's publicization of her work at Caney Creek featured stereotypical portrayals of mountain residents that fellow reformers resented. See Searles, *College for Appalachia*; Stoddart, *Challenge and Change*.

75. EC meeting minutes, September 14, 1926, FNSCUK, box 2, folder 16.

76. EC meeting minutes, October 5, 1925, FNSCUK, box 2, folder 6; EC meeting minutes, December 30, 1925, FNSCUK, box 2, folder 10; EC meeting minutes, February 9, 1926, FNSCUK, box 2, folder 11; semiannual meeting minutes, May 12, 1926, FNSCUK, box 2, folder 13; "Maternity Work in Leslie County to Be Shown in Film," *Louisville Herald-Post*, November 28, 1926, WPAR, box 11, folder 38.

77. "Primitive America on Screen," *New York Times*, December 12, 1926, FNSCUK, box 39, folder 1.

78. M. C. Roarke, "The New York Women Missed the Trail," *Thousandsticks*, January 20, 1927, 1, FNSCUK, box 39, folder 1.

79. W. Raleigh Hall to MB, January 10, 1927, FNSCUK, box 51, folder 16.

80. Elizabeth Perkins, "Response," *Thousandsticks*, April 7, 1927, FNSCUK, box 39, folder 1.

81. W. Raleigh Hall to MB, January 10, 1927, FNSCUK, box 51, folder 16.

82. Mary Swain Routzhan, "Presenting Mountain Work to the Public," *Mountain Life and Work*, July 1928, 29.

83. For biographical information on Caffin, see MB to Elizabeth Bruce, September 23, 1926, FNSCUK, box 337, folder 8; Catherine S. Gaines, "A Finding Aid to the Charles Henry Caffin Papers, circa 1883–1973," <http://www.aaa.si.edu/collections/findingaids/caffchar.htm>, accessed December 7, 2006.

84. Freda Caffin and Caroline Caffin, "Experiences of the Nurse-Midwife in the Kentucky Mountains," reprinted from *Nation's Health* 8 (December 1926), FNSCBC, box 1, folder 4.

85. Freda Caffin to Annie S. Humphrey, December 30, 1926, FNSCUK, box 52, folder 3.

86. Freda Caffin to C. N. Manning, February 16, 1927, FNSCUK, box 52, folder 4. Caffin wrote to Manning, treasurer of the FNS, for advice because she did not want to bother Breckinridge, who was recovering from a recent hysterectomy.

87. Ed C. Huff to Freda M. Caffin, January 9, 1927, Freda M. Caffin to Ed Huff, January 13, 1927, FNSCUK, box 52, folder 4.

88. Freda Caffin to Mrs. McAllister, February 15, 1927, FNSCUK, box 52, folder 4.

89. Elizabeth Bruce to Gladys Peacock, August 24, 1926, FNSCUK, box 337, folder 8; Wendover guest book, March 1926–May 1934, FNSCUK, box 42, folder 1.

90. Elizabeth Bruce to Gladys Peacock, August 24, 1926, FNSCUK, box 337, folder 8.

91. Elizabeth Bruce to MB, August 24, 1926, FNSCUK, box 337, folder 8.

92. MB to Elizabeth Bruce, September 23, 1926, FNSCUK, box 337, folder 8.

93. Ibid.

94. Elizabeth Bruce to MB, October 4, 1926, FNSCUK, box 337, folder 8; board of directors roster, *FNSQB* 3 (August 1927): 54.

95. It is unclear why Caffin left Leslie County. She apparently left with Rockstroh, the other original FNS nurse. Rockstroh claimed that Breckinridge forced her to leave because she had chronic bronchitis. See Edna Rockstroh, interview by Betty Lester, September 22, 1977, 83OH40FNS193, FNSOHC. In another source, Breckinridge suggests that Caffin had "personal relations" with a local physician and left for that reason (MB to Al [Alice Logan], January 26, 1928, FNSCUK, box 338, folder 2).

96. Committee on Records, *Record Routine*, 2nd rev. ed., FNSCUK, box 27, folder 7, marginal annotation in Dorothy Buck's private copy of the *Record Routine*.

97. MB, memorandum for midwifery records, [October 19, 1929], FNSCUK, box 51, folder 16.

98. MB to MacAlpen, January 11, 1929, FNSCUK, box 338, folder 3.

99. MB, memorandum for midwifery records. The FNS would make an exception if the nurses were called for "humanitarian reasons," but these were not booked and instead were designated as "emergency" cases. The FNS was trying to demonstrate the link between thorough prenatal care and successful outcomes and wanted to be sure that the records truly reflected that link.

100. MB, "Nurse-Midwife," 11.

101. Freda Caffin to Annie S. Humphrey, December 30, 1926, FNSCUK, box 52, folder 3. See also "For the Last Quarter," *FNSQB* 2 (October 1926): 2.

102. Altizer, "Establishment," 41.

103. Whisnant, *All That Is Native and Fine*, 260.

104. Ibid., 261.

105. Ibid., 12.

106. *WN*, 241.

107. Quoted in Whisnant, *All That Is Native and Fine*, 29.

108. Forderhase, "Eve Returns to the Garden," 253. In fact, Mary Rose McCord, who ran the Presbyterian mission at Wooten when the FNS began operation, was an outspoken critic of alcohol. See Mary Rose McCord, "A Letter," *Thousandsticks*, February 1, 1940. For more information on McCord, see Brewer, *Rugged Trail*, 52–54.

109. Allyn J. Shepherd, interview by Marian Barrett, January 18, 1979, 79OH141FNS48, FNSOHC.

110. Quoted in Poole, *Nurses on Horseback*, 41–42.

111. "Rounds," *FNSQB* 5 (September 1929): 13; "Sayings of the Children," *FNSQB* 3 (Winter 1934): 2.

112. MB to Maud Cashmore, August 14, 1929, FNSCUK, box 338, folder 4.

113. Della Int-Hout, "Tales of Old Kentucky," FNSCUK-2005MS47, box 41, folder 4.

114. My understanding of the relationship between FNS nurses and patients is shaped by Leavitt's discussion of American women's response to the shift to a medicalized model of childbirth (*Brought to Bed*, 84) and by Odem's study of turn-of-the-century attempts to control young women's sexuality. Odem usefully points out that reformers' efforts cannot be seen as a "top-down model of class control" but instead must be viewed as "a triangulated network of struggles and negotiations among working-class parents, their teenage daughters, and court officials" (*Delinquent Daughters*, 158).

115. Cavender, *Folk Medicine*, 147.

116. Barney, *Authorized to Heal*, 116–19. Barney notes that although patients had the power to choose from the care options available, no "free market" existed for medicine because scientific "regular" medicine had the weight of the state behind it and mechanisms existed to punish traditional practitioners.

117. Wilma Duvall, "Kentucky's National Demonstration," *Kentucky Progress Magazine* 6 (Spring 1934): 148.

118. Stoddart, *Challenge and Change*, 30, argues that Katherine Pettit and May Stone, founders of Hindman Settlement School, similarly developed a more sophisticated understanding of their mountain neighbors as time went on.

119. Dammann, *Social History*, 28.

120. Artemus Campbell, interview by Dale Deaton, October 30, 1978, 79OH30FNS31, FNSOHC.

121. "Ninth Annual Report," *FNSQB* 10 (Summer 1934): 3.

Chapter Seven

1. Poole, "Nurse on Horseback," 210.

2. Louis I. Dublin to MB, May 4, 1932, published in *FNSQB* 8 (Summer 1932): 7–9.

3. Committee on the Costs of Medical Care, *Medical Care*, 143. This committee, funded by the U.S. Public Health Service and eight philanthropies, was established in 1926 to study the rising cost of medical care. For more information on this study, see Starr, *Social Transformation*, 261–66.

4. Poole, "Nurse on Horseback," 210.

5. *WN*, 345.

6. MB, "The Rural Family and Its Mother," reprinted from *The Mother*, April 1944, FNSCBC, box 1, folder 4.

7. "Annual Report of the Frontier Nursing Service, May 1, 1935 to April 30, 1936," *FNSQB* 12 (Summer 1936): 6; "Fourth Annual Report," *FNSQB* 5 (June 1929): 2.

8. "Ozarks," *FNSQB* 6 (Autumn 1930): 13.

9. "Sixth Annual Report," *FNSQB* 7 (Summer 1931): 4; *WN*, 228.

10. Many charities experienced a similar struggle to remain solvent during this period. A study of great interest to Breckinridge, published in 1941, found that philanthropic giving in the United States declined by 53 percent between 1928 and 1933 (Raymond Rich Associates, "Tax-Exempt Contributions and Philanthropic Organizations," September 15, 1941, FNSCUK, box 64, folder 1). According to Melosh, the depression hit public health nursing services especially hard, as "private contributions evaporated." The crisis, she explains, accelerated the transition from privately funded services to government-funded agencies ("*Physician's Hand*," 144–46).

11. EC meeting minutes, April 2, 1931, FNSCUK, box 3, folder 1; general fund ledger, FNSCUK, box 240, folders 3, 7, 8; articles of incorporation, October 9, 1925, FNSCUK, box 1, folder 1; MB to Mr. Booth, May 4, 1931, FNSCUK, box 1, folder 5.

12. "Annual Report," *FNSQB* 8 (Summer 1932): 3.

13. Dammann, *Social History*, 39. In 1967, for example, all four of the Cincinnati Committee's new officers were former couriers (list of Cincinnati Committee's new officers, November 9, 1967, FNSCUK, box 330, folder 3). When the FNS launched its capital campaign to build the new Mary Breckinridge Hospital in 1966, more than 450 former couriers provided

an important support network. For more details, see Marts and Lundy, "Fund Raising Survey Report Made for Frontier Nursing Service, Wendover, Kentucky," October 5, 1966, 6, FNSCUK, box 158, folder 5.

14. Dammann, *Social History*, 39.

15. On letters of recommendation, see Mardi B. Perry and Susan M. Putnam, interview by Anne Campbell, January 25, 1979, 79OH146FNS53, FNSOHC. See also "Chicago Debs Work in Hills," *Louisville Courier-Journal*, March 13, 1932, WPAR, box 11, folder 39; *WN*, 272–77. In *Wide Neighborhoods*, Breckinridge notes that enough couriers-to-be were registered as to make it hard for applicants "without ancestry in the Frontier Nursing Service" to be accepted.

16. "F.N.S. Benefits," *FNSQB* 9 (Spring 1934): 18.

17. *WN*, 281.

18. See Baltzell, *Protestant Establishment*, 118–19.

19. "Activities of Our Various Committees," *FNSQB* 7 (Winter 1932): 6.

20. Zaydee DeJonge to Thompy [MB], December 2, 1932, November 17, 1931, FNSCUK, box 329, folder 1; "Activities of Our Various Committees," *FNSQB* 7 (Winter 1932): 6; "February 27: The Britannic Sails Away to Southern Climes for 16 Days," FNSCUK, box 333, folder 41.

21. James Parton, interview by Anne Campbell, May 25, 1979, 79OH226FNS118, FNSOHC; MB to Zaydee DeJonge, February 7, 1933, FNSCUK, box 329, folder 3; *WN*, 281.

22. Zaydee DeJonge to Thompy [MB], February 2, 1932, FNSCUK, box 329, folder 2.

23. "Annual Report," *FNSQB* 8 (Summer 1932): 3.

24. Anne Winslow to Zaydee DeJonge, February 2, 1933, FNSCUK, box 333, folder 3.

25. "The West Indies Cruise . . . ," *FNSQB* 9 (Summer 1933): 8.

26. *WN*, 283–85; MB to Clifton Breckinridge, December 9, 1931, PC.

27. "New York Writes Words of Praise for Frontier Nurses," *Lexington Herald*, December 21, 1931, WPAR, box 11, folder 39; *WN*, 285; MB to C. E. A. Winslow, December 5, 1931, FNSCUK, box 329, folder 1.

28. *WN*, 286.

29. MB to Adeline Cashmore, January 28, 1932, FNSCUK, box 343A, folder 9.

30. Mrs. S. Thruston Ballard, Kate H. Alexander, and C. N. Manning to "Friend," December 8, 1931, FNSCBC, box 1, folder 1; "Special Appeal, 1931," FNSCUK, box 29, folder 3.

31. MB to Adeline Cashmore, Maud Cashmore, and Lillian, January 19, 1932, FNSCUK, box 343A, folder 9.

32. "Open Letter," *FNSQB* 9 (Spring 1934): 3.

33. MB, "Amateur Editor," *FNSQB* 16 (Winter 1941): 26.

34. MB to Mrs. Codman, December 15, 1936, FNSCUK, box 328, folder 11.

35. EC meeting minutes, April 2, 1931, FNSCUK, box 3, folder 1; "Annual Report," *FNSQB* 21 (Summer 1945): 7. The service finally repaid these loans in 1945.

36. "Annual Report," *FNSQB* 8 (Summer 1932): 2.

37. Betty Lester, for example, went from earning $175 per month in December 1931 to

earning as little as $25 during some months in 1932 and 1933 (nurses' salaries, FNSCUK, box 263, folder 1). Even Dr. John Kooser, the first medical director, hired in 1932, took a reduction in salary, receiving only $100 per month instead of the $250 owed him (EC meeting minutes, October 16, 1934, FNSCUK, box 3, folder 21).

38. "Annual Report," *FNSQB* 8 (Summer 1932): 2. Nurses' responses are located in FNSCUK, box 51, folder 17. Even at the lower salaries, most of Breckinridge's nurses were relieved simply to be employed. For years, nursing schools had been creating an oversupply of nurses. Clients seeking private-duty nurses to care for sick relatives in their homes employed most graduate nurses. During the depression, however, many people viewed private nurses as an unaffordable luxury, and unemployment among nurses skyrocketed. In 1932, 60 percent of all nurses were unable to find work. See "Unemployment Relief," *American Journal of Nursing* 32 (October 1932): 1053; Reverby, *Ordered to Care*, 177.

39. MB to Zaydee DeJonge, June 13, 1932, FNSCUK, box 329, folder 2.

40. EC meeting minutes, May 11, 1933, FNSCUK, box 3, folder 12; report on benefits and books, FNSCUK, box 51, folder 5. In 1929, before the onset of the depression, the FNS spent less than 4 percent of its income on fund-raising expenses. During the depression, the percentage of the budget spent on fund-raising increased to between 10 and 15 percent. Breckinridge assured patrons that she would not be content until the organization returned to its predepression record. Compare "Annual Report," *FSNQB* 6 (Summer 1930): 1, with "Annual Report," *FNSQB* 8 (Summer 1932): 2.

41. However, Breckinridge encouraged city committees to continue sponsoring benefits. See "F.N.S. Benefits," *FNSQB* 9 (Spring 1934): 18.

42. MB to Zaydee DeJonge, March 29, 1932, FNSCUK, box 329, folder 2.

43. "A Suggestion to Those Who Have Only Five or Ten Cents to Give," *FNSQB* 6 (Spring 1931): 9.

44. "Statement of Cash Receipts and Disbursements, May 10, 1933 to May 10, 1934, and May 10, 1934 to May 10, 1935," FNSCUK, box 233, folders 7, 8; donors, 1934–35, FNSCUK, box 296, folder 6. Contributions and subscriptions for fiscal year 1929–30 totaled $131,680.31. For more details, see "Fifth Annual Report," *FNSQB* 6 (Summer 1930): 4.

45. EC meeting minutes, October 2, 1935, FNSCUK, box 53, folder 16; Income report, FNSCUK, box 51, folder 9.

46. See papers in FNSCUK, box 343, folder 2; "Old Staff News," *FNSQB* 41 (Summer 1965): 40; MB to Josephine Hunt, February 23, 1933, FNSCUK, box 344, folder 5.

47. Annual meeting minutes, May 23, 1936, FNSCUK, box 4, folder 4.

48. EC meeting minutes, director's report, May 11, 1933, FNSCUK, box 3, folder 13.

49. *WN*, 171.

50. Eller, *Miners, Millhands, and Mountaineers*. For an example of how subsistence agriculture became increasingly unworkable in one Appalachian community, see Billings and Blee, *Road to Poverty*.

51. Harry Caudill quoted in Billings and Blee, *Road to Poverty*, 199.

52. Poole, *Nurses on Horseback*, 134–36. Ford tenants paid very little rent and were allowed to extract coal for personal use in exchange for promising to watch over the land.

53. Eller, *Miners, Millhands, and Mountaineers*, 237–39. For more specific data concerning Leslie County, see Willeford, *Income and Health*, 31; MB, "Corn-Bread Line."

54. *WN*, 268; Salstrom, *Appalachia's Path to Dependency*, xxiii–xxiv, 94–96; Woodruff, *As Rare as Rain*, 4–5, 7.

55. MB, "Corn-Bread Line."

56. "Foreword," *FNSQB* 6 (Spring 1931): 1.

57. "What Price Famine?," *FNSQB* 6 (Winter 1931): 2.

58. Alpha Omicron Pi fund ledgers, FNSCUK, box 256, folder 1; "Sixth Annual Report," *FNSQB* 7 (Summer 1931): 2; "Sorority Aids Nursing Work," *Thousandsticks*, December 13, 1934, reprinted from the *Louisville Courier-Journal*, December 9, 1934.

59. "What Price Famine?," 3–4; MB to Alben W. Barkley, January 3, 1931, FNSCUK, box 53, folder 11. For information on the creation of the American Red Cross, see Woodruff, *As Rare as Rain*, 8.

60. According to Woodruff, *As Rare as Rain*, 140, Red Cross agents were often slow to provide assistance. Made up of prominent, wealthy members of the community, these committees consistently denied that conditions were as bad as some claimed. Appalachian relief committees saw the crisis as an opportunity to rid the mountains of the "unfit" by withholding aid.

61. *WN*, 270; MB, memorandum regarding conferences on drought relief, February 24, 1931, FNSCUK, box 53, folder 11.

62. MB to Alben W. Barkley, January 3, 1931, FNSCUK, box 53, folder 11.

63. MB, memorandum regarding conferences on drought relief.

64. Woodruff, *As Rare as Rain*, 50.

65. MB to Alben W. Barkley, February 28, 1931, FNSCUK, box 53, folder 11.

66. Alben Barkley to MB, January 23, 1932, MB to Agnes [Lewis], February 6, 1932, FNSCUK, box 54, folder 3.

67. See correspondence in FNSCUK, box 54, folder 3; "Federal Farm Loans," *FNSQB* 7 (Winter 1932): 20–21; "Personals," *FNSQB* 7 (Spring 1932): 36.

68. Poole, *Nurses on Horseback*, 29.

69. Bland Morrow, "A Study of First Causes . . . Leads to a Better Understanding of the Social Problems in the Kentucky Hills," *FNSQB* 10 (Autumn 1934): 11–17, reprinted from *To Dragma* (magazine of Alpha Omicron Pi sorority), March 1934.

70. Ibid., 13.

71. Many early-twentieth-century Appalachian reformers sought to promote community development. See Becker, *Selling Tradition*, 57.

72. "Leslie County Home Economics Pictures," *FNSQB* 13 (Autumn 1937): 22.

73. "Confluence News," *Thousandsticks*, July 26, 1934, August 9, 1934.

74. Katharine Sitton, "The Singing Class," *FNSQB* 9 (Spring 1936): 15–16; Quarles, "Comparison," 86.

75. In the 1970s, Appalachian scholars began offering new theories on why the region, located within the boundaries of the world's wealthiest nation, remained so poor. Borrowing heavily from Latin American dependency theory, they rejected the standard "culture of poverty" thesis, which

suggested that the isolation of the mountains and the inherent characteristics of the mountain's residents had led the area to resist capitalism. Instead, they claimed that the particular form modernization took in the mountains rather than a lack of modernization had brought such inequality. This new wave of scholarship focused on the ways outsiders had exploited Appalachia's riches for their own benefit. See, for example, Caudill, *Night*; Lewis, Johnson, and Askins, *Colonialism*; Eller, *Miners, Millhands, and Mountaineers*.

76. MB, "Corn-Bread Line," 423. For a recent historical interpretation of this problem, see Williams, *Appalachia*, 312–14.

77. MB to F. S. Silcox, June 3, 1935, FNSCUK, box 54, folder 1; "Frontier Nursing Service Worker Tells of Persistent Hardships," March 13, 1934, WPAR, box 11, folder 40.

78. EC meeting minutes, March 28, 1932, FNSCUK, box 3, folder 5; "Field Notes," *FNSQB* 7 (Spring 1932): 36. This road was built but was not paved until the 1950s.

79. Julia Lee and Richard D. Stevens, "A Forest Survey," *FNSQB* 7 (Spring 1932): 17–33. It is unclear why Breckinridge contacted scholars from Yale to conduct this study when the University of Kentucky had a very active agricultural department under the guidance of Thomas Poe Cooper. She may not have seen eye to eye with UK representatives, or she may have been looking for the prestige the Yale name would give to her ideas.

80. Collins, *History*, 183–200.

81. MB, memorandum regarding timberland both for forestation and reforestation in Kentucky counties east of the proposed Cumberland Purchase Unit; MB to F. S. Silcox, June 3, 1935, FNSCUK, box 54, folder 10.

82. MB to R. Y. Stuart, July 21, 1933, July 31, 1933, FNSCUK, box 54, folder 10.

83. William P. Kramer, report concerning visit to Clay, Perry, and Leslie Counties, August 28, 1933, FNSCUK, box 54, folder 10.

84. Joseph C. Kircher to MB, March 26, 1934, FNSCUK, box 54, folder 10.

85. Collins, *History*, 201; William E. Hedges, interview by Dale Deaton, April 18, 1978, 79OH179FNS79, FNSOHC.

86. MB to F. A. Silcox, April 29, 1935, June 3, 1935, FNSCUK, box 54, folder 10.

87. *WN*, 171.

88. William P. Kramer to regional forester, August 28, 1933, FNSCUK, box 54, folder 10.

89. R. M. Evans to MB, June 8, 1935, FNSCUK, box 54, folder 10.

90. MB to R. M. Evans, June 17, 1935, FNSCUK, box 54, folder 10. The U.S. Forest Service eventually added Leslie and Clay Counties to the National Forest area in 1964, when the Red Bird Purchase Unit was established. For information on the Red Bird purchase, see Collins, *History*, chapter 33.

91. Collins, *History*, 201. Breckinridge's plan would have benefited the region from an environmental standpoint but might have further undermined the area's economic base. The federal government does not pay state, county, or city taxes on national forestland, thereby reducing counties' tax bases and limiting their ability to support schools, roads, and public welfare programs. For more information on the economic ramifications of national forests, see Kahn, "Forest Service and Appalachia," 89–90; Appalachian Land Use Task Force, *Who Owns Appalachia?*

92. MB, memorandum regarding timberland, 2; MB to Anne [Dike], May 6, 1925, FNSCUK, box 337, folder 6. Katherine Pettit (Pine Mountain), May Stone (Hindman), and Lucy Furman (Hindman) served on the original Kentucky Committee for Mothers and Babies.

93. In one case, friction seems to have developed between Breckinridge's organization and various faith-based projects after an article spotlighting the Kentucky Committee for Mothers and Babies noted that the area had "no schools, no churches" ([Freda Caffin] to MB, January 14, 1926, FNSCUK, box 52, folder 2).

94. MB to Alben W. Barkley, January 3, 1931, FNSCUK, box 53, folder 11.

95. Skocpol, *Protecting Soldiers and Mothers*.

96. MB, "Outline."

97. Director's report, May 21, 1929, FNSCUK, box 2, folder 29; MB, "Memorandum Concerning a Suggested Demonstration."

98. See, for example, *WN*, 271.

99. "Beyond the Mountains," *FNSQB* 24 (Autumn 1948): 67–68.

100. "Statement in Regard to Cost of Running Nursing Service of the Kentucky Committee for Mothers and Babies," *FNSQB* 3 (November 1927): 10–11.

101. "406 Bare Feet," *FNSQB* 5 (December 1929): 4.

102. "Exceptional People," *FNSQB* 5 (Spring 1930): 7.

103. *WN*, 271.

104. For more information on Hoover's political philosophy, see Hoover, *American Individualism*, 71. See also Woodruff, *As Rare as Rain*, 39–40; Trattner, *From Poor Law to Welfare State*, 276–77.

105. EC meeting minutes, director's report, May 11, 1933, FNSCUK, box 3, folder 13; *WN*, 268.

106. MB to "People," February 28, 1931, FNSCUK, box 53, folder 11. The fear of undermining clients' initiative appears to have been particularly pronounced among Appalachian relief workers. A contributor to *Mountain Life and Work* remarked that although he believed in the necessity of securing "ample relief, one hopes there will not be any breaking down of a most commendable type of pride which has made them so self-sustaining in the past" (Maurice R. Reddy, "Red Cross Drought Relief in Kentucky," *Mountain Life and Work* 6 [January 1931]: 31).

107. Starr, *Social Transformation*.

108. Grey, *New Deal Medicine*.

109. Reflecting her family's long-standing relationship with the Democratic Party, Breckinridge voted Democrat throughout her life. See MB to Caroline Bagby, September 8, 1948, FNSCUK, box 341, folder 4; MB to Mary Armstrong, October 31, 1952, FNSCUK, box 353, folder 3.

110. For an excellent discussion of how other female Appalachian reformers used their positions as caregivers to step into traditionally male arenas, see Blackwell, "Ability 'To Do Much Larger Work.'"

111. John C. Campbell, *Southern Highlander*, 124.

112. For "whispering campaigns" on behalf of political candidates, see HEB, interview by Dale Deaton, March 27, 1979, 79OH174FNS75, FNSOHC. Breckinridge refused to support publicly any political campaign, arguing that it would be inappropriate for the leader of an organization that received funding from donors of all political persuasions to do so. See MB to Frank L. Polk, September 21, 1928, FNSCUK, box 338, folder 4; MB to Grace Abbott, July 24, 1936, FNSCUK, box 339, folder 1; MB to Eleanor Roosevelt, October 16, 1944, FNSCUK, box 346, folder 10. For road construction efforts, see "Field Notes," *FNSQB* 29 (Spring 1954): 45–46.

113. MB to Josephine Hunt, April 8, 1932, FNSCUK, box 344, folder 3.

114. Baldwin, *Cora Wilson Stewart*, 163. For a discussion of the 1920s tendency for female voluntary organizations to be co-opted, see Deutsch, "Learning to Talk More Like a Man," 379–404.

115. "Sixth Annual Report," *FNSQB* 7 (Summer 1931): 2; *WN*, 269; general meeting minutes, May 31, 1930, FNSCUK, box 2, folder 34; MB, "Corn-Bread Line," 423.

116. "Reemployment Information," *Thousandsticks*, March 22, 1934.

117. MB, "To the People Who Owe Money to the Frontier Nursing Service—," July 20, 1932, FNSCUK, box 55, folder 7.

118. MB, "Corn-Bread Line," 422.

119. Anonymous to MB, March 21, 1936, FNSCUK, box 53, folder 18.

120. MB to Mattie Norton, August 8, 1936, FNSCUK, box 53, folder 18.

121. Local residents contributed $102 to offset the cost of bringing in bloodhounds (contributions to fund for bloodhounds, FNSCUK, box 296, folder 7; MB, "Letter of Appreciation," *Thousandsticks*, July 23, 1936).

122. See letters located in FNSCUK, box 53, folder 18.

123. MB to Margaret Rogan, August 5, 1936, FNSCUK, box 53, folder 18.

124. MB to Kenneth Boyd, September 27, 1936, FNSCUK, box 53, folder 18.

125. MB to Kenneth Boyd, September 16, 1936, MB to Dorothea Blagden, September 18, 1936, MB to Margaret Rogan, August 5, 1936, MB to E. S. Jouett, August 24, 1936, MB to Kenneth Boyd, September 27, 1936, FNSCUK, box 53, folder 18.

126. Supplemental report of the director of the Frontier Nursing Service to the EC, November 5, 1936, FNSCUK, box 53, folder 18.

127. Report on benefits and books, FNSCUK, box 51, folder 5.

128. Poole, *Nurses on Horseback*, 26.

129. "Report on the Third Thousand Confinements of the Frontier Nursing Service, Inc.," FNSCUK, box 12, folder 3. For a sense of how FNS results compared with national and state figures, see Mary B. Willeford and Marion S. Ross, "How the Frontier Nurse Spends Her Time," *FNSQB* 12 (Spring 1937): 10.

130. Breckinridge of course credited the skill of her nurses for this low intervention rate, but she also credited the racial purity of the region for allowing women to have easy deliveries. She concluded that the most significant reason why Appalachian mothers delivered their babies without the aid of forceps or Cesarean sections was because they belonged to a "homogeneous population." Breckinridge contended that "the baby's head [was] racially

designed to go through the mother's pelvis"; therefore, nurses did not need to interfere with nature (*WN*, 315). See also MB to T. S. Hyland, October 14, 1949, FNSCUK, box 196, folder 3.

131. "Report on the Third Thousand Confinements." In 1915, doctors used forceps in as many as half of all deliveries. For more information on the frequency of forceps deliveries and Cesarean sections, see Antler and Fox, "Movement toward a Safe Maternity," 493. The FNS's rate of intervention was so low that some physicians, when first hearing these statistics, doubted their validity (Louis Hellman, interview by Anne Campbell, November 20, 1979, 79OH273FNS124, FNSOHC).

132. By 1939, charitable giving nationwide rose to 82 percent of its 1928 level (Raymond Rich Associates, "Tax-Exempt Contributions").

133. EC meeting minutes, May 28, 1937, March 4, 1938. Breckinridge earned $125 per month beginning in 1938. For additional information on her earnings, see director's salary accounts, FNSCUK, box 261, folder 3.

134. "Statement of Donations and Subscriptions Paid, May 1, 1928 to April 30, 1929," FNSCUK, box 233, folder 3; "Statement of Receipts and Disbursements, May 1, 1937 to April 30, 1938," FNSCUK, box 233, folder 11; "Balance Sheet as at April 30, 1939," FNSCUK, box 233, folder 12.

135. This shift becomes obvious from a comparison of the service's 1937 and 1938 annual reports. See *FNSQB* 13 (Summer 1937): 2–3; *FNSQB* 14 (Summer 1938): 2–4.

Chapter Eight

1. Director's report to the EC, January 12, 1939, FNSCUK, box 53, folder 17.

2. American Presidency Project, "Franklin Delano Roosevelt, Fireside Chat," September 3, 1939, <http://www.presidency.ucsb.edu/>, accessed January 22, 2007.

3. "War Demands Break Ranks of Frontier Nurses," *Louisville Courier-Journal*, May 29, 1940, FNSCUK, box 39, folder 3; MB to members of the EC, FNSCUK, box 53, folder 17.

4. MB to Anne Coffman, May 30, 1932, FNSCUK, box 53, folder 6.

5. EC meeting minutes, May 7, 1935, FNSCUK, box 3, folder 22; EC meeting minutes, October 2, 1935, FNSCUK, box 53, folder 16; EC meeting minutes, April 25, 1936, FNSCUK, box 53, folder 17; MB, memorandum, April 25, 1936, FNSCUK, box 53, folder 17; "Field Notes," *FNSQB* 13 (Winter 1938): 20.

6. Ettinger, *Nurse-Midwifery*, 74–75.

7. Litoff, *American Midwives*, 123–26. For statistics on the placement of early MCA graduates, see Ettinger, *Nurse-Midwifery*, 87.

8. MB to members of the EC, FNSCUK, box 53, folder 17.

9. Director's report to EC, FNSCUK, box 53, folder 17.

10. Dorothy F. Buck, "The Frontier Graduate School of Midwifery," *FNSQB* 18 (Autumn 1942): 35; director's report to EC, FNSCUK, box 53, folder 17; "Training Frontier Nurse-Midwives," *FNSQB* 15 (Autumn 1939): 25.

11. "The Frontier School of Midwifery and Family Nursing," *FNSQB* 54 (Autumn 1978): 4.

12. "Thirty Years Onward: Frontier Nursing Service, Inc., 1925–1955," 23, FNSCUK, box 29, folder 27; Dammann, *Social History*, 59; Dorothy F. Buck, "The Training of Frontier Nurse-Midwives," *FNSQB* 15 (Spring 1940): 18–20; Buck, "Frontier Graduate School." Kentucky had issued Breckinridge a certificate to practice midwifery in 1925. Lacking an established form, state officials adapted a certificate to practice medicine by crossing off "medicine" and writing in "midwifery" (FNSCUK, box 364, folder 15).

13. "Progressive Education," *FNSQB* 5 (September 1929): 18.

14. "Field Notes," *FNSQB* 12 (Summer 1936): 19. Breckinridge pointed out that one FNS nurse, Mrs. Gillis Morgan, was a member of the "mountain population," but she worked only until she married and then chose to dedicate herself to her family.

15. By 1953, graduates of the FGSM were serving in the Philippines, Japan, the Belgian Congo, Malaya, Arabia, New Zealand, India, Siam, Africa, South America, Canada, and Alaska as well as throughout the U.S. South. For more details, see "Minutes of the General Meeting," May 28, 1953," *FNSQB* 30 (Summer 1954): 37–47.

16. "Field Notes," *FNSQB* 15 (Spring 1940): 48.

17. Buck, "Nurses on Horseback," FNSCUK, box 35, folder 24; "Field Notes," *FNSQB* 15 (Winter 1940): 44.

18. HEB, interview by Dale Deaton, March 27, 1979, 79OH174FNS75, FNSOHC; "Field Notes," *FNSQB* 16 (Winter 1941): 68–69.

19. Agnes Lewis, interview by Dale Deaton, January 5, 1978, 82OH03FNS146, FNSOHC.

20. "Field Notes," *FNSQB* 16 (Winter 1941): 68–69.

21. As early as 1918, she protested the employment of untrained nurses. See MBT to C. C. Pierce, March 23, 1918, FNSCUK, box 336, folder 4; MB to Josephine Hunt, March 20, 1930, FNSCUK, box 344, folder 1.

22. HEB, interview by Deaton.

23. MB, review of "Union Now," by Clarence K. Streit, *FNSQB* 15 (Summer 1939): 29–31; Andre Maurois, "A Frenchman on Union Now," *FNSQB* 16 (Autumn 1940): 68–71.

24. MB, "A Frontier Nurse Speaks Out," *Lexington Herald-Leader*, August 11, 1940, FNSCUK, box 356, folder 12.

25. MB, Review of "Union Now with Britain," *FNSQB* 16 (Spring 1941): 19.

26. MB, "A Frontier Nurse Speaks Out."

27. MB to "Dear Friends in the Old Country," December 1941, FNSCUK, box 58, folder 4.

28. MB to Marvin Breckinridge Patterson, December 19, 1941, FNSCUK, box 63, folder 8.

29. *Appalachian Data Book*, 3–29.

30. Eller, *Uneven Ground*.

31. MB, report of the director to the EC meeting, November 28, 1944, FNSCUK, box 5, folder 20.

32. MB to Kenneth Boyd, September 27, 1936, FNSCUK, box 53, folder 18.

33. MB, report of the director, November 28, 1944.

34. HEB, interview by Deaton; director's report to the EC, November 1, 1943, FNSCUK, box 5, folder 16; director's report to the EC, November 28, 1944, FNSCUK, box 5, folder 20.

35. HEB to MB, Agnes Lewis, and Dorothy Buck, October 31, 1944, FNSCUK, box 198, folder 7; Josephine Pitman Prescott to MB, October 22, 1942, FNSCUK, box 198, folder 6.

36. Hazel Corbin quoted in Ettinger, *Nurse-Midwifery*, 110.

37. Marjorie Miller, "Babies Aren't Rationed," *Woman's Home Companion*, August 1943, FNSCUK, box 44, folder 2.

38. "The Frontier Graduate School of Midwifery, 1944," *FNSQB* 19 (Spring 1944): 4; "Kentucky Woman's Work Helps Babies Get a Start," *Louisville Courier-Journal*, July 22, 1943, FNSCUK, box 44, folder 2.

39. Roberts, *American Nursing*, 331–32.

40. Skocpol, *Protecting Soldiers and Mothers*, argues that rather than establishing a full-fledged welfare state, as European countries did, the United States created a system organized largely around gender and whether aid recipients were "deserving."

41. U.S. Cadet Nurse Corps information brochure, FNSCUK, box 58, folder 12; Bullough and Bullough, *Emergence*, 191.

42. Kalisch and Kalisch, *Advance*, 473–74.

43. MB to Anna D. Wolf, June 13, 1944, FNSCUK, box 58, folder 12.

44. Elsie Norman to Dorothy Buck, February 18, 1947, FNSCUK, box 62, folder 5.

45. MB to Elsie Norman, March 18, 1947, FNSCUK, box 62, folder 5.

46. Director's report to the EC, November 28, 1944, FNSCUK, box 5, folder 20.

47. Director's report to the EC, December 2, 1945, FNSCUK, box 5, folder 24.

48. For a discussion of the decline of eugenic rhetoric during the depression, see Gordon, *Woman's Body, Woman's Right*, 303. The FNS discontinued its use of racist descriptions later than most Appalachian organizations. By 1930, the Anglo-Saxonist rhetoric had disappeared from *Mountain Life and Work*, the journal that reported on Appalachian reform. From that point on, the publication's articles display a more professional, detached tone. Instead of describing why the mountains deserved outside aid, contributors began to focus more on systematically describing efforts to help the Appalachian people. By the mid-1930s, many authors even began to doubt that a specific mountain type existed. Paul Doran, a minister active in mountain reform, argued in 1936, "There is no type that can be said to represent the mountaineers as a whole, either as to their physical appearance, or as to their racial characteristics, any more than there is a type for New Englanders or New Yorkers" ("The Mountain Spirit," *Mountain Life and Work* 12 [April 1936]: 18). Doran's position represented a distinct shift away from that found in articles the journal printed during the 1920s.

49. MB, "Childbirth and War," *FNSQB* 18 (Autumn 1942): 5.

50. *American Appeal*, May 1942, FNSCUK, box 29, folder 14.

51. Skocpol, *Protecting Soldiers and Mothers*, 215.

52. Ibid., 23.

53. Ibid., 127.

54. Muncy, *Creating a Female Dominion*, 96–97.

55. *American Appeal*, May 1942, FNSCUK, box 29, folder 14.

56. "War Demands Break Ranks of Frontier Nurses."

57. Second reminder, [spring–summer 1942], FNSCUK, box 30, folder 5.

58. "Annual Report," *FNSQB* 17 (Summer 1941): 16.

59. See correspondence in FNSCUK, box 59, folder 4; "Childbirth and War," *FNSQB* 18 (Autumn 1942): 5.

60. Annual reports, *FNSQB* (Summer 1941–Summer 1945); MB to C. N. Manning, November 6, 1944, FNSCUK, box 282, folder 1.

61. MB to Mr. Meskey, July 24, 1945, FNSCUK, box 282, folder 1. Breckinridge did not begin to apply unrestricted endowments to operating expenses until May 1948. See resolution for annual meeting, May 28, 1948, FNSCUK, box 6, folder 14.

62. Adeline Cashmore to MB, January 23, 1944, FNSCUK, box 343B, folder 9.

63. "Field Notes," *FNSQB* 19 (Spring 1944): 91.

64. MBT, *Breckie*, 93–94; "Annual Report," *FNSQB* 19 (Summer 1943): 3.

65. "Field Notes," *FNSQB* 21 (Summer 1945): 66–67; Dammann, *Social History*, 60.

66. "Field Notes," *FNSQB* 18 (Autumn 1942): 72; "Field Notes," *FNSQB* 19 (Summer 1943): 76–77.

67. MB, report of the director of the Frontier Nursing Service, December 2, 1945, FNSCUK, box 5, folder 24.

Chapter Nine

1. Nash, *Crucial Era*, 168; Honey, *Creating Rosie the Riveter*, 20–21; Rowbotham, *Century of Women*, 249–51; Evans, *Born for Liberty*, 222. For an overview of the ways World War II disrupted traditional gender roles, see Fox-Genovese, "Mixed Messages," 235–45.

2. This is not to say that women other than FNS employees did not work outside the home before World War II. Economic need constantly forced women into the workforce. For African American women following emancipation, working outside the home was a necessity. Immigrant women, too, often contributed to their families' support. In addition, the death of a spouse or abandonment could require a woman to seek employment at any time. Around the turn of the century, as women pursued higher education in larger numbers, it became more acceptable for professional women to work after they married. Still, once they had children, society expected white women to forgo their careers. By the early 1930s, scholars estimate, nearly 29 percent of married American women were working outside the home (Kessler-Harris, *Out to Work*, 259). For a discussion of African American women's wage work, see Jones, *Labor of Love*. For more information on immigrant women's work patterns, see Ewen, *Immigrant Women*.

3. Ettinger, *Nurse-Midwifery*, 21.

4. "To Lend a Hand," *Johns Hopkins Magazine*, November 1965, 10, FNSCUK, box 40, folder 1.

5. *WN*, 308.

6. Grace Reeder, interview by Carol Crowe-Carraco, January 25, 1979, 79OH144FNS51, FNSOHC.

7. Medical Advisory Committee, *Medical Routine*, 2nd rev. ed., September 23, 1930, FNSCUK, box 27, folder 2.

8. Tirpak, "Frontier Nursing Service," 194.

9. Dorothy Caldwell, interview by Marian Barrett, January 18, 1979, 79OH142FNS49, FNSOHC.

10. Lucille Knechtly, interview by Dale Deaton, July 9, 1979, 82OH18FNS161, FNSOHC.

11. *WN*, 231.

12. Gladys Peacock, "We Built the First Outpost Nursing Center," *FNSQB* 25 (Summer 1949): 39.

13. Ibid., 42.

14. *WN*, 231; "The Districts Develop, 1925–1930," *FNSQB* 52 (Winter 1977): 4.

15. "A Tribute to Agnes Lewis," *FNSQB* 32 (Spring 1957): 48; Mardi B. Perry and Susan M. Putnam, interview by Anne Campbell, January 25, 1979, 79OH146FNS53, FNSOHC.

16. Agnes Lewis, interview by Dale Deaton, January 5, 1979, 82OH03FNS146, FNSOHC.

17. Agnes Lewis, "We Are Our Own Contractors," *FNSQB* 25 (Spring 1950): 3–14.

18. Gardner, "Frontier Nurse Chieftain," 2.

19. In 1929, the FNS had three couriers, all male (MB, "Rounds," *FNSQB* 5 [September 1929]: 4).

20. Peacock, "We Built."

21. "Wells and the Water Witch," *FNSQB* 12 (Autumn 1936): 2.

22. Betty Ann Bradbury, "Taking over a Center," *FNSQB* 29 (Autumn 1953): 9.

23. Director's report to the EC, December 2, 1945, FNSCUK, box 5, folder 24; "Field Notes," *FNSQB* 20 (Spring 1945): 58.

24. MB to Florence Stone, December 30, 1941, Florence Stone to MB, August 28, 1944, MB to Helen "Pebble" Stone, December 22, 1942, FNSCUK, box 64, folder 6.

25. Jonathan Fried, "1978 Courier Conclave, May 11–13," *FNSQB* 53 (Spring 1978): 10.

26. Marion Shouse to MB, August 30, 1942, MB to Marion Shouse, October 30, 1942 (two documents), FNSCUK, box 62, folder 6.

27. Dorothy Buck to MB, January 9, 1942, FNSCUK, box 60, folder 10.

28. Dorothy Buck to MB, January 13, 1942, FNSCUK, box 60, folder 10.

29. MB to Louis Dublin, February 11, 1942, FNSCUK, box 59, folder 4. The service lost 704 records, but much of the data were reconstructed from nurses' reports and hospital records. These cases were never tabulated.

30. Goffman, *Interaction Ritual*.

31. Ruth Boswell to Sister M. Theophane Shoemaker, October 28, 1954, quoted in Ettinger, *Nurse-Midwifery*, 179.

32. Molly Lee, interview by Carol Crowe-Carraco, February 6, 1979, 79OH149FNS56, FNSOHC; "In Memoriam," *FNSQB* 24 (Winter 1949): 7–18.

33. Dammann, *Social History*, 74. Breckinridge and her staff developed closer relationships with their neighbors as the years went on but continued to view the mountain people as culturally and economically different. The director discouraged young members of the staff from dating their Leslie County neighbors for fear that the nurses "would pick up with the wrong kind of men." She also feared that nurses and couriers who dated local men would become the subject of gossip and that their actions would reflect negatively on the service. As

Dammann, a former nurse-midwife, points out, a "definite line" existed between FNS professional staff and Leslie County natives.

34. "In Memoriam," *FNSQB* 7 (Autumn 1931): 2, 5. For details on subsequent FNS funerals, see *WN*, 299–300; *FNSQB* 41 (Summer 1965): 17.

35. Betty Lester, interview by Jonathan Fried, March 3, 1978, 78OH146FNS06, FNSOHC.

36. Buck, "Nurses on Horseback," FNSCUK, box 35, folder 24.

37. HEB, interview by Carol Crowe-Carraco, March 26, 1979, 79OH173FNS74, FNSOHC.

38. Betty Lester, interview by Dale Deaton, July 27, 1978, 82OH12FNS155, FNSOHC.

39. HEB, interview by Crowe-Carraco.

40. Nora K. Kelley, "When I Joined Up in 1930," *FNSQB* 15 (Autumn 1939): 13.

41. Lucy Ratliff, "The Shangri-La Cure," *FNSQB* 22 (Winter 1947): 27.

42. Lewis, interview by Deaton.

43. Mary B. Willeford, "Organization and Supervision of the Field Work of the Frontier Nursing Service, Inc.," *FNSQB* 10 (Winter 1935): 18–19.

44. Melosh, *"Physician's Hand,"* 5.

45. Beeber, "To Be One of the Boys," 33, describes a similar process among Red Cross nurses during World War I.

46. Melosh, *"Physician's Hand,"* 49.

47. Ibid., 63.

48. Gardner, *Clever Country*; Poole, "Nurse on Horseback," 38.

49. Holland, "Many Faces"; Brenda S. Wilson, "Nicknaming Practices."

50. Parker, "Made to Fit a Woman," 53, 56, 61.

51. Committee on Uniforms to Nurses quoted in ibid., 58.

52. Dammann, *Social History*, 73; Catherine V. Uhl, "First Impressions of a Pupil Nurse-Midwife," *FNSQB* 16 (Autumn 1940): 8; Mary Ann Quarles Hawkes, interview by Dale Deaton, June 16, 1979, 80OH34FNS132, FNSOHC; Mary Wilson Neal, interview by Anne Campbell, December 1, 1979, 79OH275FNS126, FNSOHC.

53. EC meeting minutes, October 26, 1942, FNSCUK, box 5, folder 12. For more information on Breckinridge's struggle to obtain telephone connections for Bowlington and Brutus, see FNSCUK, box 64, folder 8.

54. Lester, interview by Deaton.

55. Anne D. Mulhauser, interview by Marian Barrett, January 17, 1979, 79OH143FNS50, FNSOHC.

56. Carolyn Booth Gregory, interview by Linda Green, March 31, 1979, 79OH186FNS85, FNSOHC.

57. "From a Young Male Guest," *FNSQB* 15 (Summer 1939): 40.

58. Dammann, *Social History*, 72; Peggy G. Elmore, "Aunt Hattie's Barn," *FNSQB* 45 (Winter 1970): 9.

59. Joan Court, "Diary of a New Nurse-Midwife," *FNSQB* 27 (Winter 1952): 4.

60. Carolyn McK. Christian, "Impressions of Wendover," *FNSQB* 15 (Spring 1940): 4. For a detailed description of Wendover, see Grace A. Terrill, "The Living Room in the Big House," *FNSQB* 37 (Winter 1961): 3–10.

61. Faderman, *Surpassing*; Rupp, " 'Imagine My Surprise' "; Sahli, "Smashing"; Smith-Rosenberg, "Female World."

62. MB to Maud Cashmore, [May 15, 1944], FNSCUK, box 58, folder 13.

63. Adeline Cashmore to MB, September 29, 1940, FNSCUK, box 343B, folder 5.

64. Elizabeth Lansing, interview by Anne G. Campbell, June 6, 1980, 80OH119FNS145, FNSOHC; Lester, interview by Deaton.

65. "Annual Report," *FNSQB* 16 (Summer 1940), 5; "Field Notes," *FNSQB* 16 (Summer 1940): 67.

66. MB to Marion Shouse, April 14, 1942, FNSCUK, box 62, folder 6.

67. [Nurse] to MB, April 16, 1945, FNSCUK, box 343B, folder 10; MB to Maud Cashmore, July 26, 1948, FNSCUK, box 341, folder 4.

68. MB to Reeve Lewis, December 18, 1943, MB to Marion Shouse Lewis, August 18, 1945, FNSCUK, box 62, folder 6.

Chapter Ten

1. The FNS received 163 mentions in the *New York Times* between 1930 and 1945 (data compiled by searching for "Frontier Nursing Service" in the online historical edition of the *New York Times*).

2. Select examples include Gardner, *Clever Country*; Worden, "She Nurses Her Patients"; Poole, "Nurse on Horseback"; Poole, *Nurses on Horseback*; "Frontier Nurses Cut Maternity Deaths of 2,000 Women," *New York Times*, January 24, 1935; "The Frontier Nursing Service Brings Health to Kentucky Mountaineers," *Life*, June 1937, 32–35, FNSCUK, box 35, folder 17; Helen Riesenfield, "Frontier Nurse," *Look*, January 23, 1945, 30, FNSCUK, box 36, folder 3.

3. *WN*, 25.

4. Zaydee DeJonge to Thompy [MB], November 17, 1931, FNSCUK, box 329, folder 1.

5. Anne Winslow to Zaydee DeJonge, November 20, 1931, November 25, 1931, FNSCUK, box 333, folder 1.

6. Director's report to trustees, May 28, 1941, FNSCUK, box 5, folder 5.

7. Gardner, *Clever Country*; Poole, *Nurses on Horseback*.

8. "Beyond the Mountains," *FNSQB* 19 (Autumn 1943): 55–56.

9. *WN*, 321; MB to John H. Welsh, September 24, 1946, FNSCUK, box 56, folder 17.

10. MB to Anne Winslow, November 24, 1931, FNSCUK, box 329, folder 1.

11. Paul Cook to MB, November 1, 1950, FNSCUK, box 195, folder 6.

12. See correspondence in FNSCUK, box 62, folder 1.

13. EC meeting minutes, December 1, 1945, FNSCUK, box 5, folder 23; MB to Mrs. Henry James, October 9, 1941, FNSCUK, box 62, folder 1.

14. Arthur H. DeBra to Mrs. William K. Draper, August 6, 1941, FNSCUK, box 62, folder 1.

15. Arthur H. DeBra to MB, January 21, 1942, FNSCUK, box 62, folder 1.

16. Director's report to the EC, December 2, 1945, FNSCUK, box 5, folder 24; MB to [William Saal], July 12, 1945, William Saal to MB, July 20, 1945, FNSCUK, box 61, folder 9.

17. MB to Mr. Morgan, July 28, 1945, FNSCUK, box 61, folder 9.

18. MB to E. S. Jouett, August 3, 1945, FNSCUK, box 61, folder 9.

19. Ibid.; E. S. Jouett to MB, August 8, 1945, FNSCUK, box 61, folder 9.

20. Knechtly, *Where Else but Here?*, 73–74. Local resident Leonard Howard insisted that Breckinridge was always approachable: "She was a person that never seemed to be above you" (interview by Dale Deaton, July 9, 1979, 80OH36FNS134, FNSOHC).

21. EC meeting minutes, December 6, 1948, FNSCUK, box 6, folder 15; EC meeting minutes, June 1, 1949, FNSCUK, box 6, folder 18.

22. For biographical information on Day, see Day, *Bloody Ground*, introduction.

23. MB to John Day, May 23, 1941, FNSCUK, box 59, folder 12.

24. Contract signed by John F. Day, June 4, 1940, FNSCUK, box 59, folder 12.

25. Day, *Bloody Ground*, chapter 17.

26. MB to John Day, May 23, 1941, FNSCUK, box 59, folder 12.

27. MB, memorandum having reference to Mr. Day's chapter called "Frontier Nurses," June 4, 1941, FNSCUK, box 59, folder 12.

28. John F. Day to MB, May 30, 1941, FNSCUK, box 59, folder 12.

29. John F. Day to MB, May 16, 1941, FNSCUK, box 59, folder 12.

30. Day, *Bloody Ground*, 261.

31. T. S. Hyland, "The Fruitful Mountaineers: A Biological Joy Ride to Hell," *Life*, December 1949, 60, FNSCUK, box 85, folder 9.

32. MB to T. S. Hyland, October 14, 1949, FNSCUK, box 196, folder 3.

33. T. S. Hyland to MB, November 22, 1949, FNSCUK, box 84, folder 9.

34. MB to T. S. Hyland, November 28, 1949, T. S. Hyland to MB, November 22, 1949, Brownie to MB, November 28, 1949, T. S. Hyland to MB, December 3, 1949, FNSCUK, box 84, folder 9.

35. Thumper [Lucille Knechtly] to MB, December 16, 1949, FNSCUK, box 84, folder 9.

36. Hyland, "Fruitful Mountaineers."

37. Ibid. For a full consideration of Breckinridge's views on birth control, see chapter 11.

38. Breckinridge suggested that these women visit their doctors. If they still could not obtain information, they could visit the FNS's medical director for advice. Letters regarding employment and birth control information are located in FNSCUK, box 84, folder 9.

39. B. I. Rutledge to MB, January 7, 1950, FNSCUK, box 84, folder 9.

40. Lee Daniel, "Comment on Article Printed in *Life* Magazine," *Thousandsticks*, January 12, 1950.

41. John Richard Pack, "To the Editor," *Thousandsticks*, January 19, 1950.

42. Dammann, *Social History*, 79.

43. Hsiung, *Two Worlds*.

44. Mary Biggerstaff, interview by Dale Deaton, February 12, 1979, 79OH150FNS57, FNSOHC.

45. MB to Lavinia Sloan, March 19, 1952, FNSCUK, box 117, folder 8.

46. MB to *Hazard Herald*, January 2, 1950, FNSCUK, box 84, folder 9.

47. "Figures That Are Facts," *FNSQB* 26 (Winter 1951): 30–31. Census data reveal that

Hyland was probably not too far off base. The fertility ratio of Leslie County women in 1950 was calculated at 829 (meaning for every 1,000 women of childbearing age, there were 829 children under the age of five), much higher than the rates for nearby counties such as Bell (672), Estill (597), and Jackson (681). For more details, see James S. Brown and Ramsey, *Kentucky's Population*, 13–15.

48. MB to Mrs. Marston Allen, March 23, 1950, FNSCUK, box 65, folder 8.

49. MB to the *Hazard Herald*, January 2, 1950, FNSCUK, box 84, folder 9.

50. "Joe Creason's Kentucky," *Louisville Courier-Journal*, May 19, 1965. For more details on the *Life* request, see field report, September 1970, FNSCUK, box 8, folder 39.

51. See, for example, Anne G. Campbell, "Mary Breckinridge"; Crowe-Carraco, "Mary Breckinridge"; Klotter, *Breckinridges of Kentucky*, chapters 17, 18. Janet Wilson James, "Writing and Rewriting Nursing History," 569–70, provides the only critical scholarly interpretation of Breckinridge's autobiography, which James describes as "a remorselessly detailed travelogue through [Breckinridge's] life and opinions." According to James, "Breckinridge was not a ministering angel," as she depicts herself, "but an empire builder in the American business tradition."

52. See chapter 1 for more detail about this work. She of course had written a tremendous amount of material for the *Quarterly Bulletin*, which six thousand supporters received by 1952, but this was her first attempt at writing a longer piece. For information on the circulation of the *FNSQB*, see Thumper [Lucille Knechtly] to MB, September 14, 1954, FNSCUK, box 123, folder 6.

53. MB to Katherine Carson, September 3, 1948, FNSCUK, box 341, folder 4.

54. MB to Dorothy Breckinridge, September 1, 1948, MB to Anne Wilson, September 17, 1948, FNSCUK, box 341, folder 4.

55. MB to Gerald Heard, December 28, 1949, FNSCUK, box 352, folder 1. Breckinridge first met Gage at an FNS fund-raising event in the late 1920s. She became a dedicated contributor and eventually a member of the service's board of trustees. Breckinridge and Gage developed a close friendship when they discovered their mutual interest in spiritualism and theology. Breckinridge met Heard, who had published several books with Harper Brothers, through Gage. For more information on Breckenridge's relationship with these two individuals, see correspondence between Breckinridge and Gage, FNSCUK, box 352, folder 1.

56. According to Spender, "Confessions and Autobiography," 117, the recognition that one is his or her own historian is often the key factor that motivates individuals to write autobiographies.

57. MB to Chela [Margaret Gage], January 21, 1950, FNSCUK, box 352, folder 1.

58. MB to Dorothy Breckinridge, February 21, 1950, FNSCUK, box 342, folder 1.

59. MB to Elizabeth Lawrence, October 13, 1951, FNSCUK, box 352, folder 2. Breckinridge's refusal to talk about her marriages was not unusual. According to Wagner-Martin, *Telling Women's Lives*, 76–77, prior to 1970, silence about sexuality was a tradition in women's autobiography. For example, in her account of her life, Margaret Sanger left out her two marriages, a divorce, and her relationship with Havelock Ellis.

60. MB to Elizabeth Lawrence, October 19, 1949, FNSCUK, box 352, folder 2.

61. Mrs. Morris Belknap to trustees, February 24, 1949, FNSCUK, box 94, folder 6.

62. EC meeting minutes, October 25, 1949, FNSCUK, box 6, folder 20.

63. Agnes Lewis, interview by Dale Deaton, January 5, 1978, 82OHo3FNS146, FNSOHC.

64. MB to Chela [Margaret Gage], October 26, 1950, FNSCUK, box 352, folder 1.

65. *WN*, 49.

66. MB to Lucille "Pansy" Turner, January 2, 1951, FNSCUK, box 346, folder 13. Agnes Lewis, Breckinridge's close friend and coworker, applauded her decision to burn her personal papers: "One has a right to a private life" (interview by Deaton).

67. HEB, interview by Carol Crowe-Carraco, March 26, 1979, 79OH173FNS74, FNSOHC.

68. MB to Marvin Breckinridge Patterson, November 6, 1950, FNSCUK, box 90, folder 5.

69. MB to Eleanor Blaydes, October 3, 1950, FNSCUK, box 342, folder 1.

70. MB to Daisy Rogers, June 17, 1950, FNSCUK, box 87, folder 7.

71. MB to Marion Belknap, August 1, 1951, FNSCUK, box 101, folder 9.

72. MB to Chela [Margaret Gage], April 4, 1951, FNSCUK, box 352, folder 1.

73. MB to Chela [Margaret Gage] and Gerald Heard, August 15, 1951, FNSCUK, box 352, folder 1.

74. Chela [Margaret Gage] to MB, April 24, 1951, FNSCUK, box 352, folder 1.

75. Caroline [Gardner] to MB, July 3, 1951, FNSCUK, box 343, folder 2.

76. A copy of this poem is located in the FNS scrapbook, fall 1951–June 1954, FNSCUK, box 45.

77. Wagner-Martin, *Telling Women's Lives*, 76. Only since World War II have literary theorists seriously considered autobiography a unique genre worthy of analysis. Before the 1940s, scholars regarded autobiography as little more than a source of information on an individual (that is, where they were born, when they married). Modern readers have become more sensitive to the overall picture an author chooses to paint of his or her life instead of simply focusing on the "facts" that are included. Very recently, literary critics have begun to consider gender when analyzing autobiography. Scholars traditionally judged autobiographies according to a set of standards derived from studying men's life stories. In the past twenty years, however, scholars have begun to consider women's autobiographies separate from men's and to establish new methodologies that help to shed light on how women see their lives. See, for example, Jelinek, *Tradition*; Brownley and Kimmich, *Women and Autobiography*; Mason, "Other Voice."

78. Muncy, *Creating a Female Dominion*, 49, argues that Children's Bureau director Julia Lathrop adopted a similar "pose," lauding Lathrop for brilliantly combining "expectations for Victorian ladylike behavior and those for intelligent, public authority."

79. In her study of five female autobiographers, including Emmeline Pankhurst, Dorothy Day, Emma Goldman, Eleanor Roosevelt, and Golda Meir, Spacks, "Selves in Hiding," 112, argues that although each woman accomplished great things, all downplayed their achievements and claimed that destiny controlled the path they traveled. Most female autobiographers have claimed that God called them to perform a service to others.

80. Heilbrun, *Writing a Woman's Life*, 24.

81. *WN*, 48.

82. Ibid., 157.

83. Margaret Gage, memorandum for Mary Breckinridge on the first twelve chapters of her manuscript, November 13, 1950, FNSCUK, box, 352, folder 1.

84. MB to Chela [Margaret Gage], December 18, 1950, FNSCUK, box 352, folder 1.

85. Allyn J. Shepherd, interview by Marian Barrett, January 18, 1979, 79OH141FNS48, FNSOHC.

86. Goffman, *Presentation of Self*, 75.

87. *WN*, 186.

88. Ibid., 118.

89. Ibid., 4, 7, 11–12. On p. 118, Breckinridge suggests that slavery was a benevolent institution and that emancipation was a "tragedy" by telling the story of a midwife who "bust out cryin" when she found out she was free. Breckinridge assumed that these were tears of sorrow and never considered that they might be tears of joy.

90. John Q. Anderson, "Dr. James Green Carson," 246.

91. *WN*, 23.

92. Gage and Heard urged Breckinridge to cut references to relatives, friends, and their spouses from the story, advising that these references held up the story "rather like the 'begats' in the Bible!" See Gage, memorandum for Mary Breckinridge; Elizabeth Lawrence to MB, September 24, 1951, FNSCUK, box 352, folder 2; Ben C. Clough, "Life-Work of an Indomitable Woman," *Providence Journal*, April 20, 1952, FNS scrapbook, fall 1951–June 1954, FNSCUK, box 45.

93. Benstock, "Female Self," 9.

94. MB to Marion Belknap, September 10, 1951, FNSCUK, box 101, folder 9.

95. MB, memorandum for Miss Gage and Mr. Heard on their memorandum of November 13, 1950, December 1, 1950, FNSCUK, box, 352, folder 1. More often than male authors, women tend to credit others for helping to make their accomplishments possible because they are more accustomed to thinking of themselves in relation to others (Brownley and Kimmich, *Women and Autobiography*, 1).

96. MB to Elizabeth Lawrence, October 10, 1951, FNSCUK, box 352, folder 2; *WN*, 337.

97. Clippings from FNS scrapbook, fall 1951–June 1954, FNSCUK, box 45.

98. "Nursing Service's Mrs. Breckinridge Is Now 71 and Author of a Book," *Louisville Courier-Journal*, June 5, 1952, FNS scrapbook, fall 1951–June 1954, FNSCUK, box 45.

99. "Beyond the Mountains," *FNSQB* 28 (Summer 1952): 57.

100. "What America Is Reading," FNSCUK, box 352, folder 3; EC meeting minutes, September 24, 1952, FNSCUK, box 7, folder 5; "Wide Neighborhoods," *FNSQB* 28 (Summer 1952): 31; "Annual Report," *FNSQB* 28 (Summer 1952): 6. For information on the royalties the service received, see annual reports printed in the *Quarterly Bulletin* from 1953 to 1965. In 1981, the University Press of Kentucky reissued *Wide Neighborhoods*, assuring even more in royalties for the FNS.

101. Ellen Hart Smith, " 'That Blessed Old Gray-Haired Critter,' " *New York Herald-Tribune*, April 20, 1952, FNS scrapbook, fall 1951–June 1954, FNSCUK, box 45.

102. Sara Murphy, "A Task of Compassion," *Little Rock Gazette*, June 1, 1952, FNS scrapbook, fall 1951–June 1954, FNSCUK, box 45.

103. Clough, "Life-Work."

104. "Wide Neighborhoods," *FNSQB* 28 (Summer 1952): 32–33; Estelle Sharpe, " 'It's in My Nature to Do Things,' " *Washington Post*, April 16, 1952, FNS scrapbook, fall 1951–June 1954, FNSCUK, box 45.

105. This same individual took the liberty of contacting famed filmmaker Cecil B. DeMille about producing a film version of the book. She contended that DeMille was the only person who could "do it justice." DeMille politely declined, claiming that he already had too many projects in progress (Julia Carroll to MB, April 25, 1952, Cecil B. DeMille to Julia Carroll, May 31, 1952, FNSCUK, box 353, folder 3).

106. Ruth Waterbury Coates to Agnes Lewis, June 26, 1952, FNSCUK, box 353, folder 3.

107. Josephine Hunt to MB, April 25, 1952, FNSCUK, box 353, folder 3.

108. Lucille Knechtly to Margaret Gage, August 7, 1950, FNSCUK, box 79, folder 4.

109. MB to Elizabeth Lawrence, October 11, 1951, FNSCUK, box 350, folder 4.

110. Dammann, *Social History*, 76; MB to Mrs. Almon Abbott, January 27, 1949, FNSCUK, box 65, folder 2; "In Memoriam," *FNSQB* 24 (Winter 1949): 7–18.

111. "Many Reunions," *FNSQB* 28 (Autumn 1952): 35; "In Memoriam," *FNSQB* 28 (Winter 1953): 7, 11.

Chapter Eleven

1. "Field Notes," *FNSQB* 26 (Winter 1951): 51–52; Pansy [Lucille Turner] to MB, January 26, 1951, FNSCUK, box 346, folder 13.

2. Philip C. Gunion, "Frontier Nurse Describes Work in Kentucky," *Providence Evening Bulletin*, February 4, 1954, FNS scrapbook, fall 1951–June 1954, FNSCUK, box 45.

3. Lucille Elfenbein, "Favors Asserting Self at 70," *Providence Evening Bulletin*, April 24, 1952, FNS scrapbook, fall 1951–June 1954, FNSCUK, box 45.

4. Pauline Sterling, "Frontier Nurse Career Blossomed in Luxury," *Detroit Free Press*, November 14, 1952, FNS scrapbook, fall 1951–June 1954, FNSCUK, box 45.

5. MB to Martha Breckinridge, June 27, 1952, FNSCUK, box 353, folder 3.

6. "An Announcement," *FNSQB* 25 (Winter 1950): 38–39; MB to Elizabeth Lawrence, October 19, 1949, FNSCUK, box 352, folder 2.

7. Henry L. Stimson quoted in Hodgson, *America in Our Time*, 20.

8. For an overview of the postwar period, see Hodgson, *America in Our Time*; on manufactured goods, see 19.

9. Nash, *Crucial Era*, 182–85; Lee Anderson and Penningroth, *Complete in All Its Parts*, 101.

10. For a discussion of experts' theories on how to solve Appalachian poverty, see Whisnant, *Modernizing the Mountaineer*. For information on how the New Deal influenced Leslie County, see Dammann, *Social History*, 43.

11. See Bowman and Haynes, *Resources and People*, 50–51.

12. Ibid., 212, 240. Although school attendance was increasing, the quality of schools in Leslie County remained poor. School expenditures generated from local taxes in Leslie County for 1956–57 totaled less than $35 per child. In comparison, Fayette County, home to Lexington, collected more than $150 per child from local taxes (James S. Brown and Ramsey, *Kentucky's Population*, 39, 41).

13. "A Special Report: The Hyden Disaster," *Miner's Voice* (February–March 1971), FNSCUK, box 40, folder 3.

14. On the early coal boom, see Eller, *Miners, Millhands, and Mountaineers*. On the developments that allowed mining coal to become profitable in Leslie County, see Bowman and Haynes, *Resources and People*, 78–79, 311, 314.

15. Klotter, *Breckinridges of Kentucky*, 269. Caudill, *Night*, 254, claims that "no county was so drastically changed by the coal and lumbering industries as Leslie."

16. See 1960 census data, referenced in Eller, *Uneven Ground*. See also Sutton and Russell, *Social Dimensions*, 44.

17. Eller, *Uneven Ground*.

18. Ibid.

19. *Appalachian Data Book*, 3–29; James S. Brown and Ramsey, *Tables*, table 36; Bowman and Haynes, *Resources and People*, 420–21; "A Special Report: The Hyden Disaster."

20. Eller, *Uneven Ground*. See also James S. Brown and Ramsey, *Tables*, table 8; Bowman and Haynes, *Resources and People*, 180.

21. *Appalachian Data Book*, 3–32.

22. HEB, interview by Carol Crowe-Carraco, March 26, 1979, 79OH173FNS74, FNSOHC; MB to Dr. Zoeckler and Betty Lester, September 28, 1953, FNSCUK, box 119, folder 7; contract between the FNS and Smith Coal Company, FNSCUK, box 119, folder 7; conference minutes, May 26, 1949, FNSCUK, box 6, folder 17; EC meeting minutes, October 25, 1949, FNSCUK, box 6, folder 20; Agnes Lewis to MB, April 30, 1949, FNSCUK, box 87, folder 6.

23. Joseph A. Loftus, "2-Year Coal Feuds Go on in Kentucky," *New York Times*, September 8, 1953.

24. MB to Marion Belknap, February 27, 1952, FNSCUK, box 101, folder 10.

25. MB to Mr. Clapp, December 27, 1945, FNSCUK, box 59, folder 6.

26. For information on the UMW miners' hospitals, see Eller, *Uneven Ground*.

27. Quarles, "Comparison," 35.

28. *Appalachian Data Book*, 3–32; James S. Brown and Ramsey, *Kentucky's Population*, 74. Still, only 6 percent of Appalachian homes had telephones, compared to 71 percent of homes nationally (Ramsey and Warner, *Kentucky County Data Book*, 73, 75, 102, 105).

29. Frances E. Browne, "Statistics Are Vital," *FNSQB* 39 (Winter 1964): 20. For more details on the impact of television on American culture, see Twitchell, *AdcultUSA*, 92.

30. *WN*, 194.

31. Susan Spencer, FNS journal, fall 1948, 12, 15, 19, 28, FNSCUK-2005MS47, box 40, folder 3.

32. For a discussion of mountain settlement schools being "municipalized," see Whisnant, *All That Is Native and Fine*, 166. Cora Wilson Stewart provides a good example of a reformer

who watched as experts and government agencies took over her work (Baldwin, *Cora Wilson Stewart*).

33. Kalisch and Kalisch, *Advance*, 473–74.

34. MB to Frances Payne Bolton, May 4, 1949, FNSCUK, box 69, folder 7.

35. Starr, *Social Transformation*, 335.

36. According to Nash, *Crucial Era*, 10, by 1945, government came to play a dominant role in American society while relegating private and voluntary groups to a supporting role.

37. Dammann, *Social History*, 40.

38. HEB, interview by Crowe-Carraco; Agnes Lewis to MB, November 17, 1959, FNSCUK, box 124, folder 5; Dammann, *Social History*, 100.

39. "Stork Uses a Jeep in Rural Kentucky," *New York Times*, March 30, 1946.

40. Harris, "Constructing Colonialism," 52, discusses Breckinridge's hesitancy to switch from horses to jeeps.

41. Knechtly, *Where Else but Here?*, 10; Jim Lee Crawford, "Frontier Nurses Take Pride in Long Years of Service," *Corbin Daily Tribune*, August 12, 1968, FNSCUK, box 40, folder 1; EC meeting minutes, October 25, 1947, FNSCUK, box 6, folder 10; annual meeting minutes, May 26, 1954, FNSCUK, box 7, folder 10; director's report to the EC, October 25, 1947, FNSCUK, box 6, folder 11.

42. T. S. Hyland, "The Fruitful Mountaineers," *Life*, December 1949, FNSCUK, box 85, folder 9; MB to Margaret Boncompagni, May 16, 1963, FNSCUK, box 128, folder 5.

43. EC meeting minutes, December 5, 1950, FNSCUK, box 6, folder 23.

44. EC meeting minutes, November 30, 1955, FNSCUK, box 7, folder 15.

45. "Annual Report," *FNSQB* 32 (Summer 1956): 18.

46. HEB to MB, December 11, 1959, FNSCUK, box 210, folder 13; *Facts about Nursing*, 133.

47. EC meeting minutes, June 8, 1965, FNSCUK, box 8, folder 13; "Editor's Own Page," *FNSQB* 39 (Spring 1964): 22.

48. "Annual Report," *FNSQB* 32 (Summer 1956): 18.

49. MB to Marvin Breckinridge Patterson, January 9, 1961, FNSCUK, box 125, folder 1.

50. Leavitt, *Brought to Bed*, 171.

51. "Annual Report of the Frontier Nursing Service, May 1, 1938 to April 30, 1939," *FNSQB* 15 (Summer 1939): 8; "Summary of the Tenth Thousand Confinement Records of the Frontier Nursing Service," *FNSQB* 33 (Spring 1958): 45–55.

52. HEB, interview by Crowe-Carraco.

53. Ettinger, *Nurse-Midwifery*, 175–81. On this issue, I have relied heavily on Ettinger's study of the growth of the nurse-midwifery profession.

54. Ettinger, *Nurse-Midwifery*, 153–66. The Medical Mission Sisters founded the Catholic Maternity Institute in 1944 in Santa Fe, New Mexico. Similar to the FNS, its nuns provided prenatal, labor and delivery, and postnatal care to poor Latina women. It also sponsored a school to train nurse-midwives.

55. Ibid., 179–81.

56. Sister M. Theophane Shoemaker quoted in ibid., 179, 181.

57. Ibid., 184. Ettinger notes that it is no coincidence that the merger was proposed just months after Breckinridge died.

58. Ibid., 180.

59. Clifton R. Breckinridge speech, in Southern Society for the Promotion of the Study of Race Conditions and Problems in the South, *Race Problems of the South*, 174.

60. Ritterhouse, *Growing Up Jim Crow*, explores the connections among racial etiquette, segregation, and violence.

61. Joel Williamson, "How Black Was Rhett Butler?," 89. For Breckinridge's views on race, see MB to KCB, July 18, 1920, FNSCUK, box 336, folder 7.

62. Davis Lee, "The Negro: North and South," *Louisville Courier-Journal*, September 2, 1948, FNSCUK, box 363, folder 18.

63. "Beyond the Mountains," *FNSQB* 20 (Spring 1945): 50.

64. "Field Notes," *FNSQB* 16 (Autumn 1940): 87.

65. "Field Notes," *FNSQB* 11 (Autumn 1935): 17; "Indian Nurses," *FNSQB* 10 (Winter 1935): 7–8; "Field Notes," *FNSQB* 12 (Summer 1936): 20.

66. According to Browne, the shunned nurse responded to her rejection with a grateful letter, thanking Browne for being the first person to give her an honest reason for turning down her application. For more details on this incident, see HEB, interview by Crowe-Carraco.

67. Ibid.; HEB, interview by Dale Deaton, March 27, 1979, 79OH174FNS75, FNSOHC. Ritterhouse, *Growing Up Jim Crow*, 42, likens the white southern taboo against eating and drinking with blacks to that against interracial sex. Whites failed to acknowledge the irony that they would allow blacks to prepare their food yet adamantly opposed eating together.

68. HEB, interview by Deaton.

69. MB, "Is Birth Control the Answer?," 160.

70. "Will Rogers Relates Wish to Visit Kentucky Mountains in Letter to Mary Breckinridge," *Lexington Herald*, February 21, 1933, WPAR, box 11, folder 40.

71. According to Dr. Louise Hutchins, director of the Mountain Maternal Health League, Breckinridge never expressed much interest in family planning because the deaths of her two children made it difficult for her to identify with women who wanted to limit their families (Louise Gilman Hutchins, interview by James W. Reed, January 31, 1975, transcript, Schlesinger-Rockefeller Oral History Project, Schlesinger Library, Radcliffe College, Cambridge, Massachusetts).

72. MB, memorandum having reference to Mr. Day's chapter called "Frontier Nurses," June 4, 1941, FNSCUK, box 59, folder 12.

73. MB, "Is Birth Control the Answer?"

74. Hyland, "Fruitful Mountaineers."

75. MB, "Is Birth Control the Answer?," 162.

76. Ibid., 160.

77. HEB, interview by Deaton; Gertrude Isaacs, interview by Dale Deaton, November 15, 1978, 79OH79FNS35, FNSOHC.

78. MB, memorandum having reference to Mr. Day's chapter.

79. Hyland, "Fruitful Mountaineers," 60.

80. Gordon, *Woman's Body, Woman's Right*, 341–42.

81. Rock, *Time Has Come*, 18.

82. For more information on the history of the birth control pill, see Asbell, *Pill*. For an in-depth description of Rock's role in the development and marketing of Enovid, see McLaughlin, *Pill*. For a detailed discussion of the clinical trials of Enovid, see Vaughan, *Pill on Trial*. Reed, *From Private Vice to Public Virtue*, provides a comprehensive history of the birth control movement. The most recent and most analytical look at the pill's effects appears in Watkins, *On the Pill*.

83. Marks, " 'Cage,' " 225–26.

84. Ibid., 228. Before the mid-1960s, few regulations governed the use of human subjects in medical experiments.

85. Scientists conducted early trials on infertility patients at the Margaret Sanger Research Bureau in New York, on medical students in Puerto Rico, on schizophrenic patients at the Worcester State Hospital in Massachusetts, and on immigrant populations of Hispanic women in San Antonio and Los Angeles.

86. Katherine McCormick to Margaret Sanger, May 31, 1955, July 21, 1954, quoted in Marks, " 'Cage,' " 221.

87. Dr. John Rock, interview by Dale Deaton, June 15, 1979, 80OH31FNS129, FNSOHC.

88. HEB, interview by Deaton. The secondary literature on clinical trials of the pill makes no mention of tests in eastern Kentucky. Harris, "Constructing Colonialism," has attempted to correct this oversight. Although she overstates her contention that Breckinridge held a colonial mentality and viewed her patients in a thoroughly condescending fashion, the information Harris provides about the Enovid trials among FNS patients is very useful. The only source to mention the FNS trials is McLaughlin, *Pill*, 23, which parenthetically notes that Rock interceded with Searle Pharmaceuticals to provide a free supply of pills to the FNS in the 1960s.

89. Staff meeting minutes, March 17, 1960, FNSCUK, box 212, folder 5.

90. Elsie Maier, interview by Dale Deaton, December 5, 1978, 79OH86FNS42, FNSOHC.

91. EC meeting minutes, April 10, 1965, FNSCUK, box 8, folder 11. The FDA approved Enovid in 1960 (Watkins, *On the Pill*, 32).

92. Beasley, "After Office Hours," 156; Beasley, "Nurse-Midwife as a Mediator," 201.

93. Beasley, "After Office Hours," 156; "Annual Report," *FNSQB* 46 (Summer 1970): 17.

94. "Forty-fifth Annual Report," *FNSQB* 46 (Summer 1970): 17.

95. Carol Sutton, "FNS Looks to New Services," *Louisville Courier-Journal and Times*, November 30, 1969, FNSCUK, box 40, folder 1.

96. Beasley, "After Office Hours," 155.

Chapter Twelve

1. Mary H. Vorse quoted in Paul Thompson, Itzin, and Abendstern, *I Don't Feel Old*, 48.

2. Elsie Maier, interview by Dale Deaton, December 5, 1978, 79OH86FNS42, FNSOHC.

3. MB to Margaret Boncompagni, March 26, 1962, FNSCUK, box 128, folder 5.

4. Associate Editors, "Happy Birthday," *FNSQB* 36 (Winter 1961): 15–19.

5. EC meeting minutes, April 22, 1961, FNSCUK, box 8, folder 1.

6. MB to Marjorie C. Tyler, January 3, 1958, FNSCUK, box 125, folder 7.

7. "Before We Step into the Wings," *FNSQB* 36 (Summer 1960): 21; "Before We Step into the Wings," *FNSQB* 39 (Summer 1963): 21–22.

8. Dammann, *Social History*, 73.

9. Leonard Howard, interview by Dale Deaton, July 9, 1979, 80OH36FNS134, FNSOHC.

10. Agnes Lewis to Mrs. Henry Joy, January 21, 1957, FNSCUK, box 207, folder 7; MB to Margaret Gage, September 21, 1964, FNSCUK, box 153, folder 9.

11. Fred W. Luigart Jr., "Founder of Frontier Nursing Honored," *Louisville Courier-Journal*, September 25, 1962, FNS Scrapbook, FNSCUK, box 47; Peggy Elmore, "Mary Breckinridge Day," *FNSQB* 38 (Autumn 1962): 29; Vanda Summers, "The Shining Day," *FNSQB* 38 (Autumn 1962): 32.

12. MB to Dr. and Mrs. W. B. R. Beasley, November 23, 1962, FNSCUK, box 127, folder 7.

13. Agnes Lewis to Katherine Carson, September 18, 1962, FNSCUK, box 206, folder 10.

14. "Before We Step into the Wings," *FNSQB* 39 (Summer 1963): 21–22.

15. Knechtly, *Where Else but Here?*, 82.

16. MB to Dorothy Breckinridge, January 31, 1964, FNSCUK, box 148, folder 10.

17. HEB to Mrs. Karl Wilson, June 15, 1964, FNSCUK, box 331, folder 7.

18. Knechtly, *Where Else but Here?*, 81; "Beyond the Mountains," *FNSQB* 25 (Winter 1950): 55; Catherine T. Arpee, interview by Linda Green, December 2, 1978, 79OH153FNS60, FNSOHC.

19. *WN*, 60.

20. Eugene Field, "Little Boy Blue," reproduced in *FNSQB* 40 (Autumn 1964): 2.

21. Agnes Lewis to Mrs. Branham, August 31, 1964, FNSCUK, box 206, folder 5.

22. HEB, interview by Dale Deaton, March 27, 1979, 79OH174FNS75, FNSOHC.

23. "Beyond the Mountains," *FNSQB* 40 (Winter 1965): 46–47.

24. Agnes Lewis to Mrs. Branham, February 17, 1965, FNSCUK, box 206, folder 5.

25. Agnes Lewis to Mrs. John W. Price, May 22, 1965, FNSCUK, box 208, folder 4.

26. MB to Mrs. Walter Biddle McIlvain, May 15, 1965, FNSCUK, box 157, folder 14.

27. HEB, interview by Deaton; "Beyond the Mountains," *FNSQB* 40 (Winter 1965): 46–47; "Before We Step into the Wings," *FNSQB* 39 (Summer 1963): 21–22.

28. Agnes Lewis to Mrs. George S. Buck, June 29, 1965, FNSCUK, box 206, folder 9.

29. Kyle Vance, "Mrs. Breckinridge Rites Kept Simple," *Louisville Courier-Journal*, May 19, 1965, FNSCBC, box 1, folder 5; Klotter, *Breckinridges of Kentucky*, 368 n.36; HEB, interview by Deaton.

30. "Fortieth Annual Report," *FNSQB* 41 (Summer 1965): 4, 6, 15; forty-year total, FNSCUK, box 156, folder 11.

31. Ed Morgan, interview by Dale Deaton, July 7, 1978, 78OH143FNS03, FNSOHC.

Conclusion

1. See, for example, Weise, *Grasping at Independence*.

2. Shifflett, *Coal Towns*, 8.

3. See Artemus Campbell, interview by Dale Deaton, October 30, 1978, 79OH30FNS31, FNSOHC; Stidham, *Trails*, 159.

4. Scott, *Natural Allies*, 25.

5. George Wooten quoted in Peggy E. Baker, "The Historical Significance of Mary Breckinridge and the Foundation of the Frontier Nursing Service," unpublished paper, 1974, 8, FNSCUK-2005MS47, box 41, folder 11.

6. MB to Ella Phillips Crandall, October 20, 1923, FNSCUK, box 348, folder 3.

7. For more information on the reassessment of midwifery that occurred during the 1970s, see Rooks, "Nurse-Midwifery." The number of births conducted by nurse-midwives has increased consistently over the past three decades but remains small in proportion to total births. The Centers for Disease Control reported that in 2004, midwives attended 11.1 percent of all vaginal deliveries in the United States, nearly double the 1991 rate of 5.7 percent (Joyce A. Martin, Brady E. Hamilton, Paul D. Sutton, Stephanie J. Ventura, Fay Menacker, and Sharon Kirmeyer, "Births: Final Data for 2004," National Vital Statistics Report, September 29, 2006, <www.cdc.gov>, accessed July 20, 2007).

Epilogue

1. HEB to Marvin Breckinridge Patterson, March 22, 1966, FNSCUK, box 160, folder 4.

2. Kalisch and Kalisch, *Advance*, 621–23.

3. "Are We Needed?," *FNSQB* 41 (Autumn 1965): 7; HEB, interview by Dale Deaton, March 27, 1979, 79OH174FNS75, FNSOHC; HEB to W. B. R. Beasley, January 27, 1966, March 21, 1966, FNSCUK, box 147, folder 4.

4. Agnes Lewis to Berta Hamilton, January 11, 1966, FNSCUK, box 207, folder 2.

5. Marts and Lundy, "Fund Raising Survey Report Made for Frontier Nursing Service, Wendover, Kentucky," October 5, 1966, 35, FNSCUK, box 158, folder 5.

6. HEB, interview by Carol Crowe-Carraco, March 26, 1979, 79OH173FNS74, FNSOHC.

7. HEB to all FNS staff members, June 23, 1965, FNSCUK, box 210, folder 13; HEB to Lucille [Knechtly] and Madeline, June 23, 1965, FNSCUK, box 210, folder 13; salary scale, May 1, 1966, FNSCUK, box 210, folder 13.

8. Peggy Elmore, "Field Notes," *FNSQB* 41 (Spring 1966): 46; Ann C. Ghory, "Community Medicine Rotation," *FNSQB* 51 (Summer 1975): 50.

9. Dammann, *Social History*, 135–36; Gertrude Isaacs, "Frontier Nursing Service Continuing Development 1974," *FNSQB* 49 (Autumn 1973–Winter 1974): 15; Gertrude Isaacs, interview by Dale Deaton, November 15, 1978, 79OH79FNS35, FNSOHC.

10. Anne Standley and Rachel Buff, "The Home Health Agency," *FNSQB* 56 (Summer 1980): 21; HEB, "Frontier Nursing Service," 77.

11. "Thirty Ninth Annual Report—Last Year's Expenditures and This Year's Budget,"

FNSQB 40 (Summer 1964): 8; "Forty-fifth Annual Report—Statement of Income and Expenses," *FNSQB* 46 (Summer 1970): 6.

12. Agnes Lewis to Hope McCown, July 22, 1965, FNSCUK, box 207, folder 14; EC meeting minutes, October 8, 1965, FNSCUK, box 8, folder 14; "The Mary Breckinridge Hospital," *FNSQB* 41 (Autumn 1965): 8–9. Browne always regretted that the FNS had not built the new hospital sooner, when the facility could have been the "little community hospital" service leaders wanted rather than the big, high-tech hospital that was ultimately constructed (HEB, interview by Deaton).

13. Elsie Maier, interview by Dale Deaton, December 5, 1978, 79OH86FNS42, FNSOHC.

14. Molly Lee, interview by Carol Crowe-Carraco, February 6, 1979, 79OH149FNS56, FNSOHC.

15. Carolyn Gay, interview by Dale Deaton, January 16, 1979, 79OH139FNS46, FNSOHC.

16. Nancy Dammann, interview by Dale Deaton, n.d., 82OH40FNS183, FNSOHC.

17. Alberta Kelly, interview by Dale Deaton, April 26, 1979, 79OH187FNS86, FNSOHC.

18. Irene Nolan, "A Crack in the Image?," *Louisville Courier-Journal*, May 18, 1975, FNSCBC, box 1, folder 1. In 1972, 112 of 154 FNS employees were local citizens, but these individuals primarily held low-skill positions as aides, clerical workers, and maintenance and housekeeping personnel. In response, the service sought to enroll more local women in training programs. For more information, see Gertrude Isaacs, "The Family Nurse and Primary Health Care in Rural Areas," *FNSQB* 47 (Spring 1972): 7–8.

19. Nolan, "Crack in the Image?"; "The Advisory Committee to the FNS," *FNSQB* 51 (Winter 1976): 39–40.

20. "All about Hospitals," *FNSQB* 50 (Winter 1975): 3.

21. Agnes Lewis to Mrs. Beasley, April 15, 1966, FNSCUK, box 206, folder 1; HEB to Francis Massie, April 13, 1966, FNSCUK, box 158, folder 9; Agnes Lewis to Mrs. John Marshall Prewitt, March 9, 1966, FNSCUK, box 208, folder 2.

22. Jane Leigh Powell, "Come Blow Your Horn with Us," *FNSQB* 45 (Spring 1970): 5–6.

23. HEB, interview by Deaton.

24. Irene Nolan, "Frontier Nurses Dedicate New Hospital to Their Founder," *Louisville Courier-Journal*, January 7, 1975, FNSCUK, box 40, folder 4.

25. HEB, interview by Deaton.

26. Rooks, "Nurse-Midwifery."

27. *Current Issues in Nursing Education*, 17; "Rebirth of the Midwife," *FNSQB* 47 (Winter 1972): 4, reprinted from *Time*, November 20, 1972.

28. Leah Larkin, "Nurse Midwives: Providing New Direction in Obstetrical Care," *Louisville Courier-Journal and Times*, May 20, 1973, FNSCUK, box 40 folder 4. The University of Kentucky College of Nursing in Lexington established a master's program in midwifery in 1974.

29. Kalisch and Kalisch, *Advance*, 659–64.

30. Dammann, *Social History*, 128, 131.

31. "Family Nurse Practitioner Program: Progress Report," *FNSQB* 47 (Summer 1971): 31; "Family Nurse Practitioner Project," *FNSQB* 45 (Summer 1969): 32–33.

32. Gertrude Isaacs, "Family Nurse Practitioner Program: Program Report," *FNSQB* 46 (Winter 1971): 6.

33. Gertrude Isaacs, "In the Interest of Primary Health Service," *FNSQB* 53 (Summer 1977): 25–32.

34. "Beyond the Mountains," *FNSQB* 53 (Autumn 1977): 51.

35. "The Frontier School of Midwifery and Family Nursing," <http://www.midwives .org/home.html>, accessed February 26, 2007.

Bibliography

Primary Sources

ARCHIVAL COLLECTIONS

Austin, Texas
    Texas History Center, University of Texas
        Airlie Plantation Records (microfilm)
Berea, Kentucky
    Southern Appalachian Archives, Hutchins Library, Berea College
        Frontier Nursing Service Collection
        William Hutchins Papers
        Pine Mountain Settlement School Collection (microfilm)
        J. A. Stucky Papers
Cambridge, Massachusetts
    Schlesinger Library, Radcliffe College
        Schlesinger-Rockefeller Oral History Project (microfilm transcript)
Lexington, Kentucky
    University of Kentucky Special Collections, M. I. King Library
        Breckinridge Family Papers
        Frontier Nursing Service Collection
        Frontier Nursing Service Oral History Collection
        Linda Neville, Charles Kerr, and Neville Family Papers
        James Parton Scrapbook, ca. 1930–32
        Prewitt Collection, Mary Breckinridge Series, uncataloged
        Shaunna L. Scott, "Grannies, Mothers, and Babies: An Examination of
            Traditional Southern Appalachian Midwifery"
        Cora Wilson Stewart Papers
Louisville, Kentucky
    Filson Club
        Johnson Family Papers
        Susan S. Towles Papers
        Alice Elizabeth Trabue Papers
    Kornhauser Health Sciences Library, University of Louisville
        Works Progress Administration Research Project Records

Sleepy Hollow, New York
  Rockefeller Foundation Archives, Rockefeller Archive Center
    Commonwealth Fund Collection

JOURNALS AND NEWSPAPERS

American Journal of Nursing
Berea Quarterly for the Southern Mountains
Eureka Springs Daily Times-Echo
Fort Smith Times-Record
Frontier Nursing Service Quarterly Bulletin
Hazard Herald
Lexington Herald-Leader
Louisville Courier-Journal
Louisville Social Register
Mountain Life and Work
New York Times
Public Health Nurse Quarterly (formerly *Visiting Nurse Quarterly*)
Southern Woman's Magazine
Thousandsticks

BOOKS

Bangs, John Kendrick. *Loss or Gain: The American Committee for Devastated France in the Field*. New York: American Committee for Devastated France, 1918.
Breckinridge, Mary. *Organdie and Mull*. Wendover, Ky.: Frontier Nursing Service, 1948.
———. *Wide Neighborhoods: A Story of the Frontier Nursing Service*. 1952; Lexington: University Press of Kentucky, 1981.
Brock, Sallie A. *The Southern Amaranth*. New York: Wilcox and Rockwell, 1869.
Campbell, John C. *The Southern Highlander and His Homeland*. 1921; Lexington: University Press of Kentucky, 1969.
Child Welfare in Kentucky: An Inquiry by the National Child Labor Committee for the Kentucky Child Labor Association and the State Board of Health. New York: National Child Labor Committee, 1919.
Committee on the Costs of Medical Care. *Medical Care for the American People*. Chicago: University of Chicago Press, 1932.
Frost, William Goodell. *For the Mountains: Our Aims, Strategic Principles: Addresses at Knoxville Mountain Workers Conference*. N.p., 1921.
Gardner, Caroline. *Clever Country: Kentucky Mountain Trails*. New York: Revell, 1931.
Grant, Madison. *The Passing of the Great Race; or, The Racial Basis of European History*. New York: Scribner's, 1922.
Hoover, Herbert. *American Individualism*. New York: Doubleday, Page, 1922.

Knechtley, Lucille. *Where Else but Here?* Pippa Passes, Ky.: Pippa Valley Printing, 1989.

Poole, Ernest. *Nurses on Horseback*. New York: Macmillan, 1933.

Raine, James Watt. *The Land of Saddle-Bags: A Study of the Mountain People of Appalachia*. New York: Council of Women for Home Missions and Missionary Education Movement of the United States and Canada, [1924].

Shawe, Rosalind Gillette. *Notes for Visiting Nurses*. Philadelphia: Blakiston, 1893.

Southern Society for the Promotion of the Study of Race Conditions and Problems in the South. *Race Problems of the South: Report of the Proceedings of the First Annual Conference*. 1900; New York: Negro Universities Press, 1969.

Thompson, Mary Breckinridge. *Breckie: His First Four Years*. New York: privately published, 1918.

Willeford, Mary B. *Income and Health in Remote Rural Areas: A Study of 400 Families in Leslie County, Kentucky*. New York: n.p., 1932.

Wilson, Samuel Tyndale. *The Southern Mountaineers*. New York: Presbyterian Home Missions, 1906.

ARTICLES, PAMPHLETS, AND DISSERTATIONS

Beasley, W. B. Rogers. "After Office Hours: Coping with Family Planning in a Rural Area." *Obstetrics and Gynecology* 41 (January 1973): 155–59.

——. "The Nurse-Midwife as a Mediator of Contraception." *American Journal of Obstetrics and Gynecology* 98 (May 15, 1967): 201–7.

Bradley, William Aspenwall. "Hobnobbing with Hillbillies." *Harper's Monthly Magazine*, December 1915, 91–103.

Breckinridge, Mary. "An Adventure in Midwifery: The Nurse-on-Horseback Gets a 'Soon Start.'" *Survey Graphic*, October 1, 1926, 25–27, 47.

——. "Is Birth Control the Answer?" *Harper's Magazine*, July 1931, 157–63

——. "The Corn-Bread Line." *Survey*, August 15, 1930, 422–23.

——. "The Nurse-Midwife—A Pioneer." *American Journal of Public Health* 17 (November 1, 1927): 1147–51.

——. "Where the Frontier Lingers." *The Rotarian* 47 (September 1935): 9–12.

Bromley, Dorothy Dunbar. "What Risk Motherhood?" *Harper's Monthly Magazine*, June 1929, 11–33.

Buck, Dorothy F. "The Nurses on Horseback Ride On." *American Journal of Nursing* 40 (September 1940): 993–95.

Gardner, Caroline. "Frontier Nurse Chieftain." *Arkansas Gazette Magazine*, October 27, 1935, 2.

Hardin, E. R. "The Midwife Problem." *Southern Medical Journal* 18 (May 1925): 347.

Harney, Will Wallace. "A Strange Land and a Peculiar People." In *Appalachian Images in Folk and Popular Culture*, edited by W. K. McNeil, 429–38. Knoxville: University of Tennessee Press, 1995.

Hyland, T. S. "The Fruitful Mountaineers." *Life*, December 1949, 60–67.

MacKaye, Percy. "Untamed America: A Comment on a Sojourn in the Kentucky Mountains." *Survey*, January 1, 1924, 326–31, 360, 362–63.

Morrison, Mary Breckinridge. "The Poetry of the Southern United States." *Westminster Review*, July 1911, 61–72.

———. "The Women of Thackeray." *Westminster Review*, September 1907, 299–303.

Quarles, Mary Ann Stillman. "A Comparison of Some Aspects of Family Life between Two Areas of Leslie County, Kentucky." Master's thesis, University of Kentucky, 1952.

Pearl, Raymond. "Distribution of Physicians in the United States." *Journal of the American Medical Association* 84 (April 4, 1925): 1024–28.

Poole, Ernest Poole. "The Nurse on Horseback." *Good Housekeeping*, June 1932, 38–39, 203–9.

Robb, Isabel Hampton. "A Brief Sketch of the History of District Nursing." *Visiting Nurse Quarterly* 2 (January 1910): 11–15.

Rude, Anna E. "The Midwife Problem in the United States." *Journal of the American Medical Association* 81 (September 22, 1923): 987–92.

Semple, Ellen Churchill. "The Anglo-Saxons of the Kentucky Mountains: A Study in Anthropogeography." In *Appalachian Images in Folk and Popular Culture*, edited by W. K. McNeil, 145–74. Knoxville: University of Tennessee Press, 1995.

Thompson, Mary Breckinridge. "Motherhood—A Career." *Southern Woman's Magazine*, November 1916–June 1917.

———. "Report of the Nursing Representative of the National Organization for Public Health Nursing in Arkansas." *Public Health Nurse Quarterly* 10 (April 1918): 202–4.

Van Blarcom, Carolyn Conant. "Provisions for Maternity Care in the United States." *American Journal of Obstetrics and Gynecology* 9 (May 1925): 697–703.

Veech, Annie S. "For Blue Grass and Hill Babies." *Survey*, September 15, 1924, 625–26.

Worden, Helen. "She Nurses Her Patients for a Dollar a Year." *American Magazine* 112 (December 1931): 108.

Secondary Sources

BOOKS

Aiken, Katherine G. *Harnessing the Power of Motherhood: The National Florence Crittenden Mission, 1883–1925*. Knoxville: University of Tennessee Press, 1998.

Allard, Chester C., ed. *Who Is Who in Arkansas*. Vol. 1. Little Rock, Ark.: Allard House, 1959.

Allen, Frederick Lewis. *Only Yesterday: An Informal History of the Nineteen-Twenties*. New York: Harper and Row, 1931.

Anderson, Lee, and Kathy Penningroth. *Complete in All Its Parts: Nursing Education at the University of Iowa, 1898–1998*. Ann Arbor: University of Michigan Press, 1998.

Appalachian Data Book. Vol. 3. Washington, D.C.: Appalachian Regional Commission, 1970.

Appalachian Land Use Task Force. *Who Owns Appalachia?: Landownership and Its Impact.* Lexington: University Press of Kentucky, 1983.

Asbell, Bernard. *The Pill: A Biography of the Drug That Changed the World.* New York: Random House, 1995.

Baldwin, Yvonne Honeycutt. *Cora Wilson Stewart and Kentucky's Moonlight Schools: Fighting for Literacy in America.* Lexington: University Press of Kentucky, 2006.

Baltzell, E[dward] Digby. *The Protestant Establishment: Aristocracy and Caste in America.* New York: Random House, 1964.

Barney, Sandra Lee. *Authorized to Heal: Gender, Class, and the Transformation of Medicine in Appalachia, 1880–1930.* Chapel Hill: University of North Carolina Press, 2000.

Batteau, Allen W. *The Invention of Appalachia.* Tucson: University of Arizona Press, 1990.

Becker, Jane. *Selling Tradition: Appalachia and the Construction of an American Folk, 1930–1940.* Chapel Hill: University of North Carolina Press, 1998.

Bederman, Gail. *Manliness and Civilization: A Cultural History of Gender and Race in the United States, 1880–1917.* Chicago: University of Chicago Press, 1995.

Billings, Dwight B., and Kathleen M. Blee. *The Road to Poverty: The Making of Wealth and Hardship in Appalachia.* Cambridge: Cambridge University Press, 2000.

Blair, Emily Newell. *Bridging Two Eras: The Autobiography of Emily Newell Blair, 1877–1951.* Preface by Virginia Jeans Laas. Columbia: University of Missouri Press, 1999.

Bledstein, Burton J. *The Culture of Professionalism: The Middle Class and the Development of Higher Education in America.* New York: Norton, 1976.

Borst, Charlotte G. *Catching Babies: The Professionalization of Childbirth, 1870–1920.* Cambridge: Harvard University Press, 1995.

Boston Women's Health Book Collective. *The New Our Bodies, Ourselves: A Book by and for Women.* 2nd ed. New York: Touchstone, 1992.

Bowman, Mary Jean, and W. Warren Haynes. *Resources and People in East Kentucky: Problems and Potentials of a Lagging Economy.* Baltimore: Johns Hopkins Press for Resources for the Future, 1963.

Braude, Ann. *Radical Spirits: Spiritualism and Women's Rights in Nineteenth-Century America.* Boston: Beacon, 1989.

Brewer, Mary T. *Of Bolder Men: A History of Leslie County, Kentucky and Its People.* Wooten, Ky.: Brewer, 1978.

———. *Rugged Trail to Appalachia: A History of Leslie County, Kentucky and Its People, Celebrating Its Centennial Year, 1878–1978.* Wooten, Ky.: Brewer, 1978.

Brodhead, Richard H. *Cultures of Letters: Scenes of Reading and Writing in Nineteenth-Century America.* Chicago: University of Chicago Press, 1993.

Brown, Alexander. *The Cabells and Their Kin.* Boston: Houghton Mifflin, 1895.

Brown, E. Richard. *Rockefeller Medicine Men: Medicine and Capitalism in America.* Berkeley: University of California Press, 1979.

Brown, James S., and Ralph J. Ramsey. *Kentucky's Population in the 1960s: A County Data Book.* Lexington: University of Kentucky Agricultural Experiment Station, 1963.

———. *Tables on Population Characteristics: Eastern Kentucky Resource Development Counties.* Lexington: Kentucky Agricultural Experiment Station, 1962.

Brownley, Martine Watson, and Allison B. Kimmich, eds. *Women and Autobiography*. Wilmington, Del.: Scholarly Resources, 1999.

Brundage, W. Fitzhugh, ed. *Where These Memories Grow: History, Memory, and Southern Identity*. Chapel Hill: University of North Carolina Press, 2000.

Buhler-Wilkerson, Karen. *False Dawn: The Rise and Decline of Public Health Nursing, 1900–1930*. New York: Garland, 1989.

——. *No Place Like Home: A History of Nursing and Home Care in the United States*. Baltimore: Johns Hopkins University Press, 2001.

Bullough, Vern L., and Bonnie Bullough. *The Emergence of Modern Nursing*. London: Macmillan, 1969.

Caudill, Harry M. *Night Comes to the Cumberlands: A Biography of a Depressed Area*. Boston: Little, Brown, 1963.

Cavender, Anthony. *Folk Medicine in Southern Appalachia*. Chapel Hill: University of North Carolina Press, 2003.

Chambers, J. S., and Harry R. Lynn. *Medical Service in Kentucky*. Lexington: University of Kentucky, 1931.

Chesler, Ellen. *Woman of Valor: Margaret Sanger and the Birth Control Movement in America*. New York: Doubleday, 1992.

Collins, Robert F. *A History of the Daniel Boone National Forest, 1770–1970*. Washington, D.C.: U.S. Department of Agriculture, Forest Service, Southern Region, 1976.

Cott, Nancy F. *The Grounding of Modern Feminism*. New Haven: Yale University Press, 1987.

Current Issues in Nursing Education. New York: National League for Nursing, 1973.

Curry, Lynne. *Modern Mothers in the Heartland: Gender, Health, and Progress in Illinois, 1900–1930*. Columbus: Ohio State University Press, 1999.

Dammann, Nancy. *A Social History of the Frontier Nursing Service*. Sun City, Ariz.: Social Change, 1982.

Davis, Allen F. *American Heroine: The Life and Legend of Jane Addams*. New York: Oxford University Press, 1973.

——. *Spearheads for Reform: The Social Settlements and the Progressive Movement, 1890–1914*. New York: Oxford University Press, 1967.

Davis, Ronald L. F. *Good and Faithful Labor: From Slavery to Sharecropping in the Natchez District, 1860–1890*. Westport, Conn.: Greenwood, 1982.

Day, John F. *Bloody Ground*. Garden City, N.Y.: Doubleday, Doran, 1941.

DeJong, Gordon F. *Appalachian Fertility Decline: A Demographic and Sociological Analysis*. Lexington: University Press of Kentucky, 1968.

Donegan, Jane B. *Women and Men Midwives: Medicine, Morality, and Misogyny in Early America*. Westport, Conn.: Greenwood, 1978.

Donovan, Mary Sudman. *A Different Call: Women's Ministries in the Episcopal Church, 1850–1920*. Wilton, Conn.: Morehouse-Barlow, 1986.

Dyer, Thomas G. *Theodore Roosevelt and the Idea of Race*. Baton Rouge: Louisiana State University Press, 1980.

Ehrenreich, Barbara, and Deirdre English. *For Her Own Good: 150 Years of the Experts' Advice to Women*. Garden City, N.Y.: Anchor, 1979.

Eller, Ronald D. *Miners, Millhands, and Mountaineers: Industrialization of the Appalachian South, 1880–1930*. Knoxville: University of Tennessee Press, 1982.

——. *Uneven Ground: Appalachia since 1945*. Lexington: University Press of Kentucky, forthcoming.

Ellis, John H. *Medicine in Kentucky*. Lexington: University Press of Kentucky, 1977.

Ettinger, Laura E. *Nurse-Midwifery: The Birth of a New American Profession*. Columbus: Ohio State University Press, 2006.

Evans, Sara M. *Born for Liberty: A History of Women in America*. New York: Free Press, 1991.

Ewen, Elizabeth. *Immigrant Women in the Land of Dollars*. New York: Monthly Review Press, 1985.

Facts about Nursing: A Statistical Summary. New York: Nursing Information Bureau of the American Nurses' Association, 1960.

Faderman, Lillian. *Surpassing the Love of Men: Romantic Friendship and Love between Women from the Renaissance to the Present*. New York: Morrow, 1981.

Fitzpatrick, Ellen. *Endless Crusade: Women Social Scientists and Progressive Reform*. New York: Oxford University Press, 1990.

Fosl, Catherine. *Subversive Southerner: Anne Braden and the Struggle for Racial Justice in the Cold War South*. New York: Palgrave Macmillan, 2002.

Foster, Gaines M. *Ghosts of the Confederacy: Defeat, the Lost Cause, and the Emergence of the New South, 1865–1913*. New York: Oxford University Press, 1987.

Frankel, Noralee, and Nancy S. Dye, eds. *Gender, Class, Race, and Reform in the Progressive Era*. Lexington: University Press of Kentucky, 1991.

Freedman, Estelle B. *Maternal Justice: Miriam Van Waters and the Female Reform Tradition*. Chicago: University of Chicago Press, 1996.

Friedman, Jean E. *The Enclosed Garden: Women and Community in the Evangelical South, 1830–1900*. Chapel Hill: University of North Carolina Press, 1985.

Gaventa, John. *Power and Powerlessness: Quiescence and Rebellion in an Appalachian Valley*. Urbana: University of Illinois Press, 1980.

Goffman, Erving. *Interaction Ritual: Essays in Face-to-Face Behavior*. Chicago: Aldine, 1967.

——. *The Presentation of Self in Everyday Life*. Garden City, N.Y.: Doubleday Anchor, 1959.

Goldberg, David J. *Discontented America: The United States in the 1920s*. Baltimore: Johns Hopkins University Press, 1999.

Gordon, Linda. *Pitied but Not Entitled: Single Mothers and the History of Welfare, 1890–1935*. New York: Free Press, 1994.

——. *Woman's Body, Woman's Right: Birth Control in America*. New York: Grossman, 1974.

Grant, Julia. *Raising Baby by the Book: The Education of American Mothers*. New Haven: Yale University Press, 1998.

Greenleaf, William. *From These Beginnings: The Early Philanthropies of Henry and Edsel Ford, 1911–1936*. Detroit: Wayne State University Press, 1964.

Grey, Michael R. *New Deal Medicine: The Rural Health Programs of the Farm Security Administration*. Baltimore: Johns Hopkins University Press, 1999.

Hall, Jacquelyn Dowd. *Revolt against Chivalry: Jessie Daniel Ames and the Women's Campaign against Lynching*. New York: Columbia University Press, 1979.

Haller, Mark. *Eugenics: Hereditarian Attitudes in American Thought*. New Brunswick, N.J.: Rutgers University Press, 1963.

Harrison, Lowell H. *John Breckinridge: Jeffersonian Republican*. Louisville: Filson Club, 1969.

Harrison, Lowell H., and James C. Klotter. *A New History of Kentucky*. Lexington: University Press of Kentucky, 1997.

Heilbrun, Carolyn G. *Writing a Woman's Life*. New York: Norton, 1988.

Hess, Stephen. *America's Political Dynasties*. 2nd ed. New Brunswick, N.J.: Transaction, 1997.

Higham, John. *Strangers in the Land: Patterns of American Nativism, 1860–1925*. New Brunswick, N.J.: Rutgers University Press, 1955.

History of the St. Luke's Hospital Training School for Nurses, New York. New York: St. Luke's Alumni Association, 1938.

Hodgson, Godfrey. *America in Our Time: From World War II to Nixon, What Happened, and Why*. New York: Vintage, 1976.

Hoganson, Kristin L. *Fighting for American Manhood: How Gender Politics Provoked the Spanish-American and Philippine-American Wars*. New Haven: Yale University Press, 1998.

Honey, Maureen. *Creating Rosie the Riveter: Class, Gender, and Propaganda during World War II*. Amherst: University of Massachusetts Press, 1985.

Hsiung, David C. *Two Worlds in the Tennessee Mountains: Exploring the Origins of Appalachian Stereotypes*. Lexington: University Press of Kentucky, 1997.

Jelinek, Estelle C. *The Tradition of Women's Autobiography: From Antiquity to the Present*. Boston: Twayne, 1986.

———, ed. *Women's Autobiography: Essays in Criticism*. Bloomington: University of Indiana Press, 1980.

James, D. Clayton. *Antebellum Natchez*. Baton Rouge: Louisiana State University Press, 1968.

Jones, Jacqueline. *Labor of Love, Labor of Sorrow: Black Women, Work, and the Family from Slavery to the Present*. New York: Basic Books, 1985.

Kalisch, Philip A., and Beatrice J. Kalisch. *The Advance of American Nursing*. Boston: Little, Brown, 1978.

Katz, Michael B. *In the Shadow of the Poorhouse: A Social History of Welfare in America*. Tenth anniversary ed. New York: Basic Books, 1996.

Keeling, Arlene W. *Nursing and the Privilege of Prescription, 1893–2000*. Columbus: Ohio State University Press, 2007.

Kessler-Harris, Alice. *Out to Work: A History of Wage-Earning Women in the United States*. Oxford: Oxford University Press, 1982.

Klaus, Alisa. *Every Child a Lion: The Origins of Maternal and Infant Health Policy in the United States and France, 1890–1920*. Ithaca: Cornell University Press, 1993.

Kline, Wendy. *Building a Better Race: Gender, Sexuality, and Eugenics from the Turn of the Century to the Baby Boom*. Berkeley: University of California Press, 2001.

Klotter, James C. *The Breckinridges of Kentucky, 1760–1981*. Lexington: University Press of Kentucky, 1986.

Koven, Seth, and Sonya Michel, eds. *Mothers of a New World: Maternalist Politics and the Origins of Welfare States*. New York: Routledge, 1993.

Kraut, Alan M. *Silent Travelers: Germs, Genes, and the "Immigrant Menace."* Baltimore: Johns Hopkins University Press, 1994.

Ladd-Taylor, Molly. *Mother-Work: Women, Child Welfare, and the State, 1890–1930*. Urbana: University of Illinois Press, 1994.

——. *Raising a Baby the Government Way: Mothers' Letters to the Children's Bureau, 1915–1932*. New Brunswick, N.J.: Rutgers University Press, 1986.

Larson, Magali Sarfatti. *The Rise of Professionalism: A Sociological Analysis*. Berkeley: University of California Press, 1977.

Lears, T. J. Jackson. *No Place of Grace: Antimodernism and the Transformation of American Culture, 1880–1920*. Chicago: University of Chicago Press, 1981.

Leavitt, Judith Walzer. *Brought to Bed: Childbearing in American Society, 1750–1929*. New York: Oxford University Press, 1986.

Leavitt, Judith Walzer, and Ronald L. Numbers, eds. *Sickness and Health in America: Readings in the History of Medicine and Public Health*. Madison: University of Wisconsin Press, 1985.

Lewenson, Sandra Beth. *Taking Charge: Nursing, Suffrage, and Feminism in America, 1873–1920*. New York: National League for Nursing Press, 1996.

Lewis, Alfred Allan. *Ladies and Not-So-Gentle Women*. New York: Penguin, 2000.

Lewis, Helen Matthews, Linda Johnson, and Donald Askins, eds. *Colonialism in Modern America: The Appalachian Case*. Boone, N.C.: Appalachian Consortium, 1978.

Lindenmeyer, Kriste. *"A Right to Childhood": The U.S. Children's Bureau and Child Welfare, 1912–1946*. Urbana: University of Illinois Press, 1997.

Litoff, Judy Barrett. *The American Midwife Debate: A Sourcebook on Its Modern Origins*. Westport, Conn.: Greenwood, 1986.

——. *American Midwives: 1860 to the Present*. Westport, Conn.: Greenwood, 1978.

McGregor, Deborah Kuhn. *From Midwives to Medicine: The Birth of American Gynecology*. New Brunswick, N.J.: Rutgers University Press, 1998.

McLaughlin, Loretta. *The Pill, John Rock, and the Church: The Biography of a Revolution*. Boston: Little, Brown, 1982.

Meckel, Richard A. *Save the Babies: American Public Health Reform and the Prevention of Infant Mortality, 1850–1929*. Baltimore: Johns Hopkins University Press, 1990.

Melosh, Barbara. *"The Physician's Hand": Work Culture and Conflict in American Nursing*. Philadelphia: Temple University Press, 1982.

Menn, Joseph Karl. *The Large Slaveholders of Louisiana—1860*. New Orleans: Pelican, 1964.

Moldow, Gloria. *Women Doctors in Gilded-Age Washington: Race, Gender, and Professionalization.* Urbana: University of Illinois Press, 1987.

Morantz-Sanchez, Regina Markell. *Sympathy and Science: Women Physicians in American Medicine.* New York: Oxford University Press, 1985.

Muncy, Robyn. *Creating a Female Dominion in American Reform, 1890–1935.* Oxford: Oxford University Press, 1991.

Nash, Gerald D. *The Crucial Era: The Great Depression and World War II, 1929–1945.* New York: St. Martin's, 1992.

Odem, Mary E. *Delinquent Daughters: Protecting and Policing Adolescent Female Sexuality in the United States, 1885–1920.* Chapel Hill: University of North Carolina Press, 1995.

Olney, James, ed. *Autobiography: Essays Theoretical and Critical.* Princeton: Princeton University Press, 1980.

Pascoe, Peggy. *Relations of Rescue: The Search for Female Authority in the American West, 1874–1939.* New York: Oxford University Press, 1990.

Payne, Elizabeth Anne. *Reform, Labor, and Feminism: Margaret Dreier Robins and the Women's Trade Union League.* Urbana: University of Illinois Press, 1988.

Pickens, Donald K. *Eugenics and the Progressives.* Nashville, Tenn.: Vanderbilt University Press, 1968.

Pinkley-Call, Cora. *Pioneer Tales of Eureka Springs and Carroll County.* Eureka Springs, Ark.: n.p., 1930.

Ramsey, Ralph J., and Paul D. Warner. *Kentucky County Data Book, 1960 and 1970.* Lexington: University of Kentucky Cooperative Extension Service, 1974.

Rayburn, Otto Ernest. *The Eureka Springs Story.* 1954; Eureka Springs, Ark.: Wheeler, 1982.

Reed, James. *From Private Vice to Public Virtue: The Birth Control Movement and American Society since 1830.* New York: Basic Books, 1978.

Rehder, John B. *Appalachian Folkways.* Baltimore: Johns Hopkins University Press, 2004.

Reverby, Susan M. *Ordered to Care: The Dilemma of American Nursing, 1850–1945.* Cambridge: Cambridge University Press, 1987.

Ritterhouse, Jennifer. *Growing Up Jim Crow: How Black and White Southern Children Learned Race.* Chapel Hill: University of North Carolina Press, 2006.

Roark, James L. *Masters without Slaves: Southern Planters in the Civil War and Reconstruction.* New York: Norton, 1977.

Roberts, Mary M. *American Nursing: History and Interpretation.* New York: Macmillan, 1961.

Rock, John. *The Time Has Come: A Catholic Doctor's Proposals to End the Battle over Birth Control.* London: Longmans, Green, 1963.

Rosenzweig, Linda W. *The Anchor of My Life: Middle-Class American Mothers and Daughters, 1880–1920.* New York: New York University Press, 1993.

———. *Another Self: Middle-Class American Women and Their Friends in the Twentieth Century.* New York: New York University Press, 1999.

Rothman, Ellen K. *Hands and Hearts: A History of Courtship in America.* New York: Basic Books, 1984.

Rothstein, William G. *American Medical Schools and the Practice of Medicine: A History.*
New York: Oxford University Press, 1987.

Rowbotham, Sheila. *A Century of Women: The History of Women in Britain and the United States.* London: Viking, 1997.

Salstrom, Paul. *Appalachia's Path to Dependency: Rethinking a Region's Economic History, 1730–1940.* Lexington: University Press of Kentucky, 1994.

Sandelowski, Margarete. *Devices and Desires: Gender, Technology, and American Nursing.* Chapel Hill: University of North Carolina Press, 2000.

Schaefer, Susan. *I Didn't Know That Either!: About Eureka Springs.* Eureka Springs, Ark.: Ozark Mountain, 1993.

Scott, Anne Firor. *Natural Allies: Women's Associations in American History.* Urbana: University of Illinois Press, 1991.

——. *The Southern Lady: From Pedestal to Politics, 1830–1930.* Chicago: University of Chicago Press, 1970.

Searles, P. David. *A College for Appalachia: Alice Lloyd on Caney Creek.* Lexington: University Press of Kentucky, 1995.

Shapiro, Henry D. *Appalachia on Our Mind: The Southern Mountains and Mountaineers in the American Consciousness, 1870–1920.* Chapel Hill: University of North Carolina Press, 1978.

Shifflett, Crandall A. *Coal Towns: Life, Work, and Culture in Company Towns of Southern Appalachia, 1880–1960.* Knoxville: University of Tennessee Press, 1991.

Shorter, Edward. *Women's Bodies: A Social History of Women's Encounter with Health, Ill-Health, and Medicine.* 2nd ed. New Brunswick, N.J.: Transaction, 1997.

Sims, Anastatia. *The Power of Femininity in the New South: Women's Organizations and Politics in North Carolina, 1880–1930.* Columbia: University of South Carolina Press, 1997.

Skocpol, Theda. *Protecting Soldiers and Mothers: The Political Origins of Social Policy in the United States.* Cambridge: Harvard University Press, 1992.

Smiley, Gene. *Rethinking the Great Depression.* Chicago: Dee, 2002.

Solomon, Barbara Miller. *In the Company of Educated Women: A History of Women and Higher Education in America.* New Haven: Yale University Press, 1985.

Southard, Mary Young, ed. *Who's Who in Kentucky: A Biographic Assembly of Notable Kentuckians.* Louisville, Ky.: Standard Printing, 1936.

Starr, Paul. *The Social Transformation of American Medicine.* New York: Basic Books, 1982.

Stidham, Sadie Wells. *Trails into Cutshin Country: A History of the Pioneers of Leslie County, Kentucky.* [Corbin, Ky.]: Stidham, [1978].

Stoddart, Jess. *Challenge and Change in Appalachia: The Story of the Hindman Settlement School.* Lexington: University Press of Kentucky, 2002.

Sutton, Willis A., Jr., and Jerry Russell. *The Social Dimensions of Kentucky Counties: Data and Rankings of the State's 120 Counties on Each of 81 Characteristics.* Lexington: University of Kentucky College of Arts and Sciences, 1964.

Taney, Mary Florence. *Kentucky Pioneer Women: Columbian Poems and Prose Sketches.* Cincinnati: Clarke, 1893.

Thompson, Paul, Catherine Itzin, and Michele Abendstern. *I Don't Feel Old: The Experience of Later Life*. Oxford: Oxford University Press, 1990.

Tice, Karen W. *Tales of Wayward Girls and Immoral Women: Case Records and the Professionalization of Social Work*. Urbana: University of Illinois Press, 1998.

Trattner, Walter I. *From Poor Law to Welfare State: A History of Social Welfare in America*. 6th ed. New York: Free Press, 1999.

Twitchell, James B. *AdcultUSA: The Triumph of Advertising in American Culture*. New York: Columbia University Press, 1996.

Ulrich, Laurel Thatcher. *A Midwife's Tale: The Life of Martha Ballard, Based on Her Diary, 1785–1812*. New York: Vintage, 1990.

Van Ingen, Philip. *The Story of the American Child Health Association*. New York: American Child Health Association, 1936.

Vaughan, Paul. *The Pill on Trial*. New York: Coward-McCann, 1970.

Wagner-Martin, Linda. *Telling Women's Lives: The New Biography*. New Brunswick, N.J.: Rutgers University Press, 1994.

Waller, Altina L. *Feud: Hatfields, McCoys, and Social Change in Appalachia, 1860–1900*. Chapel Hill: University of North Carolina Press, 1988.

Watkins, Elizabeth Siegel. *On the Pill: A Social History of Oral Contraceptives, 1950–1970*. Baltimore: Johns Hopkins University Press, 1998.

Waugh, Joan. *Unsentimental Reformer: The Life of Josephine Shaw Lowell*. Cambridge: Harvard University Press, 1997.

Weise, Robert S. *Grasping at Independence: Debt, Male Authority, and Mineral Rights in Appalachian Kentucky, 1850–1915*. Knoxville: University of Tennessee Press, 2001.

Wertz, Richard W., and Dorothy C. Wertz. *Lying-In: A History of Childbirth in America*. New York: Free Press, 1977.

Whisnant, David E. *All That Is Native and Fine: The Politics of Change in an American Region*. Chapel Hill: University of North Carolina Press, 1983.

——. *Modernizing the Mountaineer: People, Planning, and Power in Appalachia*. New York: Franklin, 1980.

Wiebe, Robert H. *The Search for Order, 1877–1920*. New York: Hill and Wang, 1967.

Wilkie, Katharine Elliott, and Elizabeth R. Moseley. *Frontier Nurse: Mary Breckinridge*. New York: Messner, 1969.

Williams, John Alexander. *Appalachia: A History*. Chapel Hill: University of North Carolina Press, 2002.

Williamson, J. W. *Hillbillyland: What the Movies Did to the Mountains and What the Mountains Did to the Movies*. Chapel Hill: University of North Carolina Press, 1995.

Williamson, Joel. *The Crucible of Race: Black-White Relations in the American South since Emancipation*. New York: Oxford University Press, 1984.

Wilson, Charles Reagan. *Baptized in Blood: The Religion of the Lost Cause, 1865–1920*. Athens: University of Georgia Press, 1980.

Wolfe, Margaret Ripley. *Daughters of Canaan: A Saga of Southern Women*. Lexington: University Press of Kentucky, 1995.

Woloch, Nancy. *Women and the American Experience*. New York: Knopf, 1984.

Woodman, Harold D. *King Cotton and His Retainers: Financing and Marketing the Cotton Crop of the South, 1800–1925*. Lexington: University Press of Kentucky, 1968.

Woodruff, Nan. *As Rare as Rain: Federal Relief in the Great Southern Drought of 1930–1931*. Urbana: University of Illinois Press, 1985.

Woodward, C. Vann. *Origins of the New South, 1877–1913*. 1951; Baton Rouge: Louisiana State University Press and the Littlefield Fund for Southern History of the University of Texas, 1994.

Wyatt-Brown, Bertram. *Southern Honor: Ethics and Behavior in the Old South*. New York: Oxford University Press, 1982.

Zeiger, Susan. *In Uncle Sam's Service: Women Workers with the American Expeditionary Force, 1917–1919*. Ithaca: Cornell University Press, 1999.

ARTICLES

Abel, Emily K. "Valuing Care: Turn-of-the-Century Conflicts between Charity Workers and Women Clients." *Journal of Women's History* 10 (Autumn 1998): 32–52.

Anderson, John Q. "Dr. James Green Carson, Ante-Bellum Planter of Mississippi and Louisiana." *Journal of Mississippi History* 18 (October 1956): 243–67.

Antler, Joyce. " 'After College What?': New Graduates and the Family Claim." *American Quarterly* 32 (Autumn 1980): 409–34.

Antler, Joyce, and Daniel M. Fox. "The Movement toward a Safe Maternity: Physician Accountability in New York City, 1915–1940." In *Sickness and Health in America: Readings in the History of Medicine and Public Health*, edited by Judith Walzer Leavitt and Ronald L. Numbers, 490–506. Madison: University of Wisconsin Press, 1985.

Baker, Paula. "The Domestication of Politics: Women and American Political Society, 1780–1920." In *Unequal Sisters*, edited by Vicki L. Ruiz and Carol DuBois, 85–110. New York: Routledge, 1994.

Beeber, Linda S. "To Be One of the Boys: Aftershocks of the World War I Nursing Experience." *Advances in Nursing Science* 12 (July 1990): 32–43.

Benstock, Shari. "The Female Self Engendered: Autobiographic Writing and Theories of Selfhood." In *Women and Autobiography*, edited by Martine Watson Brownley and Allison B. Kimmich, 3–14. Wilmington, Del.: Scholarly Resources, 1999.

Bolin, James Duane. "Clifton Rodes Breckinridge: 'The Little Arkansas Giant.' " *Arkansas Historical Quarterly* 53 (Winter 1994): 407–27.

———. "The Sins of the Fathers: Clifton Rodes Breckinridge Remembers the Civil War." *Civil War History* 44 (March 1998): 35–52.

Browne, Helen E. "Frontier Nursing Service and Its Implications for Other Rural Areas." In *The Midwife in the United States: Report of a Macy Conference*, 75–79. New York: Josiah Macy Jr. Foundation, 1968.

Campbell, Anne G. "Mary Breckinridge and the American Committee for Devastated France: The Foundations of the Frontier Nursing Service." *Register of the Kentucky Historical Society* 82 (Summer 1984): 257–76.

Chuppa-Cornell, Kimberly. "The U.S. Women's Motor Corps in France, 1914–1921." *Historian* 56 (Spring 1994): 465–76.

Conti, Eugene A., Jr. "The Cultural Role of Local Elites in the Kentucky Mountains: A Retrospective Analysis." *Appalachian Journal* 7 (Autumn–Winter 1979–80): 51–68.

Crowe-Carraco, Carol. "Mary Breckinridge and the Frontier Nursing Service." *Register of the Kentucky Historical Society* 76 (July 1978): 179–91.

Davis, Mrs. Samuel Preston, Sr. "The Arkansas Society, Daughters of the American Revolution." *Arkansas Historical Quarterly* 2 (March 1943): 359–68.

Davis, William C. "John C. Breckinridge." *Register of the Kentucky Historical Society* 85 (Summer 1987): 197–212.

Deutsch, Sarah. "Learning to Talk More Like a Man: Boston Women's Class-Bridging Organizations, 1870–1940." *American Historical Review* 97 (April 1992): 379–404.

Dye, Nancy Schrom. "Mary Breckinridge, the Frontier Nursing Service, and the Introduction of Nurse-Midwifery in the United States." *Bulletin of the History of Medicine* 57 (Winter 1983): 485–507.

Dye, Nancy Schrom, and Daniel Blake Smith. "Mother Love and Infant Death, 1750–1920." *Journal of American History* 73 (September 1986): 329–53.

Forderhase, Nancy K. "Eve Returns to the Garden: Women Reformers in Appalachian Kentucky in the Early Twentieth Century." *Register of the Kentucky Historical Society* 85 (Summer 1987): 237–61.

Fox-Genovese, Elizabeth. "Mixed Messages: Women and the Impact of World War II." *Southern Humanities Review* 27 (Summer 1993): 235–45.

Freedman, Estelle B. " 'The Burning of Letters Continues': Elusive Identities and the Historical Construction of Sexuality." *Journal of Women's History* 9 (Winter 1998): 181–99.

Friedson, Eliot. "Are the Professions Necessary?" In *The Authority of Experts*, edited by Thomas Haskell, 3–25. Bloomington: Indiana University Press, 1984.

Gavit, John P. "Rural Social Settlements." *Commons*, May 1899, 5–6.

Goan, Melanie Beals. "Establishing Their Place in the Dynasty: Sophonisba and Mary Breckinridge's Paths to Public Service." *Register of the Kentucky Historical Society* 101 (Winter–Spring 2003): 45–73.

Graham, Laurel D. "Domesticating Efficiency: Lillian Gilbreth's Scientific Management of Homemakers, 1924–1930." *Signs* 24 (Spring 1999): 633–75.

Hall, Jacquelyn Dowd. " 'You Must Remember This': Autobiography as Social Critique." *Journal of American History* 85 (September 1998): 439–65.

Holland, Theodore J., Jr. "The Many Faces of Nicknames." *Names* 38 (December 1990): 255–72.

James, Janet Wilson. "Writing and Rewriting Nursing History: A Review Essay." *Bulletin of the History of Medicine* 58 (Winter 1984): 568–84.

Kahn, Si. "The Forest Service and Appalachia." In *Colonialism in Modern America: The Appalachian Case*, edited by Helen Matthews Lewis, Linda Johnson, and Donald Askins, 85–109. Boone, N.C.: Appalachian Consortium, 1978.

Klotter, James C. "Family Influences on a Progressive: The Early Years of Sophonisba P. Breckinridge." In *Kentucky Profiles: Biographical Essays in Honor of Holman Hamilton*, edited by James C. Klotter and Peter J. Sehlinger, 120–54. Frankfort: Kentucky Historical Society, 1982.

Kobrin, Frances E. "The American Midwife Controversy: A Crisis of Professionalism." In *Sickness and Health in America: Readings in the History of Medicine and Public Health*, edited by Judith Walzer Leavitt and Ronald L. Numbers, 318–26. Madison: University of Wisconsin Press, 1985.

Kornbluh, Felicia A. "The New Literature on Gender and the Welfare State: The U.S. Case." *Feminist Studies* 22 (Spring 1996): 170–97.

Ladd-Taylor Molly. " 'Grannies' and 'Spinsters': Midwife Education under the Sheppard-Towner Act." *Journal of Social History* 22 (Winter 1988): 255–75.

——. "Hull House Goes to Washington: Women and the Children's Bureau." In *Gender, Class, Race, and Reform in the Progressive Era*, edited by Noralee Frankel and Nancy S. Dye, 110–26. Lexington: University Press of Kentucky, 1991.

——. " 'My Work Came Out of Agony and Grief: Mothers and the Making of the Sheppard-Towner Act.' " In *Mothers of a New World: Maternalist Politics and the Origins of Welfare States*, edited by Seth Koven and Sonya Michel, 321–42. New York: Routledge, 1993.

——. "Toward Defining Maternalism in U.S. History." *Journal of Women's History* 5 (Fall 1993): 110–13.

Marks, Lara. "A 'Cage' of Ovulating Females: The History of the Early Oral Contraceptive Pill Clinical Trials, 1950–1959." In *Molecularizing Biology and Medicine: New Practices and Alliances, 1910s–1970s*, edited by Soraya de Chadarevian and Harmke Kamminga, 221–47. Amsterdam: Harwood Academic, 1998.

Martin, C. Brenden. "To Keep the Spirit of Mountain Culture Alive: Tourism and Historical Memory in the Southern Highlands." In *Where These Memories Grow: History, Memory, and Southern Identity*, edited by W. Fitzhugh Brundage, 249–70. Chapel Hill: University of North Carolina Press, 2000.

Mason, Mary G. "The Other Voice: Autobiographies of Women Writers." In *Autobiography: Essays Theoretical and Critical*, edited by James Olney, 207–35. Princeton: Princeton University Press, 1980.

Miller, Elissa Lane. "Arkansas Nurses, 1895–1920: A Profile." *Arkansas Historical Quarterly* 47 (Summer 1988): 154–71.

O'Neill, William L. "Divorce in the Progressive Era." In *Reform, Crisis, and Confusion, 1900–1929*, edited by R. Jackson Wilson, 151–65. New York: Random House, 1970.

Parker, Donna. "Made to Fit a Woman: Riding Uniforms of the Frontier Nursing Service." *Dress* 20 (1993): 53–64.

Phipps, Sheila Rae. " 'Their Desire to Visit the Southerners': Mary Greenhow Lee's Visiting 'Connexion.' " In *Negotiating Boundaries of Southern Womanhood: Dealing with the Powers That Be*, edited by Janet L. Coryell, Thomas H. Appleton Jr., Anastatia Sims, and Sandra Gioia Treadway, 215–33. Columbia: University of Missouri Press, 2000.

Rooks, Judith P. "Nurse-Midwifery: The Window Is Wide Open." *American Journal of Nursing* 90 (December 1990): 30–36.

Rupp, Leila J. " 'Imagine My Surprise': Women's Relationships in Historical Perspective." *Frontiers* 5 (Autumn 1980): 61–70.

Sahli, Nancy. "Smashing: Women's Relationships before the Fall." *Chrysalis* 8 (Summer 1979): 17–27.

Shelby, Anne. "The 'R' Word: What's So Funny (and Not So Funny) about Redneck Jokes." In *Back Talk from Appalachia: Confronting Stereotypes*, edited by Dwight B. Billings, Gurney Norman, and Katherine Ledford, 153–60. Lexington: University Press of Kentucky, 1999.

Simmons, Christina. "Companionate Marriage and the Lesbian Threat." In *Women and Power in American History*, vol. 2, edited by Kathryn Kish Sklar and Thomas Dublin, 183–94. Englewood Cliffs, N.J.: Prentice Hall, 1991.

Sklar, Kathryn Kish. "*Hull-House Maps and Papers*: Social Science as Women's Work in the 1890s." In *The Social Survey in Historical Perspective, 1880–1940*, edited by Martin Bulmer, Kevin Bales, and Kathryn Kish Sklar, 111–47. Cambridge: Cambridge University Press, 1991.

Smith-Rosenberg, Carroll. "The Female World of Love and Ritual: Relations between Women in Nineteenth Century America." *Signs* 1 (Autumn 1975): 1–29.

Spacks, Patricia Meyer. "Selves in Hiding." In *Women's Autobiography: Essays in Criticism*, edited by Estelle C. Jelinek, 112–32. Bloomington: University of Indiana Press, 1980.

Spender, Stephen. "Confessions and Autobiography." In *Autobiography: Essays Theoretical and Critical*, edited by James Olney, 115–22. Princeton: Princeton University Press, 1980.

Tice, Karen W. "School-Work and Mother-Work: The Interplay of Maternalism and Cultural Politics in the Educational Narratives of Kentucky Settlement Workers, 1910–1930." *Journal of Appalachian Studies* 4 (Fall 1998): 191–224.

Welter, Barbara. "The Cult of True Womanhood: 1820–1860." *American Quarterly* 18 (Summer 1966): 151–74.

Williamson, Joel. "How Black Was Rhett Butler?" In *The Evolution of Southern Culture*, edited by Numan V. Bartley, 88–107. Athens: University of Georgia Press, 1988.

Willis, James F. "An Arkansan in St. Petersburg: Clifton Rodes Breckinridge, Minister to Russia, 1894–1897." *Arkansas Historical Quarterly* 38 (Spring 1979): 3–31.

Wilson, Darlene. "The Felicitous Convergence of Mythmaking and Capital Accumulation: John Fox Jr. and the Formation of an (Other) Almost-White American Underclass." *Journal of Appalachian Studies* 1 (Fall 1995): 5–44.

THESES, DISSERTATIONS, AND UNPUBLISHED MANUSCRIPTS

Altizer, Anna L. "The Establishment of the Frontier Nursing Service." Master's thesis, University of Kentucky, 1990.

Arnett, Douglas O'Neil. "Eastern Kentucky: The Politics of Dependency and Under-Development." Ph.D. diss., Duke University, 1978.

Baldwin, Yvonne Honeycutt. "Cora Wilson Stewart and the Illiteracy Crusade: 'Moonlight Schools' and Progressive Reform." Ph.D. diss., University of Kentucky, 1996.

Barr, Nancy Ellen. "A Profession for Women: Education, Social Service Administration, and Feminism in the Life of Sophonisba Preston Breckinridge, 1886–1948." Ph.D. diss., Emory University, 1993.

Blackwell, Deborah Lynn. "The Ability 'To Do Much Larger Work': Gender and Reform in Appalachia, 1890–1935." Ph.D. diss., University of Kentucky, 1998.

Brown, Loren Nunn. "The Work of the Dawes Commission among the Choctaw and Chickasaw Indians." Ph.D. diss, University of Oklahoma, 1937.

Cook, Florence Elliott. "Growing Up White, Genteel, and Female in a Changing South, 1865–1915." Ph.D. diss., University of California, 1992.

Cornett, Judy Gail. "Angel for the Blind: The Public Triumphs and Private Tragedy of Linda Neville." Ph.D. diss., University of Kentucky, 1993.

Criss, Barbara Ann. "Culture and the Provision of Care: Frontier Nursing Service, 1925–1940." Ph.D. diss., University of Utah, 1988.

Greeley, Dawn. "Beyond Benevolence: Gender, Class, and the Development of Scientific Charity in New York City, 1882–1935." Ph.D. diss., State University of New York at Stony Brook, 1995.

Gribble, Constance J. " 'We Hope to Live through It': Nursing and the 1918 Influenza Epidemic: Lessons for This Century and the Next." Master's thesis, Gonzaga University, 1997.

Harris, Heather. "Constructing Colonialism: Medicine, Technology, and the Frontier Nursing Service." Master's thesis, Virginia Polytechnic Institute and State University, 1995.

Hudson, Karen Elaine. " 'God Held the Torch That Brought the Old House Down': Class, Gender, and the Built Environment of the Appalachian Kentucky Social Settlement House Movement, 1880s–1930s." Ph.D. diss., University of Pennsylvania, 1995.

Nies, Betsy Lee. "Eugenic Fantasies: Racial Ideology in the Literature and Popular Culture of the 1920s." Ph.D. diss., University of Florida, 1998.

Snihurowycz, Maria Zoreslawa. "The Frontier Nursing Service of Kentucky and Its Antecedents in Public Health Nursing." Ph.D. diss., Yale University, 1968.

Terry, Gail S. "Family Empires: A Frontier Elite in Virginia and Kentucky, 1740–1815." Ph.D. diss, College of William and Mary, 1992.

Tirpak, Helen. "The Frontier Nursing Service: An Adventure in the Delivery of Health Care." Ph.D. diss., University of Pittsburgh, 1972.

Wilson, Brenda S. "Nicknaming Practices of Women in a Nontraditional Occupation: Female Professional Baseball Players." Master's thesis, University of North Carolina at Greensboro, 1991.

Index

Breckinridge, Madeline McDowell, 273 (n. 48)

Breckinridge, Mary: ambition of, 73, 142, 203, 250; appearance of, 3, 103; birth of, 16, 20; birth control views of, 239–41; childhood of, 21–27; death of, 248; declining health of, 225, 244–47; depression of, 24–25, 27, 51, 56, 76, 268 (n. 52), 281 (n. 116); destruction of records by, 4, 51, 216; as "dutiful daughter," 30, 36, 56, 250; education of, 25–27, 30, 31, 33–36, 57, 270 (n. 106); fear of change, 230, 232, 243, 257; female friendships of, 93, 198, 223; French relief efforts of, 47, 53–54, 55, 60; fund-raising success of, 101, 115, 248; initial impression of Leslie County, 125, 219–20; introduction of nurse-midwifery, 62, 252–53; and jingoism, 177–78; and midwifery training, 73–74, 76; personal charisma of, 101–3, 157; racial views of, 22–24, 109–10, 236–39; religious faith of, 76–77, 218–19; riding accident of, 149–51, 157; suffrage support of, 46; work with U.S. Children's Bureau, 42, 51–52, 274 (n. 82)

Breckinridge, Mary Cyrene Burch, 18

Breckinridge, Sophonisba, 29, 30, 46, 50, 56, 269 (n. 83)

Breckinridge, Susanna Preston "Lees," 20, 24–25, 47, 268 (n. 51)

Breckinridge, W. C. P., 29–30

Breckinridge family, 213; arrival in North America, 16; and gender expectations, 16, 28, 218; and slave ownership, 220; political success of, 17–18; talent as public speakers, 102; tradition of public service, 15, 73

British Hospital for Mothers and Babies, 73, 76

Brock, Sallie A., 25

Bromley, Dorothy Dunbar, 126

Browne, Helen, 212, 216, 225, 232, 235, 238–39, 244, 246, 247; arrival in Leslie County, 194; efforts to modernize FNS, 255–60; named director of FNS, 248

Bruce, Elizabeth, 140

Buck, Dorothy, 133, 151, 192, 193, 197, 199, 223, 248

Butler, Harriet, 73

Cadet Nurse Corps, 181–82

Caffin, Freda, 83, 85, 86, 88, 90, 133, 139–41, 294 (n. 95)

Caffin, Caroline, 85

Campbell, John C., 65, 126, 167

Campbell, Olive Dame, 6

Capps, H. C., 91

Carni, Henri, 290 (n. 2)

Carni, Juliette, 290 (n. 2)

Carson, Catherine Waller, 19–20

Carson, James Green, 19–20, 220

Carson, Jessie "Kit," 101–2

Carson, Joseph, 21, 25, 32

Cashmore, Adeline, 76–77, 93, 150, 185, 187, 198–99, 218–19, 281 (n. 117)

Cashmore, Maud, 76, 93, 150, 198

Catholic Maternity Institute, 235

Caudill, Harry, 154

Cavender, Anthony, 144

Chandler, Albert B. "Happy," 103

Childbirth: as female ritual, 61; medicalization of, 61–62, 234; risks of, 42, 58–59, 60; and rural mothers, 52, 60

Child welfare movement, 40–42, 59–60

Clark, Edward, 28

Collins, Robert F., 162

Colonial Dames, 102, 109, 238

Comité Américain pour les Régions Dévastées de la France, 53–54, 61, 136, 198, 242

Committee on the Costs of Medical Care, 146, 174

Commonwealth Fund, 99–100

Corbin, Hazel, 180

Quarles, Mary Ann Stillman, 230

Raine, James Watt, 113–14
Ray Brothers Drugstore, 72
Reeder, Grace, 188
Republic Productions, 206
Reverby, Susan, 34
Ritterhouse, Jennifer, 237
Roarke, M. C., 137
Roberts, Zilpha, 83
Rock, John, 241–42
Rockstroh, Edna, 83, 85, 86, 104, 140, 294
    (n. 95)
Rogers, Will, 239
Roosevelt, Eleanor, 162, 170
Roosevelt, Franklin Delano, 160, 162, 163,
    166, 173
Roosevelt, Theodore, 42, 108, 113
Root, Elihu, 183
Rosemont, 26
Routzhan, Mary Swain, 138
Rural Health Clinic Services Act, 261

Saal, William, 206
St. Luke's Hospital School of Nursing, 34–
    36
Sanger, Margaret, 241
Scientific medicine, 9–10
Scientific motherhood, 43–44
Scott, Anne Firor, 23, 252
Scottish Highlands and Islands Medical and
    Nursing Service, 76, 83, 96
Searles, P. David, 7
Semple, Ellen Churchill, 109
Shawe, Rosalind Gillette, 129
Sheppard-Towner Maternity and Infancy
    Act, 59, 68, 163, 166
Shifflett, Crandall, 251
Shoemaker, Sister M. Theophane, 235–36
Shouse, Marion, 191
Smithsonian Institution, 255
Southern Highlander and His Homeland, 65, 126

Southern Mountain Workers, 163
Southern Woman's Magazine, 44–45
Spiritualism, 50–51, 57, 76
Stevenson, Elizabeth, 89
Stewart, Cora Wilson, 66, 67, 168
Stidham, Sadie, 131–32
Stimson, Henry, 226
Stoddart, Jess, 7
Stone, Helen, 191
Stone, May, 6–7, 66, 296 (n. 118)
Streit, Clarence, 177
Stucky, J. A., 96, 113
Summers, Vanda, 246
Swift, Gustavus, 104

Thompson, Clifton Breckinridge
    "Breckie," 45, 47, 50, 51, 54, 60, 76, 185,
    247; birth of, 39–40; death of, 48; growth
    and development of, 43–44
Thompson, Richard Ryan, 37, 50, 52, 54
Thousandsticks, 71, 72, 84, 137, 158, 211
Tice, Karen, 7–8
Turner, Lucille "Pansy," 56–57, 93, 150,
    187, 198, 224

Ulrich, Laurel Thatcher, 41
United Mine Workers, 229–30
University of Kentucky, 174
U.S. Children's Bureau, 2, 42, 49, 51, 58–
    59, 163, 180, 184, 282–83 (n. 17)
U.S. Forest Service, 160–62

Veech, Annie S., 68, 74, 99, 100, 126, 164
Vorse, Mary Heaton, 244

Wald, Lillian, 42, 63
War on Poverty, 226, 256
Weeks Act, 160
Welch, William H., 91
Wendover, 85, 86, 95, 125, 129–30, 153,
    159, 196–97, 220
Westminster Review, 33, 36

Whisnant, David, 6–8, 95–96, 101, 142, 251–52

Wide Neighborhoods, 4, 11, 213–23

Wiebe, Robert, 40

Willeford, Mary B., 132, 189

Wilson, Charles Reagan, 22

Women's Auxiliary Army Corps, 191

Women's Auxiliary Service Pilots, 191

Woodward, C. Vann, 22

Woodyard, Ella, 69

Wooten, George, 252

Yale School of Forestry, 160

York, Sergeant Alvin, 65

Zande, Ethel DeLong, 136